Obstetrics Essentials

Kate C. Arnold • Caroline J. Flint

Obstetrics Essentials

A Question-Based Review

Springer

Kate C. Arnold
Department of OB/GYN
University of Oklahoma HSC
Oklahoma City, OK
USA

Caroline J. Flint
Department of OB/GYN
University of Oklahoma HSC
Oklahoma City, OK
USA

ISBN 978-3-319-57674-9 ISBN 978-3-319-57675-6 (eBook)
DOI 10.1007/978-3-319-57675-6

Library of Congress Control Number: 2017944724

Printed on acid-free paper

This Springer imprint is published by Springer Nature
The registered company is Springer International Publishing AG
The registered company address is: Gewerbestrasse 11, 6330 Cham, Switzerland

To Isaac, Jesse, and Lexi for being patient when one or both moms were "doing practice bulletins." We love you very much. Thank you to the upcoming twins for giving us a timeline to finish this book. We look forward to meeting you.

Preface

Neither of us can remember whose idea it was to write questions based on practice bulletins; obviously, we both claim to be the inventor. Regardless, we both knew it was a great idea. The documents reviewed here are created by ACOG, which is the same organization that writes the CREOG exam and written and oral boards. Given their complexity, the documents are difficult to absorb with just the use of a highlighter. We hope that this book can serve as a resource for residents who are studying independently, for residency programs testing assigned reading, for practicing physicians wanting to test their understanding of the latest guidelines, and as a resource for licensing exams. In this book, the first part includes quizzes covering each obstetric practice bulletin, while the second part contains the same questions in random order to serve as a much broader exam. Thank you for your time, and we hope these questions help you reach your goals, no matter what they may be.

Oklahoma City, USA

Kate C. Arnold
Caroline J. Flint

Contents

Part I
Quizzes by Topic

Chapter 1
Prevention of Rh D Alloimmunization

Red cell alloimmunization refers to the production of maternal anti-red cell antibodies which can lead to fetal effects ranging from anemia to hydrops. With the use of anti-D immune globulin the incidence of red cell alloimmunization has decreased significantly. There are guidelines regarding prevention and management of pregnancies affected by the disease [1].

Recommended resource—ACOG Practice Bulletin 4: Prevention of Rh D Alloimmunization [2].

Q1: Prior to the introduction of anti-D immune globulin, hemolytic disease of the fetus and newborn affected ______ pregnancies?

A. About 10% of pregnancies
B. About 20% of pregnancies
C. About 35% of pregnancies
D. About 45% of pregnancies

Q2: In Rh-negative women who have not received immune globulin prophylaxis, the most common time to become alloimmunized is:

A. At the time of delivery
B. With third trimester bleeding
C. After therapeutic first trimester abortion
D. With amniocentesis

K.C. Arnold, C.J. Flint, *Obstetrics Essentials*,
DOI 10.1007/978-3-319-57675-6_1,

Q3: The amount of fetomaternal hemorrhage at which women can become alloimmunized is approximately:
A. 0.1 mL
B. 1 mL
C. 5 mL
D. 10 mL

Q4: Postpartum administration of a single dose of anti-D immune globulin can reduce the alloimmunization rate by 90% if given within:
A. 12 h of delivery
B. 24 h of delivery
C. 48 h of delivery
D. 72 h of delivery

Q5: The current standard prophylactic dose of anti-D immune globulin given in the United States is:
A. 50 μg
B. 100 μg
C. 200 μg
D. 300 μg

Q6: One prophylactic dose of anti-D immune globulin can prevent Rh D alloimmunization after exposure of up to ____ mL of Rh D-positive blood or ____mL of fetal cells.
A. 30 mL of Rh D-positive blood and 15 mL of fetal cells
B. 40 mL of Rh D-positive blood and 25 mL of fetal cells
C. 50 mL of Rh D-positive blood and 35 mL of fetal cells
D. 60 mL of Rh D-positive blood and 45 mL of fetal cells

Q7: A Rh-negative pregnant patient presents for her routine OB visit at 28 weeks. The father of the baby is also Rh negative. As her physician you should advise her to:

A. Receive the standard prophylactic dose of anti-D immune globulin
B. Forgo the prophylactic dose of anti-D immune globulin because it is unnecessary
C. Receive a smaller dose of anti-D immune globulin
D. Receive the prophylactic dose of anti-D immune globulin only if she has had a history of antepartum bleeding

Q8: A 28-year-old G2P1001 presents for her first prenatal visit at 12 weeks gestational age. A type and screen are performed and the patient is found to be Rh negative with a positive anti-D antibody screen. As her physician, in addition to increased antenatal surveillance, you should:

A. Administer a prophylactic dose anti-D immune globulin immediately
B. Obtain a Kleihauer-Betke test immediately and administer a sufficient amount of anti-D immune globulin accordingly
C. Administer the standard prophylactic dose of anti-D immune globulin at 28 weeks
D. Not administer anti-D immune globulin during this pregnancy

Q9: A 33-year-old Rh-negative G3P2002 with intrauterine pregnancy at 11 weeks gestational age presents for chorionic villus sampling (CVS). The patient should be given ______ prior to the procedure.

A. 50 μg anti-D immune globulin
B. 150 μg anti-D immune globulin
C. 300 μg anti-D immune globulin
D. No anti-D immune globulin

Q10: The same patient in Question #9 goes on to have a miscarriage at 15 weeks gestational age. The patient should now be given _____.

A. 50 μg anti-D immune globulin
B. 150 μg anti-D immune globulin
C. 300 μg anti-D immune globulin
D. No anti-D immune globulin

Q11: In a patient who continues to bleed after being administered prophylactic anti-D immune globulin, what test can be used to monitor persistent presence of the immune globulin?

A. Kleihauer-Betke test
B. Repeat type and screen
C. Direct Coombs test
D. Indirect Coombs test

Q12: A patient is given a dose of prophylactic anti-D immune globulin at 37 weeks gestational age due to abdominal trauma sustained during a motor vehicle accident. Patient is discharged home after extended monitoring without evidence of abruption. The patient goes on to have an uncomplicated vaginal delivery at 39/4 weeks gestational age. Does the patient need postpartum anti-D immune globulin?

A. Yes because this represents a separate event at which time fetomaternal hemorrhage can occur.
B. Yes because anti-D immune globulin half-life is only 14 days, and thus a redosing is needed.
C. No because the anti-D immune globulin half-life is 24 days, and thus a redosing is not needed.
D. No because it was an uncomplicated vaginal delivery without hemorrhage.

Q13: A G2P1001 Rh-negative patient presents for her initial prenatal visit and reports that she never received

Rh prophylaxis with her previous pregnancy. What are the chances that she is currently alloimmunized?

A. 0–5%
B. 15–20%
C. 30–40%
D. 50–70%

Q14: Rh positive refers to:

A. Presence of D antibody
B. Presence of D antigen
C. Neither
D. Both

Q15: A 34-year-old G3P2002 with intrauterine pregnancy at 32 weeks gestational age presents to labor and delivery in preterm labor with a cervical dilation of 3 cm. No vaginal bleeding is noted. She is Rh negative and received anti-D immune globulin prophylaxis at 28 weeks. Upon admission she should receive:

A. Betamethasone
B. Betamethasone and 300 μg anti-D immune globulin
C. Betamethasone and 50 μg anti-D immune globulin
D. Betamethasone and 300 μg anti-D immune globulin 12 h later

Q16: A 20-year-old known cocaine user presents to triage complaining of loss of fluid without vaginal bleeding at 30 weeks gestation and is found to have ruptured membranes. Documents show that she is Rh negative and received anti-D immune globulin at a previous triage visit at 26 weeks. Despite extensive counseling, she opts to leave the hospital AMA. Given her high risk of abruption, prior to leaving she should receive:

A. No prophylaxis
B. 300 μg anti-D immune globulin
C. 50 μg anti-D immune globulin

Q17: A Rh-negative patient should be considered a candidate for anti-D immune globulin prophylaxis after all the following events, EXCEPT:

A. External cephalic version
B. Evacuation of molar pregnancy
C. Threatened abortion
D. All of the above should be considered for prophylaxis

Q18: Which of the following is NOT an absolute indication for anti-D immune globulin in a Rh-negative woman?

A. First trimester pregnancy loss
B. Second or third trimester vaginal bleeding
C. Amniocentesis
D. Fetal blood sampling

Q19: A Rh-negative woman is postpartum day #1 after a vaginal delivery and is ready for discharge. Her baby is found to be Rh negative as well. She should receive anti-D immune globulin prior to discharge.

A. TRUE
B. FALSE

Answers

Q1: A, Q2: A, Q3: A, Q4: D, Q5: D, Q6: A, Q7: B, Q8: D, Q9: A, Q10: C, Q11: D, Q12:C, Q13: B, Q14: B, Q15: A, Q16: A, Q17: D, Q18: B, Q19:B.

Resources

1. Gabbe SG, Niebyl JR, Simpson JL, Landon MB, Galan HL, Jauniaux ERM, Driscoll DA. Obstetrics: normal and problem pregnancies. 6th ed. Philadelphia, PA: Elsevier; 2012.
2. American College of Obstetricians and Gynecologists. Practice bulletin no. 4: prevention of Rh D alloimmunization. Obstet Gynecol. 2016:1099–3630.

Chapter 2
Obstetric Analgesia and Anesthesia

Labor and delivery is associated with significant pain and it is the providers' duty to provide relief upon patient request. Available options include general, neuraxial, local, and parenteral analgesia. Each method is associated with specific indications, complications, and contraindications [1].

Recommended resource—ACOG Practice Bulletin 36: Obstetric Analgesia and Anesthesia [2].

Q1: Which of the following is FALSE regarding pain associated with labor and delivery?

A. Pain experienced with uterine contractions is mediated by T-10 through the L-1 portions of the spinal cord
B. Cervical dilation and descent of the fetal head generate somatic pain
C. The pudendal nerve is responsible for transmitting the pain felt in the pelvic floor and perineum
D. A medical indication is not necessary to provide maternal pain relief
E. None of the above

K.C. Arnold, C.J. Flint, *Obstetrics Essentials*,
DOI 10.1007/978-3-319-57675-6_2,

Q2: A patient presents for a routine prenatal visit at 34 weeks gestational age. She is wondering about the differences between parental and regional anesthesia during labor and delivery. You counsel her:

A. Regional anesthesia has been shown to be more effective at controlling pain during labor and delivery than parental agents but may have greater risks to the fetus
B. Shorter-acting parental agents may decrease some of the neonatal risks associated with longer-acting agents
C. Parental anesthesia has been shown to be as effective as regional anesthesia in providing pain relief during labor and delivery but may have greater risks to the fetus
D. A and B
E. None of the above

Q3: Which of the following is NOT a medical indication for epidural analgesia during labor and delivery?

A. History of deep vein thrombosis
B. History of malignant hyperthermia
C. Concern that the patient will be a difficult intubation
D. Prevention of autonomic hyperreflexia in patients with high spinal cord lesions

Q4: What is the typical duration of anesthesia provided with a spinal?

A. 30–60 min
B. 60–120 min
C. 30–180 min
D. 30–250 min

Q5: A patient presents to the obstetrical triage on postpartum day 3 reporting a headache that is worsened when in the sitting or standing position. Upon review of her chart, you note that she was delivered by cesarean section and had a spinal placed for analgesia. You suspect she has a postdural puncture headache. You counsel her:

A. A blood patch has minimal effectiveness in treating postdural headaches
B. A postdural puncture headache only occurs in patients who have had spinal anesthesia
C. It is reasonable to try conservative measures first including supine positioning, hydration, and analgesics
D. Having a postdural puncture headache increases her risk of having persistent back pain in the upcoming years

Q6: What is the most common side effect of regional analgesia?

A. Transient neurological symptoms
B. Pruritus
C. Postdural puncture headache
D. Hypotension

Q7: Maternal fever can be a side effect of epidural analgesia, especially in nulliparous women.

A. TRUE
B. FALSE

Q8: Which of the following is TRUE regarding inhaled anesthetic agents used during general anesthesia?

A. Some have been shown to have minimal passage across the placenta
B. They have not been associated with neonatal depression
C. They can be used as uterine relaxants in certain situations if given in high concentrations
D. Their use increases blood loss during cesarean section
E. None of the above

Q9: To decrease the potentially dangerous side effects associated with local anesthetics, it is important to take which precaution when using them?

A. First aspirate for blood prior to injection
B. Prehydrate patient with 500–1000 mL normal saline
C. Use a small caliber needle
D. Ensure normal electrolyte balance prior to use

Q10: Which of the following is FALSE regarding maternal morbidity and mortality associated with anesthesia administration during labor and delivery?

A. Regional anesthesia is preferred due to increased morbidity associated with general anesthesia
B. Complications from anesthesia account for approximately 5% of maternal deaths
C. The rate of failed intubation is higher in pregnant patients than in nonpregnant patients
D. If a patient is thought to be at increased risk for urgent cesarean delivery, it is reasonable to obtain early regional anesthesia during labor
E. None of the above

Q11: Which of the following is NOT an example of an absolute contraindication to regional anesthesia?

A. Patient with positive blood cultures for *E. coli* that resulted within the past 3 h
B. Patient with a history of an Arnold-Chiari malformation with a functioning ventricular shunt in place
C. Patient who had her last dose of low-molecular-weight heparin 10 h ago
D. Patient with a fibrinogen level of 110 micrograms/liter

Q12: Your patient presents to triage complaining of a headache at 38 weeks gestation. She is diagnosed with preeclampsia and is admitted for induction. Which of the following should be avoided?

A. Regional anesthesia
B. General anesthesia

C. Butorphanol
D. Nalbuphine
E. Fentanyl

Q13: Some of the potential benefits of using parental fentanyl for pain control during labor and delivery include:
A. Not associated with neonatal neurobehavioral depression
B. Has a short half-life
C. Associated with less nausea and vomiting
D. B and C
E. All of the above

Q14: What is the best way to administer naloxone to a neonate?
A. Intramuscularly
B. Intravenously
C. Subcutaneously
D. Orally
E. A or B

Q15: The development of chronic back pain is a known adverse outcome to epidural placement during labor and delivery.
A. TRUE
B. FALSE

Q16: Epidural-related fever is benign.
A. TRUE
B. FALSE

Q17: Which of the following is KNOWN in regard to the effect of epidural analgesia on labor?
A. May prolong labor up to 90 min
B. It doubles the need for oxytocin administration
C. Increases the rate of cesarean section
D. A and B
E. All of the above

Q18: A 36-year-old G1P0 presents to her routine prenatal visit at 36 weeks gestation with questions regarding the optimal time to obtain epidural anesthesia during labor. You counsel her:

A. Due to the increased risk of cesarean section associated with early epidural, the patient should not expect to get an epidural until at least 4–5 cm dilation
B. There is no increased risk of cesarean section associated with early epidural so the patient may have the epidural placed upon her request regardless of her cervical dilation
C. Due to evidence of early epidural increasing the risk of cesarean section, it is reasonable to try and delay epidural administration until 4–5 cm dilation if possible
D. Due to the risks of prolonging labor associated with early epidural, the patient should be encouraged to delay placement until at least 6 cm dilation
E. None of the above

Q19: Which of the following patients is at risk for developing an epidural or spinal hematoma following placement of regional anesthesia?

A. A patient who received their last dose of prophylactic low-molecular-weight heparin 8 h ago
B. A patient on unfractionated heparin with a normal activated partial thromboplastin time
C. A patient with a platelet count of 100,000/μL
D. A patient on low-dose aspirin

Q20: Depending on the type of anesthesia provided during labor and delivery, initiation of breastfeeding may need to be delayed.

A. TRUE
B. FALSE

Q21: What is the intended goal of obtaining an anesthesia consultation antepartum?
A. To help streamline the flow of patients on labor and delivery
B. To help reduce the risk of anesthesia complications in certain patients
C. To educate patients regarding their anesthesia options during labor and delivery
D. All of the above

Q22: NSAIDS used postpartum have been shown to decrease maternal opioid consumption by what percent?
A. 30%
B. 40%
C. 50%
D. 60%

Answers

Q1: B, Q2: B, Q3: A, Q4: D, Q5: C, Q6: D, Q7: A, Q8: C, Q9: A, Q10: E, Q11: C, Q12: A, Q13: E, Q14: B, Q15: B, Q16: B, Q17: D, Q18: C, Q19: A, Q20: B, Q21: B, Q22: A.

Resources

1. Gabbe SG, Niebyl JR, Simpson JL, Landon MB, Galan HL, Jauniaux ERM, Driscoll DA. Obstetrics: normal and problem pregnancies. Chapter 17. 6th ed. Philadelphia, PA: Elsevier; 2012.
2. American College of Obstetricians and Gynecologists. Obstetric analgesia and anesthesia. ACOG practice bulletin no. 36. Obstet Gynecol. 2002;100:177–91.

Chapter 3
Shoulder Dystocia

Shoulder dystocia complicates between 0.15 and 1.7% of vaginal deliveries. It is defined in one of two ways: more than 60 s from delivery of the head to the body or the need for additional obstetric maneuvers to deliver the shoulder of the fetus. Maneuvers commonly used include McRoberts, suprapubic pressure, Wood's screw, and delivery of the posterior arm [1].

Recommended resource—ACOG Practice Bulletin 40: Shoulder Dystocia [2].

Q1: Shoulder dystocia is defined as:

A. Requiring use of additional maneuvers other than downward traction on the fetal head to deliver the shoulders
B. A period of 30 s or more between delivery of the head and the shoulders
C. Use of two or more maneuvers to deliver the fetal shoulders
D. All of the above are acceptable definitions

Q2: Shoulder dystocia increases maternal risk for which of the following?

A. Postpartum hemorrhage
B. Fourth-degree laceration
C. Postpartum endometritis

K.C. Arnold, C.J. Flint, *Obstetrics Essentials*,
DOI 10.1007/978-3-319-57675-6_3,

D. A and B
E. B and C

Q3: Shoulder dystocia results in persistent brachial plexus injury in 15% of deliveries.
A. True
B. False

Q4: Which of the following increases the risk for shoulder dystocia?
A. Epidural
B. Labor induction
C. Operative vaginal delivery
D. Obesity
E. All of the above

Q5: Most cases of shoulder dystocia can be predicted.
A. True
B. False

Q6: Labor induction for suspected macrosomia is an effective strategy for decreasing the risk of shoulder dystocia.
A. True
B. False

Q7: Prophylactic cesarean section should be considered for estimated fetal weights greater than 5000 g in women without diabetes.
A. True
B. False

Q8: A 28-year-old G2P1001 presents for her first obstetrical visit in the first trimester. In review of her history, you note that her last delivery was complicated by a shoulder dystocia. The patient reports that her newborn suffered no long-term complications from the delivery. She is now asking you what mode of delivery you recommend for her current pregnancy. You counsel her:

A. Due to the increased risk of recurrence, she should undergo primary cesarean section for delivery
B. As the true risk of recurrence is unknown, depending on the factors present at her previous delivery and how this pregnancy progresses, it may be reasonable to have vaginal delivery or cesarean section
C. As the true risk of recurrence is unknown, she should undergo a vaginal delivery
D. Since there is no increased risk of recurrence, she should undergo a vaginal delivery

Answers

Q1: A, Q2: D, Q3: B, Q4: E, Q5: B, Q6: B, Q7: A, Q8: B.

Resources

1. Gabbe SG, Niebyl JR, Simpson JL, Landon MB, Galan HL, Jauniaux ERM, Driscoll DA. Obstetrics: normal and problem pregnancies. Chapter 18. 6th ed. Philadelphia, PA: Elsevier; 2012.
2. American college of obstetricians and gynecologists. ACOG practice bulletin no. 40: shoulder dystocia. Obstet Gynecol. 2002;100:1045–50.

Chapter 4
Neural Tube Defects

Neural tube defects include spina bifida and anencephaly. They are associated with maternal diabetes and use of anti-epileptic drugs as well as a history of a previous pregnancy with a neural tube defect. The defects are often due to low levels of folate at the time of neural tube closure, which is why recommended folate supplementation should begin prior to conception [1].

Recommended resource—ACOG Practice Bulletin 44: Neural Tube Defects [2].

Q1: Which of the following is TRUE in regard to neural tube defects?

A. Can be isolated or occur as part of a genetic syndrome
B. Affect the vertebral column and urogenital diaphragm
C. Most common congenital anomaly worldwide
D. Neural tube closure is normally complete by the end of the second week after conception (4 weeks after the last period)
E. All of the above

Q2: Most cranial neural tube defects are lethal.

A. TRUE
B. FALSE

K.C. Arnold, C.J. Flint, *Obstetrics Essentials*,
DOI 10.1007/978-3-319-57675-6_4,

Q3: A 23-year-old G1P0 with intrauterine pregnancy at 22 weeks has just been informed by the maternal fetal medicine specialist that her fetus has spina bifida. She calls the office wanting to know if her baby will have disabilities. In addition to referring her for additional MFM counseling, you tell her:

A. The extent of disability will depend on the level of the lesion
B. 90% of infants born with a sacral lesion will be wheelchair bound
C. Her infant will likely have some impairment of bowel and bladder function
D. Her infant will likely be severely mentally handicapped
E. A and C

Q4: Intellectual ability of patients with spina bifida is influenced by:

A. Presence of increased intracranial pressure
B. Intraoperative complications of an Arnold-Chiari malformation repair
C. Ventricular size regardless of intracranial pressure
D. A and B
E. All of the above

Q5: At least one-third of patients with a neural tube defect have a severe allergy to:

A. Penicillin
B. Latex
C. Sulfa
D. Peanuts

Q6: What percent of neural tube defects occur in families with a positive family history?

A. 5%
B. 10%
C. 30%
D. 40%

Q7: All of the following are factors that are associated with the development of neural tube defects, EXCEPT:
A. Diet
B. Maternal diabetes
C. High maternal core temperature
D. Ethnicity
E. All of the above are associated with the development of neural tube defects

Q8: Parents of a child affected by a neural tube defect are more likely to be homozygous for the ________ mutation in comparison to the unaffected population.
A. Protein C
B. Factor V Leiden
C. MTHFR
D. PKU

Q9: Which of the following is FALSE regarding folic acid supplementation?
A. It is recommended that all patients of reproductive age take 400 micrograms of folic acid daily
B. There is limited risk to taking higher levels of folic acid
C. It may interfere with some seizure medications
D. If additional folic acid supplementation is needed, it is recommended that a patient increase the dosing of their daily prenatal vitamin
E. None of the above

Q10: Which patient is at an increased risk of having a child with a neural tube defect?
A. A patient taking 400 micrograms of folic acid supplementation prior to conception and has a fasting blood glucose of 230 mg/dL at her first trimester obstetrical visit
B. A patient not taking a folic acid supplementation prior to conception and has a fasting blood glucose of 230 mg/dL at her first obstetrical visit

C. A new obstetrical patient who reports daily adherence to recommended folic acid supplementation and recent hot tub exposure while on vacation at her first obstetrical visit
D. A patient who upon review of her medications takes valproic acid and a daily prenatal vitamin
E. All of the above

Q11: What is considered to be an elevated level of maternal serum alpha-fetoprotein (MSAFP) for a single gestation?
A. More than 1.5 times the normal median
B. More than 2.0 times the normal median
C. More than 2.5 times the normal median
D. More than 3.0 times the normal median

Q12: What is considered to be diagnostic for a fetal neural tube defect?
A. Elevated MSAFP and presence of acetylcholinesterase in amniotic fluid
B. Elevated MSAFP and elevated amniotic fluid AFP
C. Presence of acetylcholinesterase in amniotic fluid
D. Elevated amniotic fluid AFP and presence of acetylcholinesterase in amniotic fluid

Q13: There is an increased relative risk of poor pregnancy outcomes associated with elevated MSAFP.
A. TRUE
B. FALSE

Q14: Decreased levels of MSAFP are independently associated with an increased risk of fetal aneuploidy.
A. TRUE
B. FALSE

Q15: Fetal spina bifida increases the risk for oligohydramnios.
A. TRUE
B. FALSE

Q16: A 33-year-old G2P1001 presents for her routine obstetrical visit at 32 weeks gestation. Diagnostic tests have previously revealed her fetus to be affected with spina bifida. She asks you about plans for delivery. You counsel her:

A. She will need a cesarean section at term
B. She will likely be able to have a vaginal delivery at term
C. She will need a cesarean section at 37 weeks
D. She will be offered induction of labor at 37 weeks

Q17: For women at higher risk of having a fetus affected with a neural tube defect, what is the daily recommended folic acid intake?

A. 400 micrograms
B. 4 milligrams
C. 40 milligrams
D. 4 grams

Q18: Your pregnant patient has epilepsy and is taking carbamazepine. What is she at an increased risk for?

A. Fetal neural tube defects
B. Increased seizure activity due to folic acid supplementation
C. Both of the above
D. None of the above

Q19: Your patient was just told that her fetus has a neural tube defect. She inquires about fetal surgery. Which of the following is FALSE?

A. It significantly raises the risk for preterm labor
B. It is currently considered investigational
C. Studies show an increased rate of hindbrain herniation
D. Patients require delivery by cesarean section if they proceed with the surgery
E. All of the above are true

Answers

Q1: A, Q2: A, Q3: E, Q4: D, Q5: B, Q6: A, Q7: E, Q8: C, Q9: D, Q10: E, Q11: C, Q12: D, Q13: A, Q14: B, Q15: B, Q16: B, Q17: B, Q18: C, Q19: C.

Resources

1. Gabbe SG, Niebyl JR, Simpson JL, Landon MB, Galan HL, Jauniaux ERM, Driscoll DA. Obstetrics: normal and problem pregnancies. Chapter 7. 6th ed. Philadelphia, PA: Elsevier; 2012.
2. American College of Obstetricians and Gynecologists. ACOG practice bulletin no. 44: neural tube defects. Obstet Gynecol. 2003;102:203–13.

Chapter 5
Pregestational Diabetes Mellitus

Diabetes mellitus is a metabolic disorder. Type 1 diabetes is caused by autoimmune destruction of the pancreas, making patients dependent on exogenous insulin; during pregnancy these patients are at increased risk for diabetic ketoacidosis and hypoglycemia. Type 2 diabetes is caused by decreased insulin sensitivity and often they can be managed with oral agents; these patients are generally older and more likely to be obese. Pregnancy outcomes for women with pregestational diabetes are improved with glucose monitoring and control [1].

Recommended resource—ACOG Practice Bulletin 60: Pregestational Diabetes Mellitus [2].

Q1: Which of the following is TRUE?
- A. Pregestational diabetes complicates 10% of all pregnancies
- B. 90% of all diabetes cases during pregnancy are pregestational
- C. Pathogenesis of type 1 diabetes includes destruction of pancreatic beta cells
- D. A and C
- E. All of the above

K.C. Arnold, C.J. Flint, *Obstetrics Essentials*,
DOI 10.1007/978-3-319-57675-6_5,

Q2: Late in the first trimester:
- A. Estrogen increases insulin sensitivity
- B. Estrogen decreases insulin sensitivity
- C. Progesterone decreases insulin sensitivity
- D. Progesterone increases insulin sensitivity

Q3: What percent of daily caloric intake should come from protein during pregnancy?
- A. 20%
- B. 30%
- C. 40%
- D. 50%

Q4: A new obstetric patient presents for her initial visit. This is her first pregnancy and review of her record reveals she is an insulin-dependent type II diabetic. She asks what changes she should expect in her insulin dosing during the pregnancy. You counsel her:
- A. Her insulin dosage will increase until 28 weeks, then return to baseline
- B. Her insulin dosage will increase throughout pregnancy, though most rapidly at about 30 weeks gestation
- C. Her insulin dosage will increase throughout pregnancy, though most rapidly at about 20 weeks gestation
- D. Her insulin dosage will gradually increase throughout pregnancy

Q5: Which of the following is an example of how regular insulin differs from insulin lispro?
- A. Regular insulin carries a greater risk of hypoglycemia
- B. Lispro should be taken 30 min prior to eating
- C. Lispro has improved compliance and patient satisfaction
- D. A and C
- E. None of the above

Q6: A type II diabetic patient brings her glucose log for review at her prenatal visit. It is noted that her pre-meal glucose values are consistently elevated. Her current insulin dosing is intermediate-acting insulin 20 units BID and lispro 10 units with meals. How should her dosing be adjusted?

A. Increase nighttime intermediate-acting insulin to 25 units
B. Increase lispro to 12 units with meals
C. Increase morning intermediate-acting insulin to 22 units
D. Increase morning intermediate-acting insulin to 24 units

Q7: When increasing a patient's insulin, it is important to warn them about the risks of hypoglycemia. How do you counsel her?

A. She should have a glass of milk if she becomes hypoglycemic
B. She should have a glass of orange juice if she becomes hypoglycemic
C. Hypoglycemia is defined as a blood sugar of less than 60 mg/dL
D. A and C
E. All of the above are reasonable

Q8: Diabetic nephropathy, when in the setting of pregnancy, can lead to end-stage renal disease particularly if:

A. Serum creatinine is above 1.0 mg/dL or 24 h protein is 300 mg per 24 h
B. Serum creatinine is above 1.5 mg/dL or 24 h protein is 3000 mg per 24 h
C. Serum creatinine is above 2.0 mg/dL or 24 h protein is 300 g per 24 h
D. Serum creatinine is above 2.5 mg/dL or 24 h protein is 3000 g per 24 h
E. Urine protein is not predictive of progression to end-stage renal disease

Q9: Diabetic ketoacidosis occurs more commonly in pregnancy and can even occur in patients who have normal blood glucose readings.

A. True
B. False

Q10: Which of the following is FALSE regarding the management of diabetic ketoacidosis in pregnancy?

A. Start an insulin drip
B. Hydrate with 4–6 L of half normal saline in the first 12 h
C. Give 5% dextrose once glucose is below 250 mg/dL
D. If fetal heart tracing is Category II, continue to treat maternal condition and anticipate improvement in fetal status

Q11: What is the leading cause of perinatal mortality in pregnancies complicated by pregestational diabetes?

A. Congenital anomalies
B. Iatrogenic preterm deliveries
C. Spontaneous preterm deliveries
D. Diabetic ketoacidosis

Q12: All of the following are known neonatal complications due to poorly controlled pregestational diabetes, EXCEPT:

A. Hypoglycemia
B. Hypobilirubinemia
C. Respiratory distress syndrome
D. Electrolyte disturbances
E. All of the above are known complications

Q13: You are taking care of a partner's patient who is a type I diabetic with nephropathy. She is concerned because her blood pressure has been increasing over the past several weeks and asks what it could mean. You counsel that her risk of developing preeclampsia is:

A. 10%
B. 20%

C. 30%
D. 40%
E. 50%

Q14: All of the following should be included in a preconception counseling visit for a woman with diabetes, EXCEPT:
A. Impact of euglycemia in decreasing risk for congenital anomalies to baseline population risk
B. 24 h urine protein collection
C. TSH if type II diabetic as 40% will have hypothyroidism
D. Counseling to take a multivitamin with folate due to increased risk for neural tube defects
E. All of the above are true

Q15: A type II diabetic patient presents for a new obstetric visit. She is currently taking glyburide and metformin and asks about the safety of those medications during pregnancy. You tell her:
A. Glyburide crosses the placenta but appears to be safe in retrospective studies
B. Glyburide has an onset of action of 3 h with a duration of 12 h
C. Metformin is a category A drug
D. The long-term effect of metformin on pregnancy is unknown
E. All of the above are true

Q16: A preterm type II diabetic patient is admitted to the hospital for elevated blood pressures and a steroid course is initiated for fetal lung maturity. She asks how long she should expect to have an increased need in her insulin dosing. You tell her:
A. 48 h
B. 72 h
C. 5 days
D. 7 days
E. 10 days

Q17: A 32-year-old patient presents for a return obstetric visit. She is worried because her cervix is closed at 36 weeks gestation. She is a type II diabetic, controlled on insulin, with glucose logs demonstrating excellent control. Assuming no other complications, what is the latest gestational age ACOG recommends delivery?

A. 37/0 weeks gestational age
B. 38/0 weeks gestational age
C. 39/0 weeks gestational age
D. 40/0 weeks gestational age
E. 41/0 weeks gestational age

Q18: What is the goal for blood glucose levels during labor?

A. Less than 140 mg/dL
B. Less than 130 mg/dL
C. Less than 120 mg/dL
D. Less than 110 mg/dL
E. Less than 100 mg/dL

Q19: The rate of primary cesarean delivery is increased in pregestational diabetics.

A. True
B. False

Answers

Q1: C, Q2: A, Q3: A, Q4: B, Q5: C, Q6: D, Q7: D, Q8: B, Q9: A, Q10: B, Q11: A, Q12: B, Q13: E, Q14: C, Q15: D, Q16: C, Q17: D, Q18: D, Q19: A.

Resources

1. Gabbe SG, Niebyl JR, Simpson JL, Landon MB, Galan HL, Jauniaux ERM, Driscoll DA. Obstetrics: normal and problem pregnancies. Chapter 39. 6th ed. Philadelphia, PA: Elsevier; 2012.
2. American College of Obstetricians and Gynecologists. ACOG practice bulletin no. 60: pregestational diabetes mellitus. Obstet Gynecol. 2005;105:675–85.

Chapter 6
Management of Alloimmunization During Pregnancy

Once alloimmunization is diagnosed during pregnancy, maternal titers must be followed unless it is known that the father is also Rh negative. Maternal levels should be followed until a critical titer is reached, after which MCA Doppler studies should be performed. In severe cases, intrauterine transfusion may be needed [1].

Recommended resource—ACOG Practice Bulletin 75: Management of Alloimmunization During Pregnancy [2].

Q1: Alloimmunization occurs when a fetal blood group factor from the ____ is not possessed by the ____.

A. Mother, father
B. Father, mother

Q2: Which of the following is TRUE regarding the Fisher-Race nomenclature?

A. Includes five genetic loci each with two major alleles
B. No antiserum specific for "e" antigen has been found; thus, testing indicates absence of allelic product
C. Each Rh gene complex is described by three letters
D. Rh positive refers to the absence of "D" antigen on erythrocytes
E. None of the above

K.C. Arnold, C.J. Flint, *Obstetrics Essentials*,
DOI 10.1007/978-3-319-57675-6_6,

Q3: Kell alloimmunization is diagnosed in a new obstetrical patient. How should she be counseled?

A. Kell alloimmunization is often caused by prior transfusions
B. Amniotic fluid analysis correlates with the severity of fetal anemia
C. Aggressive fetal assessment is unwarranted
D. A and B
E. All of the above

Q4: What percentage of Rh alloimmunization occurs due to antepartum fetomaternal hemorrhage?

A. 1%
B. 5%
C. 10%
D. 15%

Q5: Which of the following patients are candidates for anti-D immune globulin?

A. 28-year-old at 28 weeks gestation who is Rh negative, antibody negative
B. 28-year-old at 28 weeks gestation who is Rh negative, antibody positive
C. 28-year-old at 28 weeks gestation who is Rh negative, sensitized, with Kell alloimmunization
D. A and C
E. All of the above

Q6: A Rh-negative woman should be screened for antibodies at all of the following times, EXCEPT:

A. Prior to anti-D immune globulin at 28 weeks gestation
B. Postpartum
C. Abruption
D. Subsequent pregnancies
E. All of the above are recommended

Q7: A patient is Rh negative and known to be sensitized. She is counseled regarding titers. She read on the Internet about a “critical titer” and asks what it means. You tell her:

A. A critical titer is associated with a significant risk for severe erythroblastosis fetalis and hydrops
B. In most centers it is between 8:1 and 32:1
C. Titers are reported as the lowest dilution with a positive agglutination reaction
D. A and C
E. B and C

Q8: A 32-year-old G3P2002 presents to the office as a transfer of care for pregnancy. She is Rh negative and is found to be alloimmunized. She is newly married and does not know the blood type of her husband. What is the next best step?

A. Schedule serial titers
B. Order assessment of the peak systolic velocity in the fetal middle cerebral artery
C. Obtain paternal genotype
D. A and C
E. A and B

Q9: A 20-year-old G2P1001 is found to be Rh negative and is alloimmunized. She is unsure who the father is. What is the next best step in management?

A. Schedule serial titers
B. Order assessment of the peak systolic velocity in the fetal middle cerebral artery
C. Perform amniocentesis if gestational age is appropriate
D. Perform chorionic villus biopsy if gestational age is appropriate
E. A and B

Q10: A MFM physician calls regarding a patient who had middle cerebral artery Doppler testing today. The testing revealed that the measurement was two times the median for gestational age. How should the patient be counseled?

A. This test is somewhat sensitive for fetal anemia and the baby may be anemic
B. This is a very specific test for fetal anemia and shows the baby is anemic
C. This is a very sensitive test for fetal anemia and currently the baby is not anemic
D. This test is interpreted as part of a calculation; no meaningful results can be given at this time

Q11: A patient is diagnosed with alloimmunization that is non-Rh D. Which of the following is TRUE regarding this?

A. Most are due to prior incompatible blood transfusions
B. There has been a relative decrease in this due to anti-D immune globulin
C. They occur in approximately 10% of obstetric patients
D. None of the above

Q12: Which of the following tests are predictive of fetal anemia in Kell alloimmunization?

A. Amniotic fluid bilirubin measurements
B. Middle cerebral Doppler measurements
C. Antibody titers
D. A and B
E. B and C

Q13: What is the latest gestational age that pregnancies complicated by alloimmunization should be delivered?

A. 34 weeks gestational age
B. 35 weeks gestational age

C. 36 weeks gestational age
D. 37 weeks gestational age
E. 38 weeks gestational age

Answers

Q1: B, Q2: C, Q3: A, Q4: A, Q5: D, Q6: E, Q7: A, Q8: C, Q9: C, Q10: B, Q11: A, Q12: B, Q13: E.

Resources

1. Gabbe SG, Niebyl JR, Simpson JL, Landon MB, Galan HL, Jauniaux ERM, Driscoll DA. Obstetrics: normal and problem pregnancies. Chapter 32. 6th ed. Philadelphia, PA: Elsevier; 2012.
2. American College of Obstetricians and Gynecologists. ACOG practice bulletin no. 75: management of alloimmunization during pregnancy. Obstet Gynecol. 2006;108:457–64.

Chapter 7
Postpartum Hemorrhage

Postpartum hemorrhage is an obstetrical emergency which requires immediate action. Common causes include uterine atony, genital tract lacerations, retained products of conception, and invasive placentation. Initial management may include bimanual massage, use of uterotonics, and thorough exam. In severe cases, hysterectomy may be needed for control of hemorrhage [1].

Recommended resource—ACOG Practice Bulletin 76: Postpartum Hemorrhage [2].

Q1: What is the difference between primary and secondary postpartum hemorrhage?

A. Primary postpartum hemorrhage occurs within the first 12 h of delivery and secondary hemorrhage occurs between 12 h and 6–12 weeks postpartum
B. Primary postpartum hemorrhage occurs within the first 24 h of delivery and secondary hemorrhage occurs between 24 h and 6–12 weeks postpartum
C. Primary postpartum hemorrhage occurs within the first 48 h of delivery and secondary hemorrhage occurs between 48 h and 6–12 weeks postpartum

K.C. Arnold, C.J. Flint, *Obstetrics Essentials*,
DOI 10.1007/978-3-319-57675-6_7,

D. Primary postpartum hemorrhage occurs within the first 72 h of delivery and secondary hemorrhage occurs between 72 h and 6–12 weeks postpartum

Q2: What is the most common cause of primary postpartum hemorrhage?

A. Retained placenta
B. Defects in coagulation
C. Vaginal laceration
D. Uterine atony

Q3: Examples of causes of secondary postpartum hemorrhage include all of the following, EXCEPT:

A. Infection
B. Subinvolution of placental site
C. Inherited coagulation defects
D. Retained products of conception
E. All of the above are causes of secondary postpartum hemorrhage

Q4: A 24-year-old G2P1001 is status post-spontaneous vaginal delivery 5 min ago. The placenta has delivered without issue. The patient begins to have heavy vaginal bleeding. What FIRST steps should be taken to evaluate the patient?

A. Lacerations should be ruled out with thorough visual assessment of vaginal area
B. The vagina should be packed immediately
C. The bladder should be emptied and a bimanual pelvic exam should be performed
D. Ultrasound should be performed to assess for retained placenta

Q5: Which of the following is FALSE regarding a genital tract hematoma?

A. Interventional radiology should be considered for management
B. Often times a single source of bleeding will be identified when the hematoma is incised

C. It may be appropriate to place a drain in situ after a hematoma is drained
D. Can lead to large blood loss
E. Can occur in the absence of a vaginal laceration

Q6: Which of the following makes the diagnosis of a retained placenta less likely?
A. Echogenic mass within the uterus visualized on ultrasound
B. History of previous uterine surgery
C. Manual extraction of the placenta
D. All of the above increase the likelihood of retained placenta

Q7: An amniotic fluid embolism can be associated with clotting abnormalities leading to hemorrhage.
A. True
B. False

Q8: Which of the following is TRUE regarding a clot observation test?
A. Can provide a rough estimate of fibrinogen level within 10 min
B. The blood will not clot within 10 min if fibrinogen level is less than 200 mg/dL
C. Blood with normal levels of fibrinogen will clot within 10 min and remain intact
D. A and C
E. All of the above

For the following questions, choose the uterotonic drug which best matches the description given.

Q9: Should be avoided in asthmatics.
A. Pitocin
B. Methergine
C. Hemabate
D. Misoprostol

Q10: Can cause diarrhea.
A. Pitocin
B. Methergine
C. Hemabate
D. Misoprostol

Q11: Can cause hypotension.
A. Pitocin
B. Methergine
C. Hemabate
D. Misoprostol

Q12: Dosing is 0.2 mg IM q 2–4 h
A. Pitocin
B. Methergine
C. Hemabate
D. Misoprostol

Q13: A maximum of eight doses may be given.
A. Pitocin
B. Methergine
C. Hemabate
D. Misoprostol

Q14: Should be avoided in hypertensive patients.
A. Pitocin
B. Methergine
C. Hemabate
D. Misoprostol

Q15: What step should be employed next following continued bleeding in the setting of uterine atony despite use of adequate uterotonics?
A. Tamponade of the uterus
B. Exploratory laparotomy
C. Uterine artery embolization by interventional radiology
D. Bilateral uterine artery ligation

Q16: Hypogastric artery ligation is the most effective surgical technique to control uterine bleeding.
A. True
B. False

Q17: What are the two most common indications for postpartum hysterectomy?
A. Uterine atony and uterine inversion
B. Coagulation abnormalities and uterine atony
C. Placenta accreta and uterine atony
D. Coagulation abnormalities and placenta accreta

Q18: Which of the following is FALSE in regard to placenta accreta?
A. Antepartum ultrasound can aid in diagnosis
B. Risk is related to a history of a cesarean delivery but not the number of previous cesarean sections
C. Associated with an increased risk of postpartum hemorrhage
D. Maternal age older than 35 years is a risk factor
E. None of the above

Q19: Under which circumstances should a uterine artery embolization be considered in a postpartum patient with hemorrhage?
A. Continued bleeding after hysterectomy
B. In a patient with a history of a tubal ligation
C. In a patient with persistent bleeding but stable vital signs
D. A and C
E. All of the above

Q20: Transfusion of 50 mL of platelets increases the platelet count by ________.
A. 5000–10,000/mm^3 per unit
B. 10,000–15,000/mm^3 per unit
C. 15,000–20,000/mm^3 per unit
D. 20,000–25,000/mm^3 per unit

Q21: Transfusion with fresh frozen plasma involves a greater replacement of volume than cryoprecipitate.
A. True
B. False

Q22: Two units of packed red blood cells will increase hematocrit by ______ percentage points.
A. Three
B. Four
C. Five
D. Six

Q23: Which procedure performed to reverse uterine inversion involves incising the cervical ring posteriorly?
A. Friedman procedure
B. Haultain procedure
D. Huntington procedure
E. Hasselbalch procedure

Q24: What is the recurrence risk of postpartum hemorrhage in a subsequent pregnancy?
A. 1%
B. 5%
C. 10%
D. 15%
E. 20%

Q25: Which of the following agents can be used to aid in uterine relaxation when managing a uterine inversion?
A. Magnesium sulfate
B. Halogenated general anesthetics
C. Terbutaline
D. B and C
E. All of the above

Q26: You notice on the labor and delivery schedule there is a patient for a repeat cesarean who has had six previous cesarean deliveries. What is the risk that she will need a hysterectomy?

A. 1%
B. 3%
C. 4%
D. 5%
E. 9%

Answers

Q1: B, Q2: D, Q3: E, Q4: C, Q5: B, Q6: D, Q7: A, Q8: D, Q9: C, Q10: C, Q11: A, Q12: B, Q13: C, Q14: B, Q15: A, Q16: B, Q17: C, Q18: B, Q19: D, Q20: A, Q21: A, Q22: D, Q23: B, Q24: C, Q25: E, Q26: E.

Resources

1. Gabbe SG, Niebyl JR, Simpson JL, Landon MB, Galan HL, Jauniaux ERM, Driscoll DA. Obstetrics: normal and problem pregnancies. Chapter 19. 6th ed. Philadelphia, PA: Elsevier; 2012.
2. American College of Obstetricians and Gynecologists. ACOG practice bulletin no. 76: postpartum hemorrhage. Obstet Gynecol. 2006;108:1039–47.

Chapter 8
Hemoglobinopathies in Pregnancy

Adult hemoglobin is composed of two alpha and two beta chains. Hemoglobinopathies result when there is an alteration in these chains. The two most salient diagnoses are the thalassemias and sickle cell disease. Pregnant patients with sickle cell disease are at high risk for poor outcomes and should have antenatal surveillance [1].

Recommended resource—ACOG Practice Bulletin 78: Hemoglobinopathies in Pregnancy [2].

Q1: Sickle cell disease:

A. Is an autosomal dominant disorder
B. Occurs most commonly in people of Caucasian descent
C. Involves a single nucleotide substitution on the alpha globin gene
D. A and C
E. None of the above

Q2: Hemoglobin A is composed of:

A. Two alpha and two beta chains
B. Two beta and two delta chains
C. Two alpha and two gamma chains
D. Four beta chains
E. Four alpha chains

K.C. Arnold, C.J. Flint, *Obstetrics Essentials*,
DOI 10.1007/978-3-319-57675-6_8,

Q3: Acute chest syndrome includes all of the following, EXCEPT:

A. Pulmonary infiltrates
B. Fever
C. Hypoxemia
D. Infection
E. All of the above are present in acute chest syndrome

Q4: Which of the following will NOT have clinical implications?

A. Hb SC disease
B. Hb SS
C. Hb S/beta-thalassemia
D. Deletion of one alpha globin gene
E. All of the above have clinical consequences

Q5: What is the genotype of alpha-thalassemia carriers?

A. $\alpha-/\alpha\alpha$
B. $\alpha\alpha/--$
C. $\alpha-/\alpha-$
D. B and C
E. All of the above

Q6: Hb Bart is:

A. Associated with abnormalities on the beta globin
B. Associated with hydrops fetalis
C. More common in patients of African origin
D. B and C
E. All of the above are true

Q7: Which of the following is a feature of beta-thalassemia major?

A. Precocious sexual development
B. Rapid growth
C. Extramedullary erythropoiesis
D. Decreased levels of Hb F
E. Death by age 30

Q8: Which of the following is TRUE regarding beta-thalassemia minor?
A. Severity depends on the amount of beta chain production
B. Commonly associated with HB S
C. Common in individuals of Mediterranean descent
D. All of the above
E. None of the above

Q9: A 19-year-old African American G1P0 presents for her first obstetrical visit. She denies any known history of hemoglobinopathies in her family. What initial testing should be obtained?
A. CBC
B. Hemoglobin electrophoresis
C. Solubility tests
D. A and B
E. A and C

Q10: How is alpha-thalassemia diagnosed?
A. Hemoglobin electrophoresis
B. Solubility testing
C. Molecular genetic testing
D. MCV
E. A or C

Q11: How can thalassemias be diagnosed prenatally?
A. Preimplantation genetic diagnosis
B. Chorionic villus sampling
C. Amniocentesis
D. B and C
E. All of the above

Q12: Patients with sickle cell anemia are at increased risk for:
A. Gestational diabetes
B. Preterm labor
C. Macrosomia
D. Multifetal gestations
E. All of the above

Q13: Which of the following therapies is recommended in pregnant patients with sickle cell disease?

A. 1 mg folate a day
B. 4 mg folate a day
C. Prophylactic cesarean section
D. Avoidance of regional anesthesia
E. Hydroxyurea

Q14: Which of the following accurately describes the care of a pregnant patient with a sickle cell pain crisis?

A. Diagnosis of medical problems causing predisposition
B. Control of pain while avoiding opiates
C. Oxygen to keep O_2 saturation 90% or more
D. A and B
E. B and C

Q15: What is the goal of transfusion in pregnant patients with sickle cell disease?

A. Lower the Hb S to 30% and raise the total hemoglobin to 8 g/dL
B. Lower the Hb S to 40% and raise the total hemoglobin to 10 g/dL
C. Lower the Hb S to 30% and raise the total hemoglobin to 10 g/dL
D. Lower the Hb S to 40% and raise the total hemoglobin to 8 g/dL

Q16: Monitoring of fetal growth is recommended for which of the following disorders?

A. Sickle cell disease
B. Beta-thalassemia major
C. Alpha-thalassemia trait
D. B and B
E. All of the above

Answers

Q1: E, Q2: A, Q3: D, Q4: D, Q5: D, Q6: B, Q7: C, Q8: D, Q9: D, Q10: C, Q11: E, Q12: B, Q13: B, Q14: A, Q15: B, Q16: D.

Resources

1. Gabbe SG, Niebyl JR, Simpson JL, Landon MB, Galan HL, Jauniaux ERM, Driscoll DA. Obstetrics: normal and problem pregnancies. Chapter 42. 6th ed. Philadelphia, PA: Elsevier; 2012.
2. American College of Obstetricians and Gynecologists. ACOG practice bulletin no. 78: hemoglobinopathies in pregnancy. Obstet Gynecol. 2007;109:229–37.

Chapter 9
Management of Herpes in Pregnancy

Herpes virus causes painful vesicles with HSV-1 primarily causing oral lesions and HSV-2 causing genital lesions on the vagina, vulva, or cervix. Diagnosis is made either by viral culture or nucleic acid detection. Primary outbreaks are associated with much higher rates of neonatal HSV infection than recurrent outbreaks. If there are any active lesions or prodromal symptoms present during labor, delivery should be performed by cesarean section [1].

Recommended resource—ACOG Practice Bulletin 82: Management of Herpes in Pregnancy [2].

Q1: Which of the following is FALSE regarding the herpes simplex virus?

A. Is transmitted through direct contact
B. Most people who are infected with HSV are unaware that they have the virus
C. Antibodies to HSV can be detected within 2–3 weeks after infection
D. Genital lesions caused by HSV-1 are becoming more common
E. All of the above are true

K.C. Arnold, C.J. Flint, *Obstetrics Essentials*,
DOI 10.1007/978-3-319-57675-6_9,

Q2: Which of the following is an example of a nonprimary first episode?
A. HSV-2 is isolated from a genital lesion and HSV-2 antibodies are present in the blood
B. HSV-2 is isolated from a genital lesion and no HSV-1 or HSV-2 antibodies are present in the blood
C. No genital lesions are present and HSV-1 antibodies are present in the blood
D. HSV-1 is isolated from a genital lesion and HSV-2 antibodies are present in the blood

Q3: Which of the following accurately describes the timing of new HSV-2 infections in pregnant patients?
A. Most occur in the first trimester
B. Most occur in the second trimester
C. Most occur in the third trimester
D. Approximately 1/3 occur in each trimester

Q4: The majority of HSV-infected infants are born to mothers who reported no history of HSV infection.
A TRUE
B FALSE

Q5: Which of the following is TRUE regarding neonatal herpes infection?
A. Usually acquired during the intrapartum period
B. Over half of all cases are caused by HSV-1
C. Approximately 70% of survivors will have long-term neurologic sequelae
D. Risk of development is equivalent with recurrent and nonprimary first episodes of infections
E. None of the above

Q6: Which of the following is FALSE in regard to the techniques used to diagnose herpes?
A. May include viral detection and antibody detection techniques
B. Polymerase chain reaction (PCR) techniques have increased sensitivity over cultures

C. The presence of HSV-1 antibodies alone may be indicative of either genital or orolabial infection
D. A negative genital culture excludes the presence of an infection

Q7: It is possible to differentiate between a primary herpes infection and a nonprimary first episode during pregnancy based on clinical findings alone.
A. TRUE
B. FALSE

Q8: What is the risk of vertical transmission to the neonate with a primary genital HSV outbreak at the time of delivery?
A. Less than 3%
B. 10–20%
C. 20–40%
D. 30–60%
E. As high as 80%

Q9: What are the possible reasons for increased vertical transmission of genital HSV at the time of delivery associated with primary compared to recurrent outbreaks?
A. There is increased transplacental passage of protective HSV-2-specific antibodies with recurrent outbreaks
B. Cervical shedding may be increased with primary outbreaks
C. Primary outbreaks are associated with shorter duration yet higher concentrations of viral shedding
D. A and B
E. All the above

Q10: Cesarean delivery is indicated in any woman with a history of genital HSV, regardless of current outbreak status.
A. TRUE
B. FALSE

Q11: At what gestational age should women with active recurrent genital herpes be offered suppressive viral therapy?

A. 36 weeks
B. 34 weeks
C. 32 weeks
D. 28 weeks

Q12: The three antiviral agents most commonly used to treat HSV infection in pregnancy are FDA pregnancy category A medications.

A. TRUE
B. FALSE

Q13: Routine HSV screening of pregnant women is not recommended.

A. TRUE
B. FALSE

Q14: A 34-year-old G1P0 at 39 weeks gestational age presents to labor and delivery in active labor. On exam the patient is noted to have a painful ulcer on her outer thigh. When the patient is questioned about this, she says that she has had such lesions "come and go" on her thigh previously. She denies ever having genital lesions. What is the next best step in her management?

A. Due to likely HSV infection, proceed with cesarean section for delivery
B. Due to unlikely HSV infection, proceed with vaginal delivery if otherwise indicated
C. Due to concern for HSV infection, perform thorough vaginal and cervical examination to rule out presence of additional lesions. If exam is negative, proceed with vaginal delivery if otherwise indicated
D. Start IV acyclovir immediately and proceed with cesarean section for delivery

Q15: Which of the following is TRUE regarding active herpes simplex virus infection and preterm premature rupture of membranes in a pregnant patient?

A. Expectant management is reasonable depending upon gestational age and associated risk of prematurity
B. Treatment with an antiviral medication is contraindicated
C. Administering corticosteroids for fetal lung maturity is contraindicated due to increased risk of worsening infection
D. Immediate cesarean section should be performed as long as fetus is greater than 24 weeks gestational age
E. None of the above

Q16: Breastfeeding is contraindicated in the following scenario:

A. Active primary HSV genital lesions
B. Mother is currently taking valacyclovir
C. Recurrent HSV genital lesions
D. Active HSV breast lesions
E. All of the above

Q17: What percent of pregnant women with recurrent genital HSV have at least one recurrence during pregnancy?

A. 25%
B. 40%
C. 50%
D. 75%
E. 90%

Q18: Your patient presents for a postpartum visit. She had recurrent genital HSV, used suppression therapy, and delivered vaginally after having an exam showing no lesions. She presents upset because her baby was readmitted at 2 weeks age due to neonatal HSV. She wonders if she may have infected her baby. How do you counsel her?

A. Intrapartum infection is extremely unlikely given the above scenario
B. The infection may have been acquired from a family member through oropharyngeal disease
C. The infection may have been acquired from a family member through cutaneous disease
D. A and B
E. All of the above

Answers

Q1: E, Q2: D, Q3: D, Q4: A, Q5: A, Q6: D, Q7: B, Q8: D, Q9: D, Q10: B, Q11: A, Q12: B, Q13: A, Q14: C, Q15: A, Q16: D, Q17: D, Q18: E.

Resources

1. Gabbe SG, Niebyl JR, Simpson JL, Landon MB, Galan HL, ERM J, Driscoll DA. Obstetrics: normal and problem pregnancies. Chapter 50. 6th ed. Philadelphia, PA: Elsevier; 2012.
2. American College of Obstetricians and Gynecologists. ACOG practice bulletin no. 82: management of herpes in pregnancy. Obstet Gynecol. 2007;109:1489–98.

Chapter 10
Viral Hepatitis in Pregnancy

Viral hepatitis during pregnancy in the acute setting presents with nausea, right upper quadrant pain, and decreased appetite. Laboratory results can show high aminotransferase levels. In the case of chronic hepatitis, vertical transmission to the neonate may occur at delivery; however, cesarean section is not recommended for prevention [1].

Recommended resource—ACOG Practice Bulletin 86: Viral Hepatitis in Pregnancy [2].

Q1: Transmission of this virus is generally through the use of IV drugs or through blood products and is associated with B cell lymphomas, and its association with hepatocellular carcinoma is uncertain.

A. Hepatitis A
B. Hepatitis B
C. Hepatitis C
D. Hepatitis D
E. Hepatitis B and D

Q2: This virus is transmitted through fecal-oral transmission, is an RNA virus, and does not lead to chronic infection:

A. Hepatitis A
B. Hepatitis B
C. Hepatitis C

K.C. Arnold, C.J. Flint, *Obstetrics Essentials*,
DOI 10.1007/978-3-319-57675-6_10,

D. Hepatitis D
E. Hepatitis B and D

Q3: This virus is transmitted through sexual partners or needle sharing, and the intact virus is called the Dane particle:
A. Hepatitis A
B. Hepatitis B
C. Hepatitis C
D. Hepatitis D
E. Hepatitis B and D

Q4: Which types of viral hepatitis can be prevented through vaccination?
A. Hepatitis A and B
B. Hepatitis B and C
C. Hepatitis A and C
D. Hepatitis C and D
E. Only Hepatitis B

Q5: A former sex worker presents as a new patient. A viral hepatitis panel is obtained and results as positive for the viral hepatitis most associated with sexual transmission. What is her risk for long-term consequences?
A. Chronic infection is not a feature of this hepatitis
B. Her risk for chronic infection is 10–15%
C. It is associated with increased risk for hepatocellular carcinoma
D. A and C
E. B and C

Q6: Hepatitis ____ can only cause disease if the patient is coinfected with hepatitis ___.
A. A; B
B. A; C
C. D; B
D. D; C
E. E; C

Q7: This viral hepatitis, when chronic, is associated with a mortality rate of 25% due to hepatic failure.
A. Hepatitis A
B. Hepatitis B
C. Hepatitis C
D. Hepatitis D
E. Hepatitis B and D

Q8: A pregnant patient has heard about the hepatitis A vaccine and asks if she should receive it. She is an IV drug user and has fatty liver disease. You counsel her:
A. Yes, it is recommended because of her drug use
B. Yes, it is recommended for all pregnant women
C. No, it is contraindicated during pregnancy. She may receive it at her postpartum visit
D. No, because it is contraindicated in patients who have chronic liver disease

Q9: A general surgery resident is panicked because she just had a needle stick during a surgical case on a patient with known hepatitis B. What should she receive to reduce the risk of transmission?
A. Hepatitis B vaccine
B. Immune globulin
C. Hepatitis B vaccine and immune globulin as soon as possible
D. Hepatitis B vaccine and then immune globulin in 14 days
E. No prophylaxis is shown to decrease transmission rates

Q10: All of the following are symptoms of acute viral hepatitis, EXCEPT:
A. Fatigue
B. Fever
C. Nausea
D. Darkened urine
E. Malaise

Q11: This viral hepatitis progresses to a chronic infection in 50% of infected individuals:

A. Hepatitis A
B. Hepatitis B
C. Hepatitis C
D. Hepatitis D
E. Hepatitis B and D

Q12: Which types of hepatitis are associated with travel?

A. Hepatitis A and B
B. Hepatitis B and D
C. Hepatitis D and E
D. Hepatitis A and E
E. Hepatitis B and D

Q13: What is the leading cause of chronic liver disease in the United States?

A. Pancreatitis
B. Hepatitis B
C. Hepatitis C
D. Alcoholism
E. Gallstones

Q14: A pregnant patient is positive for HBsAg. What is most likely regarding her symptoms?

A. She may not have clinical symptoms yet
B. She may have acute symptoms currently
C. She may be a chronic carrier
D. A and B
E. All of the above

Q15: Which of the following is TRUE regarding the hepatitis B core antibody?

A. Indicates a natural infection
B. Results in immunity to hepatitis B
C. Signals a chronic infection
D. Signifies evidence of prior vaccination
E. B and D

Q16: How long after symptoms start do antibodies to hepatitis C usually appear?

A. 3–5 days
B. 2 weeks
C. 4 weeks
D. 6 weeks
E. 12 weeks

Q17: A pregnant patient has recently been diagnosed with hepatitis B. She asks about long-term consequences. You inform her:

A. Perinatal infection carries a decreased risk for chronic disease of approximately 5%
B. Perinatal infection carries an increased risk for chronic disease of approximately 90%
C. The risk for chronic disease in adults is 30%
D. HBeAg decreases the risk for vertical transmission
E. Vertical transmission risk is greatest if the mother is acutely infected in the first trimester

Q18: Babies born to mothers who are HBsAg positive should receive:

A. Hepatitis B vaccine IM immediately
B. Immune globulin IM immediately
C. Hepatitis B vaccine and immune globulin immediately
D. Hepatitis B vaccine and then immune globulin in 14 days
E. No prophylaxis is shown to decrease transmission rates

Q19: All of the following are associated with an increased risk for vertical transmission of hepatitis C, EXCEPT:

A. HIV infection
B. Detectable viremia
C. Prolonged membrane rupture
D. Use of internal fetal monitoring
E. Vaginal delivery

Q20: Which of the following patients should be screened for hepatitis C?

A. A 19-year-old being treated for her first chlamydia infection
B. A 45-year-old who has been happily married for 20 years but confesses to use of heroin once at age 19
C. A 25-year-old who reports a postpartum hemorrhage with her first baby requiring massive transfusion protocol
D. Any pregnant patient
E. All of the above should be screened

Q21: To decrease risk of perinatal vertical transmission, cesarean delivery should be considered in patients with:

A. Hepatitis A
B. Hepatitis B
C. Hepatitis C
D. All of the above
E. None of the above

Q22: To decrease the risk of perinatal vertical transmission, breastfeeding should be avoided in patients with:

A. Hepatitis A
B. Hepatitis B
C. Hepatitis C
D. All of the above
E. None of the above

Q23: Which of the following is contraindicated during pregnancy?

A. Hepatitis A vaccine
B. Hepatitis A immune globulin
C. Hepatitis B vaccine
D. Hepatitis B immune globulin
E. None of the above

Q24: Which of the following carries the highest risk of transmission by occupational exposure?
A. Hepatitis A
B. Hepatitis B
C. Hepatitis C
D. Hepatitis D
E. HIV

Answers

Q1: C, Q2: A, Q3: B, Q4: A, Q5: E, Q6: C, Q7: D, Q8: A, Q9: C, Q10: B, Q11: C, Q12: D, Q13: C, Q14: E, Q15: A, Q16: D, Q17: B, Q18: C, Q19: E, Q20: B, Q21: E, Q22: E, Q23: E, Q24: B.

References

1. Gabbe SG, Niebyl JR, Simpson JL, Landon MB, Galan HL, Jauniaux ERM, Driscoll DA. Obstetrics: normal and problem pregnancies, Chapter 45. 6th ed. Philadelphia, PA: Elsevier; 2012.
2. American College of Obstetricians and Gynecologists. ACOG practice bulletin no. 86: viral hepatitis in pregnancy. Obstet Gynecol. 2007;110:941–55.

Chapter 11
Asthma in Pregnancy

Asthma is associated with chronic airway inflammation in which patients may experience as fluctuating symptoms of cough, wheezing, and feeling short of breath. The general principle guiding treatment during pregnancy relates to the benefits of prevention taking precedence over the potential risks of asthma medication usage. Treatment should be assessed using objective measures and should include patient education as an integral component [1].

Recommended resource—ACOG Practice Bulletin 90: Asthma in Pregnancy [2].

Q1: Which of the following is FALSE regarding asthma?
- A. Airway obstruction is at least partially reversible
- B. Characterized by decreased responsiveness to stimuli
- C. Characterized by chronic airway inflammation
- D. None of the above

Q2: A 33-year-old G1P0 presents for her new obstetrical visit at 6 weeks gestation. She has a history of moderate persistent asthma and is currently on two different medications to control her symptoms. She is concerned

K.C. Arnold, C.J. Flint, *Obstetrics Essentials*,
DOI 10.1007/978-3-319-57675-6_11,

about how the medications will interfere with the development of her fetus. You counsel her:

A. She should stop taking all medications due to known fetal risks and that her symptoms will be treated as they arise
B. She should continue to take her current medications because there is no known fetal risk associated with them
C. She should discontinue her medications because the teratogenic risks far outweigh the risks of an asthma exacerbation
D. She should continue her current medication regimen as the benefits of well-controlled asthma symptoms clearly outweigh the potential teratogenic risks to her fetus

Q3: Severe and poorly controlled asthma is associated with all of the following, EXCEPT:

A. Maternal morbidity and mortality
B. Prematurity
C. Cesarean delivery
D. Growth restriction
E. None of the above

Q4: Which of the following medications can potentially worsen asthma symptoms during labor and delivery?

A. Indomethacin
B. Magnesium
C. Hemabate
D. A and C
E. All the above

Q5: What are the most commonly used objective pulmonary function parameters used in pregnant patients with asthma?

A. Pulse oximetry and peak expiratory flow rate
B. Pulse oximetry and forced expiratory volume in the first second of inspiration

C. Methacholine challenge testing and peak expiratory flow rate
D. Forced expiratory volume in the first second of inspiration and peak expiratory flow rate

For the following questions (6–11), designate the classification of asthma severity:

Q6: Patient reports daily symptoms and nighttime awakening more than once per week.
A. Intermittent (well controlled)
B. Mild persistent (not well controlled)
C. Moderate persistent (not well controlled)
D. Severe persistent (very poorly controlled)

Q7: Patient reports nighttime awakening twice per month and no interference with normal activity.
A. Intermittent (well controlled)
B. Mild persistent (not well controlled)
C. Moderate persistent (not well controlled)
D. Severe persistent (very poorly controlled)

Q8: Patient reports symptoms more than 2 days per week and has minor limitation with normal activity.
A. Intermittent (well controlled)
B. Mild persistent (not well controlled)
C. Moderate persistent (not well controlled)
D. Severe persistent (very poorly controlled)

Q9: Patient only requires albuterol as needed to control symptoms.
A. Intermittent (well controlled)
B. Mild persistent (not well controlled)
C. Moderate persistent (not well controlled)
D. Severe persistent (very poorly controlled)

Q10: Patient reports being prescribed high-dose inhaled corticosteroid and salmeterol in an effort to control symptoms.

A. Intermittent (well controlled)
B. Mild persistent (not well controlled)
C. Moderate persistent (not well controlled)
D. Severe persistent (very poorly controlled)

Q11: Patient reports daily symptoms and awakens at night with symptoms more than once per week but only reports some limitation on normal activity.

A. Intermittent (well controlled)
B. Mild persistent (not well controlled)
C. Moderate persistent (not well controlled)
D. Severe persistent (very poorly controlled)

Q12: Asthma symptoms consistently worsen with pregnancy.

A. TRUE
B. FALSE

Q13: Which of the following does NOT point toward a new diagnosis of asthma in pregnancy?

A. Symptoms fluctuate in intensity and are often worse at night
B. Symptoms do not respond to typical asthma therapy
C. Symptoms are triggered by allergens
D. Wheezing can be heard on auscultation
E. FEV1 improves after bronchodilator

Q14: How can dyspnea of pregnancy be differentiated from a new diagnosis of asthma during pregnancy?

A. Dyspnea of pregnancy is not associated with a cough
B. Dyspnea of pregnancy often has evidence of airway obstruction

C. Dyspnea of pregnancy does not exhibit wheezing on auscultation
D. A and C
E. All of the above

Q15: How should a patient be counseled regarding the use of allergen immunotherapy during pregnancy?
A. Allergen immunotherapy should be immediately discontinued upon confirmation of pregnancy due to risk of anaphylaxis
B. If a patient is tolerating allergen immunotherapy prior to pregnancy, increasing the dose generally provides improve control
C. Due to the benefit of allergen immunotherapy, it is reasonable to start therapy while pregnant
D. The risk of anaphylaxis associated with allergen immunotherapy is a reason not to initiate therapy during pregnancy

Q16: What is the recommended rescue therapy for asthma during pregnancy?
A. Short-acting beta-2 agonists
B. Short-acting beta-2 antagonists
C. Inhaled mild corticosteroids
D. Oral corticosteroids

Q17: A 28-year-old G2P1001 with intrauterine gestation at 28 weeks calls the triage phone stating that she has had an acute exacerbation of her asthma symptoms. She has used her rescue treatment as her physician advised in the office and now her peak expiratory flow rate (PEFR) has reached 60% of her personal best and her symptoms have overall improved. You counsel her:
A. To continue to monitor her symptoms from home and reinitiate rescue therapy as needed
B. To lay on her left side and monitor for appropriate fetal movement

C. Her asthma exacerbation has resolved appropriately and to follow up in clinic as previously scheduled
D. To come into the hospital for medical attention as soon as possible

Q18: What is the preferred inhaled corticosteroid for use during pregnancy?
A. Budesonide
B. Salmeterol
C. Fluticasone
D. Theophylline

Q19: A 22-year-old G1P0 presents for her first obstetrical visit. In review of her history, she has a diagnosis of moderate asthma with a history of intubation secondary to acute asthma attack about 3 years ago. When discussing the necessary fetal surveillance for this patient, you counsel her:
A. She will need a first-trimester scan for dating and Level II ultrasound to assess for any structural abnormalities
B. She will need a first-trimester scan for dating and serial growth ultrasounds with antenatal testing to start at approximately 32 weeks
C. She will need a first-trimester scan for dating and only serial growth ultrasounds if an abnormality is found on her Level II scan
D. She will need a first-trimester scan for dating and only serial growth ultrasounds if her symptoms worsen during the course of her pregnancy

Q20: Asthma medications should be continued during labor and delivery, and fluids should be given sparingly to decrease the risk of bronchospasm.
A. TRUE
B. FALSE

Q21: Pregnant patients receiving systemic corticosteroids require additional IV dosing of steroids during labor and after delivery to prevent adrenal crisis.
A. TRUE
B. FALSE

Q22: Which of the following asthma medications are contraindicated with breastfeeding?
A. Prednisone
B. Cromolyn
C. Theophylline
D. Inhaled corticosteroids
E. None of the above

Answers

Q1: B, Q2: D, Q3: E, Q4: D, Q5: D, Q6: C, Q7: A, Q8: B, Q9: A, Q10: D, Q11: C, Q12: B, Q13: B, Q14: D, Q15: D, Q16: A, Q17: D, Q18: A, Q19: B, Q20: B, Q21: A, Q22: E.

Resources

1. Gabbe SG, Niebyl JR, Simpson JL, Landon MB, Galan HL, Jauniaux ERM, Driscoll DA. Obstetrics: normal and problem pregnancies. Chapter 37. 6th ed. Philadelphia, PA: Elsevier; 2012.
2. American College of Obstetricians and Gynecologists. ACOG practice bulletin no. 90: asthma in pregnancy. Obstet Gynecol. 2008;111:457–64.

Chapter 12
Use of Psychiatric Medications During Pregnancy and Lactation

Mental health disorders have the potential to profoundly impact maternal and fetal outcomes. Major depression can be screened for using the Edinburgh Postnatal Depression Scale. Bipolar disorder is characterized by depression and mania [1].

Recommended resource—ACOG Practice Bulletin 92: Use of Psychiatric Medications During Pregnancy and Lactation [2].

Q1: What proportion of pregnant women take a psychotropic medication at some point during their pregnancy?

A. 1/10
B. 1/5
C. 1/4
D. 1/3
E. None of the above

Q2: What proportion of psychotropic medications are present in amniotic fluid?

A. 1/10
B. 1/5
C. 1/4
D. 1/3
E. None of the above

K.C. Arnold, C.J. Flint, *Obstetrics Essentials*,
DOI 10.1007/978-3-319-57675-6_12,

Q3: Antidepressants, psychotherapy, and electroconvulsive therapy are all treatment options for pregnant women suffering from:
- A. Anxiety disorders
- B. Major depression
- C. Bipolar disorder
- D. Schizophrenia
- E. All of the above

Q4: Which psychiatric illness is associated with an increased risk of postnatal death?
- A. Anxiety disorders
- B. Major depression
- C. Bipolar disorder
- D. Schizophrenia
- E. All of the above

Q5: A patient has bipolar disorder and asks which medication is safest for her to take during pregnancy. You counsel her toward:
- A. Lithium
- B. Valproic acid
- C. Carbamazepine
- D. Lamotrigine
- E. All of the above have equal risks and benefits

Q6: Which selective serotonin reuptake inhibitor (SSRI) has a pregnancy risk category of D?
- A. Paroxetine
- B. Escitalopram
- C. Citalopram
- D. A and B
- E. B and C

Q7: Which of the following principles are recommended when prescribing psychotropic medications to pregnant patients?

A. Prescribe multiple medications at their lowest doses to avoid possible teratogenic consequences of higher doses
B. Prescribe medications with higher protein-binding properties to decrease placental passage
C. Continue to change medications as needed if the lowest dose is ineffective
D. Prioritize medications with more metabolites to increase efficacy at lower doses

Q8: Which class of drugs is associated with floppy infant syndrome and neonatal withdrawal syndrome?
A. Benzodiazepines
B. SSRIs
C. Lithium
D. Antiepileptic drugs
E. Antipsychotic medications

Q9: A patient presents for her first prenatal visit. She reports a history of depression and is currently taking an antidepressant. She asks about her overall risk of depression during pregnancy if she were to continue versus discontinue the medication. You counsel her that ______ % of women who discontinued their medications reported a relapse in depression compared to _______% of women who continued their medications.
A. 39%, 15%
B. 49%, 10%
C. 59%, 20%
D. 69%, 25%

Q10: Untreated depression during pregnancy is associated with:
A. Premature birth
B. Low birthweight
C. Fetal growth restriction
D. B and C
E. All of the above

Q11: Bipolar disorder:

A. Affects men and women equally
B. Typically first manifests itself in women in their early thirties
C. Carries an increased risk for postpartum psychosis of 20%
D. A and B
E. All of the above

Q12: When do most exacerbations of panic disorders occur?

A. First trimester
B. Second trimester
C. Third trimester
D. Postpartum

Q13: A woman who is pregnant for the first time presents with her husband. He reports that she has developed a flat affect, has stopped functioning well at work, and even seems paranoid at times. What is the most likely diagnosis?

A. Anxiety disorder
B. Major depression
C. Bipolar disorder
D. Schizophrenia
E. Pregnancy associated mood changes

Q14: A 28-year-old G1P0 presents for her first obstetrical visit at 8 weeks gestation. In review of her medications, it is noted that she is currently taking paroxetine for depression. What is your recommendation regarding the use of this medication?

A. Continue use given the risk of relapse
B. Discontinue use as it is associated with fetal cardiac malformations
C. Taper the medication to avoid withdrawal
D. A and C
E. B and C

Q15: Which of the following is NOT an example of an atypical antidepressant?
- A. Bupropion
- B. Duloxetine
- C. Mirtazapine
- D. Nefazodone
- E. All of the above are atypical antidepressants

Q16: A patient presents for a well-woman exam who has a history of bipolar disorder. She is currently well controlled on lithium. Prior to starting the medication, she had severe episodes, though they were infrequent. What would you recommend she do prior to attempting to conceive?
- A. Stop lithium immediately given teratogenicity
- B. Taper off of lithium given teratogenicity
- C. Taper off of lithium, then restart it after organogenesis
- D. Taper off of lithium, then restart it in the third trimester
- E. Continue throughout pregnancy due to high risk of relapse

Q17: Which of the following are included in fetal valproate syndrome?
- A. Asperger's syndrome
- B. Developmental delay
- C. Facial dysmorphology
- D. B and C
- E. All of the above

Q18: Carbamazepine has been shown to be associated with which of the following fetal anomalies?
- A. Growth restriction
- B. Neural tube defects
- C. Developmental delay
- D. Fingernail hypoplasia
- E. All of the above

Q19: Which of the following are TRUE regarding lamotrigine?

A. It is effective at managing depressive episodes of bipolar depression
B. It should be avoided in the first trimester
C. Folate supplementation of 4 g/day should be offered preconceptually
D. Studies are lacking regarding its efficacy during pregnancy
E. None of the above

Q20: A patient has been unable to stop her benzodiazepine during pregnancy. Which potential neonatal syndromes should she be counseled about?

A. Floppy infant syndrome, particularly if she used benzodiazepines during the first trimester
B. Floppy infant syndrome, which is associated with feeding issues and hypothermia
C. Neonatal withdrawal syndrome, which is characterized by hyporeflexia and somnolence
D. Neonatal withdrawal syndrome, which may last up to 3 months postpartum
E. B and D

Q21: A patient is currently taking risperidone for schizophrenia. Which of the following is TRUE regarding this medication?

A. It is a typical antipsychotic
B. It is not associated with teratogenic effects
C. It is associated with an increase in low birth weight of exposed infants
D. It has a long reproductive safety profile
E. B and D

Q22: Which of the following is TRUE regarding the fetal and neonatal effects of typical antipsychotics?

A. Their use is associated with minimal risk
B. Oral clefts are associated with their use

C. Hypertonia may persist up to one year of age
D. Their use is associated with floppy infant syndrome

Q23: Higher levels of SSRI medications are found in breast milk than the fetus was exposed to by transplacental exposure during pregnancy.
A. True
B. False

Q24: Which of the following medication is associated with fetal cholestatic hepatitis and hyperbilirubinemia?
A. Lithium
B. Valproate
C. Carbamazepine
D. Doxepin

Answers

Q1: D, Q2: E, Q3: B, Q4: D, Q5: D, Q6: A, Q7: B, Q8: A, Q9: D, Q10: E, Q11: A, Q12: D, Q13: D, Q14: E, Q15: E, Q16: C, Q17: E, Q18: D, Q19: A, Q20: E, Q21: C, Q22: A, Q23: B, Q24: C.

Resources

1. Gabbe SG, Niebyl JR, Simpson JL, Landon MB, Galan HL, Jauniaux ERM, Driscoll DA. Obstetrics: normal and problem pregnancies. Chapter 52. 6th ed. Philadelphia, PA: Elsevier; 2012.
2. American College of Obstetricians and Gynecologists. ACOG practice bulletin no. 92: use of psychiatric medications during pregnancy and lactation. Obstet Gynecol. 2008;111:1001–20.

Chapter 13
Anemia in Pregnancy

Anemia during pregnancy is common. In specific populations, it is important to screen hemoglobinopathies and vitamin deficiencies. Treatment is important as it can decrease the risk of transfusion associated with blood loss at time of delivery [1].

Recommended resource for review of this topic—ACOG Practice Bulletin 95: Anemia in Pregnancy [2].

Q1: What are the two most common causes of anemia in pregnancy and the puerperium period?

A. Hemoglobinopathies and iron deficiency
B. Iron deficiency and hemolysis
C. Acute blood loss and sickle cell anemia
D. Iron deficiency and acute blood loss

Q2: Which of the following is FALSE regarding macrocytic anemia?

A. Reticulocytosis may be decreased
B. Associated with a mean corpuscular volume greater than 100 fL
C. May be associated with folic acid deficiency
D. May be associated with liver disease
E. None of the above

K.C. Arnold, C.J. Flint, *Obstetrics Essentials*,
DOI 10.1007/978-3-319-57675-6_13,

Q3: What is the most common cause of microcytic anemia?

A. Acute blood loss
B. Iron deficiency
C. Sickle cell anemia
D. Thalassemia

Q4: A 33-year-old G1P0 is noted to have a hemoglobin of 9.8 g/dL in the second trimester. Her mean corpuscular volume (MCV) is 88 fL. Which of the following is NOT a possible cause of her anemia?

A. Early iron deficiency
B. Chronic disease
C. Autoimmune hemolysis
D. Lead poisoning

Q5: Why are hemoglobin and hematocrit levels typically decreased in a pregnant woman?

A. Due to blood volume expansion
B. Due to a decrease in red blood cell production
C. Due to increased iron requirement
D. A and C
E. All of the above

Q6: How is "iron deficiency" defined?

A. Increases of hemoglobin concentrations of more than 2 g/dL after iron supplementation
B. Absent bone marrow iron stores on bone marrow biopsy
C. Low total iron-binding capacity
D. None of the above
E. All the above

Q7: What measurement has the highest sensitivity and specificity for diagnosing iron deficiency anemia?

A. Serum ferritin levels
B. Plasma total iron-binding capacity
C. Plasma iron level

D. Transferrin saturation
E. None of the above

Q8: A 28-year-old G3P2002 presents for her first obstetrical visit. Her hemoglobin is 12.2 g/dL. You counsel her that the recommended daily dietary allowance of ferrous iron during pregnancy is:
A. 20 mg
B. 24 mg
C. 27 mg
D. 30 mg

Q9: Supplemental sustained-release iron preparations may be less effective because they dissolve poorly.
A. TRUE
B. FALSE

Q10: Of all races, which group has the highest prevalence of anemia in pregnancy?
A. Mothers of advanced maternal age
B. Mothers of low income
C. Multiparous mothers
D. Teenaged mothers

Q11: Iron deficiency anemia during pregnancy has been associated with all of the following, EXCEPT:
A. Increased risk of perinatal mortality
B. Increased risk of structural abnormalities
C. Increased risk of low birth weight
D. Increased risk of preterm delivery

Q12: A 33-year-old G1P0 presents to the office for her first obstetrical visit. In reviewing her history, you note a history of Crohn's disease. You counsel her that she is most at risk for which kind of anemia?
A. Macrocytic anemia caused by folate deficiency
B. Macrocytic anemia caused by vitamin B12 deficiency

C. Microcytic anemia caused by iron deficiency
D. Normocytic anemia caused by bone marrow suppression

Q13: Not all women should be screened for anemia during pregnancy.
A. TRUE
B. FALSE

Q14: A 22-year-old G2P1001 Caucasian patient is found to have a hemoglobin of 9.8 g/dL in the second trimester. She has no known medical issues. Which of the following is a reasonable next step in her management?
A. Obtain iron studies
B. Treat empirically with iron supplementation and monitor for improvement
C. Screen for hemoglobinopathies
D. A or B
E. All of the above are reasonable options

Q15: What is the most likely diagnosis in an anemic pregnant patient based on the following lab indices? Iron level: decreased. Total iron-binding capacity: decreased. Ferritin level: increased
A. Iron deficiency anemia
B. Thalassemia
C. Anemia of chronic disease
D. None of the above

Q16: Due to the association of abnormal fetal oxygenation, maternal blood transfusion is recommended in a pregnant woman with a hemoglobin below which level?
A. 8 g/dL
B. 7 g/dL
C. 6 g/dL
D. 5 g/dL

Q17: Which of the following is TRUE regarding parental iron?
- A. May be useful in patients with malabsorption syndromes
- B. Associated with about a 1% rate of anaphylaxis
- C. No significant difference between levels of hemoglobin after 40 days compared to those taking oral supplementation
- D. All the above are true

Q18: Iron supplementation does not decrease the prevalence of maternal anemia at the time of delivery.
- A. TRUE
- B. FALSE

Answers

Q1: D, Q2: A, Q3: B, Q4: D, Q5: D, Q6: B, Q7: A, Q8: C, Q9: A, Q10: D, Q11: B, Q12: B, Q13: B, Q14: D, Q15: C, Q16: C, Q17: D, Q18: B.

Resources

1. Gabbe SG, Niebyl JR, Simpson JL, Landon MB, Galan HL, Jauniaux ERM, Driscoll DA. Obstetrics: normal and problem pregnancies. Chapter 42. 6th ed. Philadelphia, PA: Elsevier; 2012.
2. American College of Obstetricians and Gynecologists. ACOG practice bulletin no. 95: anemia in pregnancy. Obstet Gynecol. 2008;112:201–7.

Chapter 14
Management of Stillbirth

Risk factors for stillbirth include obesity, multiple gestations, infections, diabetes, hypertensive disorders, renal and thyroid disease, and autoimmune disorders. The highest risk is in growth-restricted infants before 32 weeks gestation [1].

Recommended resource—ACOG Practice Bulletin 102: Management of Stillbirth [2].

Q1: It is suggested that a stillbirth include fetal deaths that occur at _______ weeks gestation or greater, or if gestational age is unknown, then in a fetus with a weight greater than or equal to _____ grams.

A. 20 weeks; 250 grams
B. 20 weeks; 350 grams
C. 24 weeks; 350 grams
D. 24 weeks; 450 grams

Q2: All of the following are known risk factors for stillbirth, EXCEPT:

A. Hispanic race
B. Advanced maternal age
C. Multiple gestation
D. Nulliparity
E. All of the above are known risk factors

K.C. Arnold, C.J. Flint, *Obstetrics Essentials*,
DOI 10.1007/978-3-319-57675-6_14,

Q3: Which of the following is FALSE regarding obesity and the associated risk of stillbirth?

A. The risk of obesity-related stillbirth may increase with gestational age
B. Is often related to placental dysfunction
C. Is not related to early fetal loss
D. Risk may be greater with BMI greater than 30

Q4: A 32-year-old G2P0101 presents for her first obstetrical visit. In reviewing her OB history, you note that her first delivery was at 31 weeks gestational age due to intrauterine growth restriction. She asks you about the risks associated with her current pregnancy. You counsel her:

A. Her risk for stillbirth is equal to the general population risk
B. Her risk for stillbirth is greater than the general population but less than a patient who has a history of prior stillbirth
C. Her risk for stillbirth is equal to a patient who has a history of a previous stillbirth
D. Her risk for stillbirth is greater than a patient who has a history of a previous stillbirth

Q5: If an abnormal karyotype is found in association with a stillbirth, the most common abnormalities include all of the following, EXCEPT:

A. Monosomy X
B. Trisomy 13
C. Trisomy 18
D. Trisomy 21
E. All of the above are common abnormalities in association with stillbirth

Q6: Fetal tissue sampling after birth has a greater tissue culture rate than amniocentesis before delivery.

A. TRUE
B. FALSE

Q7: Which of the following is TRUE regarding infection as it relates to stillbirth?
A. May be caused by malaria in developing countries
B. More likely to occur before the 3rd trimester in developed countries
C. May be associated with the pathogens parvovirus and syphilis
D. A and B
E. All the above

Q8: In order to report a stillbirth as being caused by a cord accident, there must be evidence of:
A. Obstruction on umbilical cord examination
B. Circulatory compromise on umbilical cord examination
C. A nuchal cord upon delivery of fetus
D. A or B
E. All of the above

Q9: What measurement can be useful to help estimate gestational age, especially before 23 weeks?
A. Humerus length
B. Foot length
C. Chest circumference
D. Femur length

Q10: Following a stillbirth in one of your patients, you offer her a fetal autopsy explaining it is the most important test in evaluation of the cause of stillbirth. She declines and wants to know what other alternatives can be offered. You counsel her:
A. A head sparing autopsy has the same benefits of a full autopsy
B. An MRI of the fetus following delivery will aid in identification of CNS, cardiac, and infectious pathology

C. Gross and microscopic placenta examination and external examination with selected biopsies will be helpful in identifying fetal infections
D. The best alternative is a fetal ultrasound performed after birth in conjunction with an external exanimation by a perinatal pathologist

Q11: Routine maternal evaluation at the time of demise may include the following labs, EXCEPT:
A. Antithrombin III deficiency
B. Anticardiolipin antibodies
C. Syphilis testing
D. Human parvovirus B-19 immunoglobulin G and M antibody
E. Fetal-maternal hemorrhage screen

Q12: The risk of recurrent stillbirth is greatest after 37 weeks gestational age.
A. TRUE
B. FALSE

Q13: Fetal kick counting can decrease the incidence of stillbirth.
A. TRUE
B. FALSE

Q14: Management of a subsequent pregnancy in a patient with a history of prior stillbirth may include all of the following, EXCEPT:
A. Antepartum fetal surveillance starting at 34 weeks gestational age or 1–2 weeks earlier than prior stillbirth
B. Support and reassurance
C. Kick counts starting at 28 weeks gestational age
D. Screening for fetal growth restriction by ultrasound after 28 weeks gestation
E. None of the above

Q15: A 34-year-old G2P1000 presents for her routine prenatal visit at 30 weeks gestation. She has an obstetrical history significant for a stillbirth in her previous pregnancy at 37 weeks gestational age with unknown cause. She has no current medical issues. Patient is asking at what gestational age she will be delivered this pregnancy. You counsel her:

A. She will be scheduled for an elective induction at 39 weeks gestation
B. She will be scheduled for an elective induction at 37 weeks gestation
C. She will be scheduled for an elective induction at 35 weeks gestation
D. A or B
E. Any of the above are reasonable given her history

Q16: What is the most efficient method of induction at less than 28 weeks if second trimester dilation and evacuation is unavailable?

A. Pitocin regardless of Bishop score and previous cesarean section history
B. Misoprostol regardless of Bishop score and previous cesarean section history
C. Misoprostol regardless of Bishop score and in patients without a previous history of cesarean section
D. Transcervical Foley catheter regardless of Bishop score and previous cesarean section history

Q17: Timing of delivery is critical following diagnosis of stillbirth due to the association of coagulopathies with prolonged fetal retention being common.

A. TRUE
B. FALSE

Q18: The rate of early stillbirth has ______ and the rate of late stillbirth has ______ since 1990.

A. Increased; decreased
B. Increased; increased
C. Decreased; decreased
D. Remained stable; decreased

Answers

Q1: B, Q2: A, Q3: C, Q4: D, Q5: E, Q6: B, Q7: E, Q8: D, Q9: B, Q10: C, Q11: A, Q12: B, Q13: B, Q14: A, Q15: A, Q16: B, Q17: B, Q18: D.

Resources

1. Gabbe SG, Niebyl JR, Simpson JL, Landon MB, Galan HL, Jauniaux ERM, Driscoll DA. Obstetrics: normal and problem pregnancies. Chapter 26. 6th ed. Philadelphia, PA: Elsevier; 2012.
2. American College of Obstetricians and Gynecologists. ACOG practice bulletin no. 102: management of stillbirth. Obstet Gynecol. 2009;113:748–61.

Chapter 15
Bariatric Surgery and Pregnancy

Sixty percent of reproductive aged women are overweight or obese. Overweight is defined as having a BMI of more than 25, obesity is defined as a BMI of greater than 30, and class 3 obesity is defined as a BMI greater than 40. Pregnant women who have undergone bariatric surgery should be monitored for nutritional deficiencies [1].

Recommended resources—ACOG Practice Bulletin 205: Bariatric Surgery and Pregnancy [2].

Q1: The prevalence of obesity has increased in reproductive aged women with the greatest proportion affecting Mexican Americans.
A. TRUE
B. FALSE

Q2: Define obesity:
A. BMI of 25 or more
B. BMI of 30 or more
C. BMI of 35 or more
D. BMI of 40 or more

Q3: Obesity affects fertility in all of the following ways EXCEPT:
A. Oligoovulation
B. Anovulation

K.C. Arnold, C.J. Flint, *Obstetrics Essentials*,
DOI 10.1007/978-3-319-57675-6_15,

C. Decreased response to ovulation induction
D. Anatomic barriers
E. All of the above are causes of infertility

Q4: Obesity during pregnancy is associated with having a higher risk of all the following EXCEPT:
A. Gestational diabetes
B. Preeclampsia
C. Long labor with more oxytocin use
D. Operative morbidity
E. Spontaneous preterm birth

Q5: Which of the following is TRUE regarding the fetal risks associated with obese patients?
A. Higher risk for fetal cardiac defects in relation to increased risk of maternal diabetes
B. Increased risk of abnormal fetal growth, most commonly, small for gestational age
C. The risk for stillbirth is eightfold greater in obese women
D. Infants born to obese women are at an increased risk for future childhood obesity
E. All of the above

Q6: A 17-year-old patient is 6 weeks postpartum from a cesarean section. She had a pregnancy complicated by class III obesity and asks what the best treatment is. You tell her:
A. Bariatric surgery is the most effective treatment for morbid obesity but is contraindicated in adolescents
B. Gastric banding is a malabsorptive procedure that may be an option for her
C. Roux-en-Y is a common procedure and can result in improved quality of life
D. Bariatric surgery is indicated for anyone with a BMI of 35 or more
E. All of the above

Q7: Pregnancies in women who have had bariatric surgery are at decreased risk for gestational diabetes and pre-eclampsia only if their postsurgery BMI is below 30.

A. TRUE
B. FALSE

Q8: A 40-year-old G2P1001 presents at 28 weeks gestation with complaints of acute abdominal pain. Upon review of her surgical history, it is noted that she has had bariatric surgery and a previous cesarean section. Which of the following is she at increased risk for?

A. Uterine rupture
B. Gastrointestinal hemorrhage
C. Intestinal obstruction
D. A and C
E. All of the above

Q9: A 17-year-old patient recently underwent bariatric surgery. At her annual exam, you counsel her:

A. Expert opinion recommends waiting 6 months after surgery before attempting pregnancy
B. Oral contraceptives are safe and effective in the absence of uncontrolled hypertension
C. Were she to become pregnant, growth ultrasounds should be considered
D. Adolescents after bariatric surgery are still at lower risk for pregnancy than the general adolescent population
E. All of the above

Q10: In pregnancies achieved after bariatric surgery, micronutrients should be tested at the beginning of pregnancy. If normal, no further laboratory testing is indicated.

A. True
B. False

Q11: How should pregnant patients who have had bariatric surgery be counseled in regard to nutrition and vitamin intake?

A. They should take two prenatal vitamins per day
B. They should double their protein intake
C. Breastfed infants should be closely monitored by their pediatrician as they may have nutritional deficiencies
D. All repletion should be parenteral due to decreased absorption
E. None of the above

Q12: Dumping syndrome:

A. Is caused by ingestion of protein
B. May cause patients to not tolerate the 50 g glucose screen
C. Causes hypoinsulinemia and hyperglycemia
D. A and B
E. B and C

Q13: Which of the following medications should be avoided in patients who have had malabsorptive procedures?

A. NSAIDs
B. Multivitamins
C. Extended release formulations
D. A and B
E. A and C

Q14: Bariatric surgery lowers the rate of cesarean sections.

A. True
B. False

Answers

Q1: B, Q2: B, Q3: D, Q4: E, Q5: D, Q6: C, Q7: B, Q8: E, Q9: C, Q10: B, Q11: E, Q12: B, Q13: E, Q14: B.

Resources

1. Gabbe SG, Niebyl JR, Simpson JL, Landon MB, Galan HL, Jauniaux ERM, Driscoll DA. Obstetrics: normal and problem pregnancies. Chapter 7. 6th ed. Philadelphia, PA: Elsevier; 2012.
2. American College of Obstetricians and Gynecologists. ACOG practice bulletin No. 105: bariatric surgery and pregnancy. Obstet Gynecol. 2009;113:1405–13.

Chapter 16
Intrapartum Fetal Heart Rate Monitoring: Nomenclature, Interpretation, and General Management Principles

Intrapartum monitoring is designed to detect fetal metabolic acidosis and to prevent hypoxia. Prior to its implementation, intrapartum fetal death rates were between 3 and 4 per 1000. A normal tracing reliably predicts a well-oxygenated fetus; however, an abnormal tracing is less predictive of fetal status. The three-tiered fetal heart rate interpretation system should be used to assist in determining fetal status [1].

Recommended resource—ACOG Practice Bulletin 106: Intrapartum Fetal Heart Rate Monitoring: Nomenclature, Interpretation, and General Management Principles [2].

Q1: Which of the following is FALSE regarding electronic fetal monitoring (EFM)?

A. Has poor interobserver and intraobserver reliability
B. Has uncertain efficacy
C. Fetal heart rate tracing patterns provide information on current acid-base status of fetus
D. Has low false-positive rates

K.C. Arnold, C.J. Flint, *Obstetrics Essentials*,
DOI 10.1007/978-3-319-57675-6_16,

Q2: When describing uterine contractions, it is important to do which of the following:

A. To note whether the contractions are associated with fetal decelerations
B. To describe whether or not hyperstimulation is occurring
C. To quantify the number of contractions in a 10-min window, averaged over a 60-min period
D. A and C
E. All of the above

Q3: Which of the following are TRUE regarding the baseline of electronic fetal monitoring?

A. Baseline must be a minimum of 4 min over any 10-min segment
B. Normal fetal heart rate baseline includes 120–160 beats per minute
C. Tachycardia is defined as baseline rate greater than 160 beats per minute
D. B and C
E. All of the above

Q4: Minimal baseline variability refers to when:

A. Amplitude range is undetectable
B. Amplitude range is detectable, but 5 beats per minute or fewer
C. Amplitude range is 6–25 beats per minute
D. Amplitude range is greater than 25 beats per minute

Q5: Which of the following is FALSE regarding a gradual fetal heart rate decrease?

A. Includes early decelerations
B. Defined as from the onset of the fetal heart rate nadir of 30 s or more
C. Includes late decelerations
D. All of the above are false
E. All of the above are true

Q6: Which of the following are TRUE as regards to fetal heart rate accelerations?
A. Onset is gradual
B. Prior to 34 weeks gestation, an acceleration has a peak of 10 beats per minute above baseline
C. If it lasts greater than 10 min, then it represents a change in baseline
D. B and C
E. All of the above are true

For questions 7–14, designate which fetal heart rate tracing category is being described:

Q7: Recurrent late decelerations with moderate baseline variability
A. Category I
B. Category II
C. Category III

Q8: Recurrent variable decelerations with absent fetal heart rate variability
A. Category I
B. Category II
C. Category III

Q9: Bradycardia with minimal baseline variability
A. Category I
B. Category II
C. Category III

Q10: Moderate baseline variability with accelerations and early decelerations
A. Category I
B. Category II
C. Category III

Q11: Baseline tachycardia
A. Category I
B. Category II
C. Category III

Q12: Sinusoidal pattern
- A. Category I
- B. Category II
- C. Category III

Q13: Moderate baseline variability without decelerations or accelerations
- A. Category I
- B. Category II
- C. Category III

Q14: Tracing that requires prompt evaluation due to association with abnormal fetal acid-base status
- A. Category I
- B. Category II
- C. Category III
- D. Category II and III

Q15: When comparing electronic fetal monitoring (EFM) with intermittent auscultation of fetal heart tones, which of the following is TRUE?
- A. Use of EFM decreases the risk of vacuum and forceps operative vaginal delivery
- B. Use of EFM reduces perinatal mortality
- C. Use of EFM reduces risk of neonatal seizures
- D. Use of EFM reduces risk of cerebral palsy
- E. All the above are TRUE

Q16: The sensitivity of EFM for predicting cerebral palsy is high.
- A. TRUE
- B. FALSE

Q17: Variable decelerations are equally likely to occur among preterm deliveries and term deliveries.
- A. TRUE
- B. FALSE

Q18: A 23-year-old G1P0 at 39 weeks gestational age is currently in labor with a cervical exam of 5 cm. She is painfully contracting and interested in regional anesthesia, but she is concerned about how this may affect her fetus and labor course. You counsel her:

A. She is at an increased risk of cesarean delivery due to fetal heart rate abnormalities associated with regional anesthesia use
B. She may experience fewer fetal heart rate abnormalities if she has a combined spinal-epidural versus epidural
C. She may develop hypotension secondary to regional anesthesia which can lead to fetal heart rate abnormalities
D. A and C
E. All the above

Q19: Decreased variability seen with use of magnesium sulfate is related to early gestational age not the serum magnesium level.

A. TRUE
B. FALSE

Q20: Use of which medication during labor can cause a transient sinusoidal fetal heart rate pattern?

A. Butorphanol
B. Morphine
C. Bupivacaine
D. Magnesium

Q21: Fetal heart rate findings which are strongly reassuring of a normal acid-base status include:

A. Moderate variability with decelerations
B. Moderate variability with no decelerations
C. Presence of accelerations
D. All the above
E. B and C

Q22: A 42-year-old G3P2002 at term is currently laboring on the maternal care unit. Her most recent cervical exam is 8/90/-1. Review of her fetal heart rate tracing reveals minimal variability without accelerations. Which of the following techniques can be performed to illicit an acceleration to give reassurance that academia is unlikely?

A. Allis clamp stimulation
B. Vibroacoustic stimulation
C. Digital scalp stimulation
D. All of the above

Q23: Maternal supplemental oxygen has been shown to be effective in improving fetal heart rate tracings.

A. TRUE
B. FALSE

Q24: Transcervical amnioinfusion has been shown to be effective at reducing which of the following fetal heart rate abnormalities:

A. Recurrent late decelerations
B. Recurrent variable decelerations
C. Recurrent early decelerations
D. A and B
E. All the above

Q25: In which scenario is tocolytic therapy thought to be most appropriate?

A. With any fetal heart rate abnormality
B. When tachysystole is present with associated fetal heart rate changes
C. When pitocin is currently being administered and a Category II tracing is noted
D. There is not an appropriate scenario for tocolytic therapy

Q26: Initial evaluation of Category II or Category III fetal heart tracing should include all the following, EXCEPT:

A. Monitoring of maternal blood pressure
B. Placement of intrauterine pressure catheter
C. Evaluation for umbilical cord prolapse
D. Cessation of labor inducing agent
E. All of the above are appropriate initial evaluations

Answers

Q1: D, Q2: A, Q3: C, Q4: B, Q5: E, Q6: C, Q7: B, Q8: C, Q9: B, Q10: A, Q11: B, Q12: C, Q13: A, Q14: C, Q15: C, Q16: B, Q17: B, Q18: C, Q19: A, Q20: A, Q21: D, Q22: D, Q23: B, Q24: B, Q25: B, Q26: B.

Resources

1. Gabbe SG, Niebyl JR, Simpson JL, Landon MB, Galan HL, Jauniaux ERM, Driscoll DA. Obstetrics: normal and problem pregnancies. Chapter 16. 6th ed. Philadelphia, PA: Elsevier; 2012.
2. American College of Obstetricians and Gynecologists. ACOG practice bulletin no. 106: intrapartum fetal heart rate monitoring: nomenclature, interpretation, and general management principles. Obstet Gynecol. 2009;114:192–202.

Chapter 17
Induction of Labor

Induction of labor is defined as stimulation of contractions in contrast to augmentation which is defined as causing an increase in contractions. Both are intended to result in a vaginal delivery. Labor induction has absolute and relative indications; it is also occasionally undertaken for elective reasons. Success can be estimated using the Bishop score; if high, the risk of cesarean delivery is similar to that of spontaneous labor [1].

Recommended resource—ACOG Practice Bulletin 107: Induction of Labor [2].

Q1: What percent of gravid women undergo induction of labor in the United States?
- A. 12%
- B. 17%
- C. 22%
- D. 33%
- E. 37%

Q2: All of the following are purposes of cervical ripening EXCEPT:
- A. Cervical thinning
- B. Decrease in time to painful contractions
- C. Cervical dilation
- D. Decrease in rate of failed induction
- E. Decrease in induction to delivery time

K.C. Arnold, C.J. Flint, *Obstetrics Essentials*,
DOI 10.1007/978-3-319-57675-6_17,

Q3: Cervical remodeling includes which of the following changes?

A. Collagen breakdown and rearrangement
B. Decreased production of cytokines
C. Red blood cell infiltration
D. All of the above

Q4: At which Bishop score is the probability of a vaginal delivery similar to that of spontaneous labor?

A. 4
B. 6
C. 8
D. Induction never obtains the same probability as spontaneous labor

Q5: Your 19-year-old primigravida presents for induction. You recommend a Foley catheter and she is nervous. What do you tell her the advantages are in comparison to other ripening agents?

A. Reduced risk of tachysystole without fetal heart rate changes
B. Painless placement
C. Associated with decreased risk of cesarean when compared to misoprostol
D. Low cost
E. A and D
F. All of the above

Q6: Misoprostol is a synthetic PGE 2 analogue with published evidence to support its efficacy and safety when used appropriately.

A. True
B. False

Q7: Your 19-year-old primigravida presents for induction. You recommend a prostaglandin and she is nervous. What do you tell her the advantages are?

A. Likelihood of delivery within 24 h is increased compared with oxytocin alone
B. Decreased risk of cesarean section

C. Decreased risk of tachysystole with fetal heart rate changes
D. A and B
E. All of the above

Q8: Uterine response to pitocin starts ________ after infusion of oxytocin and a steady state is reached at __________.
A. 1–2 min, 10 min
B. 2–3 min, 20 min
C. 2–3 min, 30 min
D. 3–5 min, 30 min
E. 3–5 min, 40 min

Q9: Membrane stripping is commonly practiced but is not supported by evidence.
A. True
B. False

Q10: Your 21-year-old G1P0 presents in active labor. At 7 cm dilation she is noted to have tachysystole. Her fetus is Category 1. How is this defined?
A. 5 contractions or more per 10 min, averaged over 20 min
B. 5 contractions or more per 10 min, averaged over 30 min
C. More than 5 contractions per 10 min, averaged over 20 min
D. More than 5 contractions per 10 min, averaged over 30 min
E. Tachysystole is only diagnosed in induced or augmented labor

Q11: Your patient requests to be induced as she lives 4 h away from the hospital. How do you counsel her?
A. This is not an indication supported by ACOG
B. This is reasonable if an ultrasound done prior to 20 weeks confirms a gestational age of 37 weeks or greater

C. This is reasonable if it has been 36 weeks since a positive urine pregnancy test
D. This is reasonable if fetal heart tones have been documented for 20 weeks by Doppler
E. None of the above are true

Q12: Your G1P0 patient has a Bishop score of 4 and requests induction. You counsel her that her risk for a cesarean section if induced as opposed to waiting for spontaneous labor is threefold. Is this:
A. True
B. False

Q13: Your patient presents for a medically indicated induction and is found to have an unfavorable cervix. Which of the following is true regarding methods of cervical ripening?
A. Foley catheter placement would significantly reduce the duration of labor
B. PGE2 gel is significantly more effective at decreasing the cesarean rate than Foley catheter placement
C. When oxytocin is added to the use of the Foley catheter, time to delivery is decreased
D. Dinoprostone is associated with more tachysystole than vaginal misoprostol
E. All of the above are false

Q14: Which of the following describes the correct administration of misoprostol?
A. One quarter of a tablet as the initial dose, placed every 6 h, starting oxytocin 4 h after last dose.
B. One quarter of a tablet as the initial dose, placed every 2–4 h, starting oxytocin 3 h after last dose.
C. One half of a tablet as the initial dose, placed every 3–6 h, starting oxytocin 4 h after the last dose.

D. One half of a tablet as the initial dose, placed every 2–4 h, starting oxytocin 4 h after the last dose.
E. One quarter of a tablet as the initial dose, placed every 3–6 h, starting oxytocin 4 h after the last dose.

Q15: Which of the following is FALSE regarding the PGE2 vaginal insert?
A. It should be used with caution in patients with asthma and hepatic or renal dysfunction
B. Removing the insert will usually reverse tachysystole
C. It has a 1% rate of uterine tachysystole with associated fetal heart rate changes
D. Maternal side effects are uncommon

Q16: Outpatient cervical ripening with a PGE2 controlled release in the outpatient setting is currently not supported by ACOG as more research needs to be done.
A. True
B. False

Q17: You are just starting an induction on your G3P002 patient. Her cervix is 4/80/-1 and you tell her your plans to start oxytocin at 2 mU/min and increase by 2 every half hour. She asks about a high-dose protocol and mentions her nurse friend told her about it. How do you counsel her?
A. High-dose regimens are associated with shorter labor and less frequent cases of chorioamnionitis
B. High-dose regimens are associated with increased rates of cesarean section for dystocia
C. High-dose protocol is not currently recommended
D. A and C
E. All of the above

Q18: Your 32-year-old G2P1001 presents at term, SROM, and is found to be 2 cm dilated. All of the following EXCEPT which are reasonable:
A. Misoprostol
B. Oxytocin
C. Intravaginal PGE2
D. Expectant management
E. All of the above are reasonable

Q19: In women with a previous uterine incision with an intrauterine fetal demise, 800 mcg every 6 h up to 28 weeks gestation does not appear to be associated with an increase in complications.
A. True
B. False

Answers

Q1: C, Q2: B, Q3: A, Q4: C, Q5: E, Q6: B, Q7: A, Q8: E, Q9: B, Q10: D, Q11: C, Q12: B, Q13: A, Q14: E, Q15: C, Q16: B, Q17: A, Q18: D, Q19: B.

Resources

1. Gabbe SG, Niebyl JR, Simpson JL, Landon MB, Galan HL, Jauniaux ERM, Driscoll DA. Obstetrics: normal and problem pregnancies. Chapter 14. 6th ed. Philadelphia, PA: Elsevier; 2012.
2. American College of Obstetricians and Gynecologists. ACOG practice bulletin no. 107: induction of labor. Obstet Gynecol. 2009;114:386–97.

Chapter 18
Vaginal Birth After Previous Cesarean Delivery

Trial of labor after cesarean section (TOLAC) has fluctuated in acceptance among the medical community. Approximately two thirds of women with a previous cesarean section are candidates for a TOLAC and its use may decrease the cesarean rate in the United States. Overall success rates are estimated to be between 60 and 80 percent with an approximate 1% risk for uterine rupture in women with one previous low transverse cesarean section [1].

Recommended resource—ACOG Practice Bulletin 115: Vaginal Birth After Previous Cesarean Delivery [2].

Q1: When counseling a patient, it is important to stress which of the following in regards to maternal morbidity and mode of delivery:

A. A VBAC carries the greatest risk to maternal morbidity
B. A scheduled repeat cesarean section carries the greatest risk to maternal morbidity
C. A scheduled repeat cesarean section has a greater risk to maternal morbidity than a failed TOLAC
D. A failed TOLAC carries the greatest risk to maternal morbidity

K.C. Arnold, C.J. Flint, *Obstetrics Essentials*,
DOI 10.1007/978-3-319-57675-6_18,

Q2: The outcome associated with TOLAC that most greatly increases the risk of neonatal and maternal morbidity is:

A. Endometritis
B. Arrest of descent
C. Uterine rupture
D. Cord prolapse
E. None of the above

Q3: A successful VBAC can have several advantages for patients in comparison to a scheduled repeat cesarean section, including:

A. Lower rates of hemorrhage
B. Shorter recovery period
C. Lower rates of infection
D. B and C
E. All of the above

Q4: A patient presents to your clinic requesting information regarding the success rates of TOLAC. Without knowing anything about the patient, it would be reasonable to tell her that success rate ranges between:

A. 40 and 50%
B. 50 and 70%
C. 60 and 80%
D. 70 and 90%

Q5: Which of the following factors make having a successful TOLAC LESS likely?

A. Indication for previous primary low transverse cesarean section was for non-reassuring fetal heart tones
B. African American ethnicity
C. Short pregnancy interval
D. B and C
E. All the above

Q6: A patient presents to your office requesting information on TOLAC. She informs you of her previous obstetric history and gives pertinent factors regarding her current pregnancy. Using all this information, you quote her a TOLAC success rate of 55%. Given this, the best way to counsel her is:

A. Inform her that she would be a great candidate to attempt TOLAC
B. Recommend she have a repeat cesarean section given her low chance of success and greater chance of morbidity
C. Inform her that everybody has the same success rate regardless of their past history and she should make her own decision
D. None of the above

Q7: Which of the following patients should NOT be offered a TOLAC?

A. Patient with a history of an extensive abdominal myomectomy
B. Patient with a current twin gestation pregnancy
C. Patient with a history of a previous low vertical incision
D. A and D
E. All the above

Q8: A patient with a previous cesarean section of unknown scar type may still be offered a TOLAC.

A. TRUE
B. FALSE

Q9: The risk of uterine rupture is greater when induction of labor is started on an unfavorable cervix versus a favorable cervix.

A. TRUE
B. FALSE

Q10: Studies have revealed that higher doses of oxytocin are associated with a dose-response effect with increasing risks of uterine rupture. Due to this, the following recommendation has been made:

A. The maximum pitocin dosage for a patient attempting TOLAC is 32 mu/min
B. Unless location of previous uterine incision is clearly documented, pitocin levels above 16 mu/min should not be used
C. There is not enough evidence to recommend an upper limit of oxytocin dosing in patients attempting TOLAC
D. In a patient with a history of two previous lower uterine segment incisions, pitocin is clearly contraindicated

Q11: In a patient attempting a TOLAC, which of the following is TRUE?

A. Misoprostol should not be used for cervical ripening or labor induction in the third trimester
B. Misoprostol should not be used as a cervical ripening or labor induction agent in the second trimester
C. Misoprostol is never safe for a patient with a previous cesarean section
D. Misoprostol may be safe for term inductions when used at lower doses in a tertiary care facility
E. None of the above are true.

Q12: What is the most common sign associated with uterine rupture?

A. Fetal heart rate abnormality
B. Increased uterine contractions
C. Vaginal bleeding
D. Loss of fetal station
E. New onset intense uterine pain

Q13: Which of the following is FALSE regarding a patient wanting to attempt a TOLAC?
- A. External cephalic version is not contraindicated; however the chances of success are lower
- B. Regional anesthesia is not recommended due to it decreasing the chances of a successful TOLAC
- C. Regional anesthesia is not recommended due to the concern it may mask the symptoms of uterine rupture
- D. None of the above
- E. All of the above

Q14: Following successful VBAC, it is important to vaginally palpate the integrity of previous lower uterine incision.
- A. TRUE
- B. FALSE

Use the following scenario for Q15–16:

A 36-year-old G4P3003 presents for her new OB visit. In reviewing her records, you note a history of a term vaginal delivery followed by a primary low transverse cesarean section for non-reassuring fetal heart tones. The patient's last delivery was complicated by an attempted TOLAC with uterine rupture necessitating an emergent cesarean delivery.

Q15: She is contemplating TOLAC with her current gestation, you counsel her:
- A. Given her history of having had a successful vaginal delivery previously, she is a reasonable candidate to attempt TOLAC
- B. If her uterine rupture was located at the level of the previous uterine incision, then her risk of repeat rupture during labor is approximately 3%
- C. If her uterine rupture extended to the upper segment of the uterus, then her risk of repeat rupture during labor may be as high as 32%
- D. B and C

Q16: Based on her history, you recommend delivery before ______ weeks gestation.

A. 41
B. 40
C. 39
D. 34

Q17: In a patient attempting TOLAC, cervical ripening with a transcervical Foley catheter has been associated with uterine rupture rates similar to spontaneous labor.

A. TRUE
B. FALSE

Q18: In a patient attempting TOLAC, cervical ripening with misoprostol for an intrauterine fetal demise in the third trimester is recommended.

A. TRUE
B. FALSE

Q19: Your 32-year-old patient had planned for a TOLAC. She presents in spontaneous labor at term and her fetus is estimated to be 4500 g. She has an otherwise uncomplicated pregnancy. How do you counsel her?

A. If her fetus is macrosomic, her likelihood of a successful VBAC is lower and her risk for uterine rupture is higher
B. If her fetus is macrosomic, her likelihood of a successful VBAC is unchanged and her risk for uterine rupture is higher
C. If her fetus is macrosomic, her likelihood of a successful VBAC is unchanged as is her risk for uterine rupture
D. If her fetus is macrosomic, her likelihood of a successful VBAC is lower, but her risk for uterine rupture is unchanged

Answers

Q1: D, Q2: C, Q3: E, Q4: C, Q5: D, Q6: B, Q7: A, Q8: A, Q9: B, Q10: C, Q11: A, Q12: A, Q13: E, Q14: B, Q15: C, Q16:C, Q17: A, Q18: B, Q19: D.

Resources

1. Gabbe SG, Niebyl JR, Simpson JL, Landon MB, Galan HL, Jauniaux ERM, Driscoll DA. Obstetrics: normal and problem pregnancies. Chapter 20. 6th ed. Philadelphia, PA: Elsevier; 2012.
2. American College of Obstetricians and Gynecologists. Practice bulletin no. 115: vaginal birth after previous cesarean delivery. Obstet Gynecol. 2010;116:450–63.

Chapter 19
Management of Intrapartum Fetal Heart Rate Tracings

Management of non-reassuring fetal heart rate patterns requires an understanding of the pathophysiology that can lead to abnormalities. Although abnormalities suggest fetal distress, false-positives are common. When aberrations are detected, other means of assessing fetal status and nonsurgical interventions should be used when possible [1].

Recommended resource—ACOG Practice Bulletin 116: Management of Intrapartum Fetal Heart Rate Tracings [2].

Q1: A nurse calls because she is concerned that a patient's contractions are too frequent. The patient is in spontaneous labor at term with 5 contractions in 10 min for the past 30 min. The fetus is currently Category I. How would you classify her pattern of uterine contractions?

A. Normal uterine activity
B. Tachysystole
C. Uterine hyperstimulation
D. Uterine hypercontractility
E. B and C

K.C. Arnold, C.J. Flint, *Obstetrics Essentials*,
DOI 10.1007/978-3-319-57675-6_19,

Q2: How often should a fetal heart rate tracing be reviewed during labor?

A. Every 30 min during the first phase and every 15 min during the second phase by a nurse or physician
B. Every 30 min during the first phase and every 15 min during the second phase by a physician
C. Every 60 min during the first phase and every 30 min during the second phase by a nurse or physician
D. Every 60 min during the first phase and every 30 min during the second phase by a physician

Q3: You are monitoring fetal heart tones on labor and delivery when you notice a deceleration. It coincides with the uterine contraction and is abrupt, and the total deceleration is noted to be 45 s. What type of deceleration is this?

A. Early deceleration
B. Late deceleration
C. Variable deceleration
D. Prolonged deceleration
E. Unable to classify based on the information given

Q4: A medical student on labor and delivery asks how baseline fetal heart rate is defined and what value is considered to be normal. You explain:

A. The baseline is given in increments of 10 beats per minute and must be present for a minimum of 3 min in a 10 min segment. Normal is defined as 120–160
B. The baseline is given in increments of 5 beats per minute and must be present for a minimum of 2 min in a 10 min segment. Normal is defined as 120–160
C. The baseline is given in increments of 10 beats per minute and must be present for a minimum of 3 min in a 10 min segment. Normal is defined as 110–160
D. The baseline is given in increments of 5 beats per minute and must be present for a minimum of 2 min in a 10 min segment. Normal is defined as 110–160

Q5: A patient presents to triage in active labor. Review of fetal heart tones reveals a baseline of 110, moderate variability, accelerations, early decelerations, and no late or variable decelerations. What category does this tracing represent?

A. Category I
B. Category II
C. Category III
D. Unable to determine

Q6: A term patient is currently laboring. Upon review of the fetal heart tracing, it is noted that the baseline is 100 with moderate variability and recurrent late decelerations. What category does this tracing represent?

A. Category I
B. Category II
C. Category III
D. Unable to determine

Q7: What is the most common fetal heart rate anomaly during labor?

A. Intermittent variable decelerations
B. Recurrent variable decelerations
C. Intermittent late decelerations
D. Recurrent late decelerations
E. Minimal variability

Q8: Which of the following is FALSE regarding recurrent variable decelerations?

A. They are defined by occurring with more than 50% of contractions
B. Moderate variability or accelerations suggests the fetus is not academic
C. Management involves relieving the compression
D. Amnioinfusion decreases their recurrence and the rate of cesarean delivery
E. None of the above

Q9: A medical student expresses concern that a fetal heart tracing shows recurrent late decelerations. Which of the following is TRUE regarding recurrent late decelerations?

A. Maneuvers to promote uteroplacental perfusion should be initiated
B. Late decelerations are highly predictive of academia
C. If variability becomes absent, the tracing is Category III
D. A and B
E. A and C
F. All of the above are true

Q10: Which of the following is FALSE regarding fetal tachycardia?

A. In isolation, it is poorly predictive of fetal academia
B. Treatment should be directed at the underlying cause
C. Infection is a common cause
D. It is defined as a rate greater than 160 for 5 min or more.
E. None of the above

Q11: A laboring patient is suddenly noted to have fetal heart tones at 100 beats per minute for 2 min. All of the following could be causative factors, EXCEPT?

A. Maternal hypertension
B. Umbilical cord prolapse
C. Uterine rupture
D. Abruption
E. Tachysystole

Q12: A prolonged deceleration is defined as:

A. A decrease in fetal heart rate of 10 beats per minute from baseline for 5 min
B. A decrease in fetal heart rate of 15 beats per minute from baseline for 2 min

C. A fetal heart rate below 110 beats per minute for 2 min
D. A fetal heart rate below 110 beats per minute for 5 min
E. A fetal heart rate below 110 beats per minute for 10 min

Q13: A 32-year-old G2P0101 at 27 weeks gestation is admitted for suspected preterm labor as a transfer. She has received butorphanol, betamethasone, and magnesium at the outside hospital. On initial monitor, the fetus has a baseline of 140 with minimal variability, no accelerations, and no decelerations. You suspect the minimal variability is likely due to maternal medications or a fetal sleep cycle. How do you proceed?
A. Expectant management for up to 60 min
B. Proceed with scalp stimulation
C. Proceed with maternal repositioning and administration of oxygen and IV fluids
D. B and C
E. Any of the above are appropriate

Q14: Tachysystole is defined as:
A. Five or more contractions over 10 min averaged over 20 min
B. More than five contractions over 10 min averaged over 20 min
C. Five or more contractions over 10 min averaged over 30 min
D. More than five contractions over 10 min averaged over 30 min

Q15: Which of the following would be classified as a Category III fetal heart tracing?
A. Baseline 100, minimal variability, recurrent late decelerations
B. Baseline 120, absent variability, intermittent variable decelerations

C. Baseline 120, absent variability, recurrent late decelerations
D. All of the above
E. None of the above

Q16: A 22-year-old G1P0 presents for a late-term induction of labor. She is initiated on oxytocin and develops a Category III fetal heart tracing. Resuscitative measures are unsuccessful and decision is made to proceed with cesarean delivery. All of the following is true EXCEPT:

A. Historically, the time frame from decision to incision had been 30 min
B. Expedient delivery may not improve fetal outcomes if injury has already been sustained
C. Neonatal outcomes are best when delivery can be accomplished within 15 min
D. Additional surgical preparation for maternal conditions such as morbid obesity should be accomplished
E. None

Answers

Q1: A, Q2: A, Q3: C, Q4: D, Q5: A, Q6: B, Q7: A, Q8: E, Q9: E, Q10: D, Q11: A, Q12: B, Q13: A, Q14: D, Q15: C, Q16: C.

Resources

1. Gabbe SG, Niebyl JR, Simpson JL, Landon MB, Galan HL, Jauniaux ERM, Driscoll DA. Obstetrics: normal and problem pregnancies. Chapter 16. 6th ed. Philadelphia, PA: Elsevier; 2012.
2. American College of Obstetricians and Gynecologists. Practice bulletin no. 116: management of intrapartum fetal heart rate tracings. Obstet Gynecol. 2010;116:1232–40.

Chapter 20
Use of Prophylactic Antibiotics in Labor and Delivery

Bacterial infections are a common complication in obstetrics. Some infections may be life-threatening to the mother or the fetus or both. Prophylaxis, in some instances, may help prevent these infections [1].

Recommended resource – ACOG Practice Bulletin 120: Use of Prophylactic Antibiotics in Labor and Delivery [2].

Q1: Which of the following is TRUE regarding antibiotic prophylaxis?
- A. May need to administered for an extended period of time
- B. Ideal to achieve therapeutic tissue levels prior to the end of the procedure
- C. Agent chosen should be short acting and broadly focused on multiple different types of bacteria
- D. Use may increase the risk of resistant flora seen postoperatively

Q2: Increases in *E.coli* sepsis and resistance is mainly seen in the preterm and low birth weight infant population.
- A. TRUE
- B. FALSE

K.C. Arnold, C.J. Flint, *Obstetrics Essentials*,
DOI 10.1007/978-3-319-57675-6_20,

Q3: Anaphylaxis to penicillin is rare. The risk of a less severe reaction to penicillin is more common, estimated to be about: _____%.
A. 5%
B. 10%
C. 20%
D. 30%

Q4: Lower serum levels of antibiotics may be seen in the pregnant patient due to all of the following physiologic changes associated with pregnancy, EXCEPT:
A. Increases in glomerular filtration rate
B. Increases in plasma volume
C. Decreases in binding proteins
D. Decreases in gastric emptying time

Q5: Which of the following antibiotics do not cross the placenta adequately?
A. Aminoglycosides and azithromycin
B. Clindamycin and ampicillin
C. Erythromycin and cephalosporin
D. Azithromycin and erythromycin

Q6: It is reasonable to increase single-dose preoperative antibiotic prophylaxis in patients with a BMI of:
A. BMI > 25
B. BMI > 30
C. BMI > 35
D. BMI > 40

Q7: What is the single most important risk factor for infection in the postpartum period?
A. Obesity
B. Prolonged rupture of membranes
C. Group B strep positive status
D. Cesarean delivery

Q8: Why would cefazolin, a first-generation cephalosporin, be a better choice for single-dose antibiotic prophylaxis for cesarean section than a second-generation cephalosporin or ampicillin?

A. Cefazolin has greater efficacy compared to the other drugs
B. Cefazolin is cheaper than a second-generation cephalosporin
C. Cefazolin has a much longer-half life than ampicillin
D. B and C
E. All of the above

Q9: A 33-year-old G1P0 is scheduled for a primary low transverse cesarean section at 38 weeks gestation due to breech presentation of twin A. In reviewing her history, it is noted that she has a severe penicillin allergy. What alternative antibiotic(s) should she receive for prophylaxis?

A. Cefazolin and clindamycin
B. An aminoglycoside and clindamycin
C. An aminoglycoside
D. Vancomycin and clindamycin

Q10: Ideally, when should antibiotic prophylaxis for cesarean section be administered?

A. More than an hour before skin incision
B. Before clamping of the umbilical cord
C. Prior to skin closure
D. Within an hour prior to skin incision

Q11: In which of the following scenario(s) should a patient receive an additional intraoperative dose of prophylactic antibiotics?

A. A cesarean section that is lengthy
B. A cesarean section with excessive blood loss
C. A cesarean section with meconium noted at time of delivery

D. A and B
E. All of the above

Q12: Routine screening of obstetric patients for MRSA colonization and subsequent treatment is recommended.
A. TRUE
B. FALSE

Q13: In which of the following scenarios is antibiotic prophylaxis appropriate?
A. To prolong labor in patients with preterm labor and intact membranes
B. For GBS prophylaxis in patients with preterm labor and intact membranes with unknown GBS status
C. For GBS prophylaxis in patients with preterm labor and intact membranes and known GBS negative status six weeks ago.
D. B and C
E. All of the above

Q14: Prophylactic antibiotic therapy for endocarditis may be considered for vaginal delivery in patients with the highest risk of adverse outcomes from endocarditis. These patients may include:
A. Patients with mitral valve prolapse
B. Patients with cyanotic cardiac disease
C. Patients with supraventricular tachycardia
D. Patients with atrial fibrillation
E. None of the above because prophylactic antibiotic therapy for endocarditis is no longer recommended in any patient undergoing a vaginal delivery

Q15: Perioperative antibiotic prophylaxis is not recommended at time of prophylactic or emergent cerclage placement.
A. TRUE
B. FALSE

Q16: What dose of prophylactic antibiotic is recommended at time of manual placenta extraction following a vaginal delivery?
A. 2 grams cefazolin
B. 1 gram cefazolin
C. 2 grams ampicillin
D. No data supports prophylactic antibiotic usage in this scenario

Answers

Q1: D, Q2: A, Q3: B, Q4: C, Q5: D, Q6: B, Q7: D, Q8: D, Q9: B, Q10: D, Q11: D, Q12: B, Q13: D, Q14: B, Q15: A, Q16: D.

Resources

1. Gabbe SG, Niebyl JR, Simpson JL, Landon MB, Galan HL, Jauniaux ERM, Driscoll DA. Obstetrics: normal and problem pregnancies. Chapter 51. 6th ed. Philadelphia, PA: Elsevier; 2012.
2. American College of Obstetricians and Gynecologists. Practice bulletin no. 120: use of prophylactic antibiotics in labor and delivery. Obstet Gynecol. 2011;117:1472–83.

Chapter 21
Thromboembolism in Pregnancy

Pregnancy and the postpartum period are associated with an increased risk for thromboembolic events. Women with thrombophilias particularly are at an increased risk. Treatment often includes use of unfractionated heparin and low-molecular-weight heparin; more rarely fondaparinux and warfarin may be used [1].

Recommended resources—ACOG Practice Bulletin 123: Thromboembolism in Pregnancy [2].

Q1: Which of the following is TRUE regarding the risk for thromboembolic events associated with pregnancy?

A. All trimesters carry increased risk
B. Third trimester has a higher risk than any trimester or postpartum
C. The risk of thromboembolic event begins to increase in the second trimester
D. Approximately 75% of thromboembolic events associated with pregnancy occur during pregnancy, with 35% occurring postpartum
E. B and C

K.C. Arnold, C.J. Flint, *Obstetrics Essentials*,
DOI 10.1007/978-3-319-57675-6_21,

Q2: All of the following EXCEPT which increase the potential for thromboembolic events during pregnancy?

A. Increased venous stasis
B. Compression of the pelvic arteries
C. Compression of the inferior vena cava
D. Decreased mobility
E. All of the above contribute to an increased risk

Q3: What percent of women who have venous thromboembolism have a thrombophilia?

A. 5–10%
B. 10–20%
C. 20–50%
D. 50–70%

Q4: Dosing of heparin compounds in pregnancy is impacted by the following:

A. Crosses the placenta but appears to be safe during pregnancy
B. Renal excretion is increased
C. Protein bound fraction is decreased
D. B and C
E. All of the above

Q5: What are the two most common symptoms of a DVT?

A. Pain and swelling at the extremity
B. Shortness of breath and pain at the extremity
C. Shortness of breath and swelling at the extremity
D. Tachycardia and swelling at the extremity
E. Tachycardia and pain at the extremity

Q6: A 38-year-old patient presents at 38 weeks gestation with complaints concerning for a DVT. What diagnostic testing do you order?

A. Ultrasound. If negative and suspect iliac vein thrombosis, proceed with CT angiogram to evaluate for pulmonary embolism
B. D-Dimer then ultrasound if elevated
C. Ultrasound. If negative and suspect iliac vein thrombosis, proceed with anticoagulation

D. Ultrasound. If negative and suspect iliac vein thrombosis, proceed with MRI
E. C and D

Q7: A 30-year-old G1P0 presents to your office for a new obstetric visit. She reports a history of a DVT when she was 17 and was on oral contraceptives. She asks what you recommend for her in terms of anticoagulation. You recommend:
A. Prophylactic anticoagulation to continue postpartum
B. Therapeutic anticoagulation to continue postpartum
C. Prophylactic anticoagulation to stop postpartum
D. Therapeutic anticoagulation to stop postpartum
E. No anticoagulation indicated

Q8: While working in triage on labor and delivery, a patient at 20 weeks gestation presents and lists warfarin as one of her medications. Which of the following is TRUE of warfarin?
A. It is associated with embryopathy if used in the second trimester
B. All patients on warfarin should be transitioned to heparin compounds if pregnant
C. Most patients on warfarin should be transitioned to heparin compounds if pregnant
D. A and B
E. A and C

Q9: You counsel your patient that because of her high-risk thrombophilia, she will need to be on prophylactic anticoagulation. Which of the following are acceptable options for her?
A. Enoxaparin 40 mg daily
B. Unfractionated heparin 10,000 units every 6 h in the third trimester
C. Unfractionated heparin 10,000 units every 12 h in the second trimester
D. A and C
E. All the above are acceptable

Q10: A 35-year-old G5P3013 presents reporting that she is currently on therapeutic doses of unfractionated heparin. You are concerned that it may not be therapeutic. When do you measure an aPTT and what is your goal?

A. Check an aPTT 4 h after the injection, goal between 2 and 3
B. Check an aPTT 6 h after the injection, goal between 1.5 and 2.5
C. Check an aPTT just prior to the next injection, goal between 2 and 3
D. Check an aPTT 4 h after the injection, goal between 1.5 and 2.5
E. Check an aPTT 6 h after the injection, goal between 2 and 3

Q11: Dosing for unfractionated heparin in pregnancy should be twice daily.

A. True
B. False

Q12: What anticoagulation should be used in the case of a patient with heparin-induced thrombocytopenia in pregnancy?

A. Warfarin
B. Low-molecular-weight heparin
C. Fondaparinux
D. B or C
E. Any of the above are reasonable

Q13: You diagnose a patient at 30 weeks gestation with a new DVT. Which of the following are indications for initiating therapeutic anticoagulation as an inpatient?

A. Large clots
B. Patients who are past 35 weeks gestation
C. All patients should be hospitalized for initiation
D. A and B

Q14: When is monitoring labs recommended for pregnancy and anticoagulation?

A. Monitor platelet counts if using unfractionated or low-molecular-weight heparin.
B. Xa should be monitored for prophylactic low-molecular-weight heparin dosing
C. Xa levels should be monitored for prophylactic unfractionated heparin dosing
D. aPTT should be monitored for therapeutic heparin dosing
E. All of the above

Q15: A 20-year-old G1P0 is at 34 weeks gestation and asks what adjustments will need to be made in preparation for delivery. You counsel her:

A. At 40 weeks she will be changed from low-molecular-weight heparin to unfractionated heparin
B. That neuraxial anesthesia generally needs to be done 12 h after the last prophylactic dose or 24 h after the last therapeutic dose
C. In cases of planned delivery, therapeutic anticoagulation may be stopped and labor may be induced within 48 h
D. If there is concern for delivery, recommendation is for low-molecular-weight heparin as it has a shorter half-life and can be reversed
E. A and C

Q16: What is the soonest anticoagulation that can be restarted following delivery?

A. 4 h after a vaginal delivery, 6 h after a cesarean delivery
B. 6 h after a vaginal delivery, 12 h after a cesarean delivery
C. 12 h after a vaginal delivery, 24 h after a cesarean delivery
D. 24 h after a vaginal delivery or a cesarean delivery
E. 12 h after if using enoxaparin, 24 h after if heparin

Q17: All of the following anticoagulants are compatible with breastfeeding, EXCEPT:
A. Low-molecular-weight heparin
B. Unfractionated heparin
C. Warfarin
D. None of the above are safe with breastfeeding
E. All of the above are safe with breastfeeding

Q18: Women who are heterozygous for Factor V Leiden are candidates for all of the following contraceptive methods, EXCEPT:
A. Progestin only pills
B. Intrauterine devices
C. Barrier methods
D. Progestin only implant
E. All of the above are acceptable

Answers

Q1: A, Q2: B, Q3: C, Q4: B, Q5: A, Q6: E, Q7: A, Q8: C, Q9: D, Q10: B, Q11: A, Q12: C, Q13: A, Q14: D, Q15: B, Q16: A, Q17: E, Q18: E.

Resources

1. Gabbe SG, Niebyl JR, Simpson JL, Landon MB, Galan HL, Jauniaux ERM, Driscoll DA. Obstetrics: normal and problem pregnancies. Chapter 43. 6th ed. Philadelphia, PA: Elsevier; 2012.
2. American College of Obstetricians and Gynecologists. Practice bulletin no. 123: thromboembolism in pregnancy. Obstet Gynecol. 2011;118:718–29.

Chapter 22
Prediction and Prevention of Preterm Birth

Preterm birth is defined as delivery between 20 and 37 weeks gestation. Neonatal mortality and short- and long-term morbidity are significant complications of preterm birth. Preterm birth can be spontaneous or iatrogenic. Gestational ages are the most significant prognostic predictor of fetal outcomes [1].

Recommended resources—ACOG Practice Bulletin 130: Prediction and Prevention of Preterm Birth [2].

Q1: Which of the following is TRUE regarding preterm birth?

A. Spontaneous preterm birth does not include birth that follows cervical insufficiency
B. After the first year of life, infants born prematurely have similar outcomes as those born at term
C. Preterm labor precedes approximately 20% of preterm birth
D. The risk of poor birth outcomes generally increases with advancing gestational age
E. None of the above

Q2: Which of the following interventions could decrease a patients' risk for preterm birth?

A. Smoking cessation
B. Improved dental care during pregnancy
C. Having an interpregnancy interval of 36 months

K.C. Arnold, C.J. Flint, *Obstetrics Essentials*,
DOI 10.1007/978-3-319-57675-6_22,

D. A and B
E. All of the above

Q3: A 34-year-old G3P1103 presents for her new OB visit. She has a past surgical history significant for a LEEP procedure. Her pregnancy history includes a term singleton vaginal delivery followed by a 28-week vaginal delivery of twins due to preterm labor. The patient is concerned about her risk of having a preterm birth with her current pregnancy. You counsel her:

A. Her risk is only increased due to her history of LEEP and not her previous preterm delivery because it was a twin gestation
B. The evidence is not clear whether or not a LEEP procedure puts her at risk of having a preterm birth
C. She is at an increased risk for preterm birth due to her pregnancy history
D. She is not at an increased risk for preterm birth, especially since her first pregnancy delivered at term
E. B and C

Q4: What is the most reliable and reproducible way to assess cervical length?

A. Digital examination
B. Transvaginal ultrasound
C. Transabdominal ultrasound
D. Magnetic resonance imaging (MRI)

Q5: Which of the following describes the correct way to measure a cervical length?

A. Patient should have a full bladder
B. The shortest of three measurements should be used
C. Calipers should be placed at the internal and external os
D. B and C
E. All the above are correct

For the following scenarios (Q6–12), pick the best option for management:

Q6: A 27-year-old G1P0 who is found to have a cervical length of 25 mm on her Level I ultrasound at 18 weeks.

A. Start 200 mg vaginal progesterone
B. Start weekly IM progesterone injections
C. Place cerclage
D. Remeasure cervical length in 2 weeks

Q7: A 32-year-old G2P0101 with history of preterm birth at 32 weeks who is found to have a cervical length of 30 mm on her growth ultrasound at 24 weeks.

A. Continue weekly IM progesterone injections
B. Place cerclage
C. Remeasure cervical length in 2 weeks
D. A and B

Q8: A 25-year-old G2P0102 with a history of preterm birth of twin gestation at 34 weeks who is found to have a cervical length of 40 mm on her Level I ultrasound at 18 weeks.

A. Continue weekly IM progesterone injections
B. Remeasure cervical length in 2 weeks
C. Continue routine obstetrical care
D. Place cerclage
E. A and D

Q9: A 26-year-old G2P0101 with a history of preterm birth at 28 weeks due to severe preeclampsia who is found to have a cervical length of 25 mm on her Level I ultrasound at 18 weeks.

A. Start 200 mg vaginal progesterone
B. Continue weekly IM progesterone injections
C. Place cerclage
D. Remeasure cervical length in 2 weeks

Q10: A 27-year-old G3P1101 with a history of preterm birth at 26 weeks who is found to have a cervical length of 24 mm on her Level I ultrasound at 18 weeks.

A. Continue weekly IM progesterone injections
B. Place cerclage
C. Remeasure length in 2 weeks
D. A and B
E. A and C

Q11: A 32-year-old G2P1001 who is found to have a cervical length of 20 mm on her Level I ultrasound at 18 weeks.

A. Start 200 mg vaginal progesterone
B. Place cerclage
C. Remeasure length in 2 weeks
D. Continue routine obstetrical care
E. A and B

Q12: A 33-year-old G1P0 with a twin gestation who is found to have a cervical length of 25 mm on her Level II ultrasound at 18 weeks.

A. Start 200 mg vaginal progesterone
B. Place cerclage
C. Remeasure length in 2 weeks
D. Continue routine obstetrical care for twin gestation
E. A and B

Q13: During what time frame should a woman with a history of preterm birth be initiated on progesterone?

A. Between 12 and 24 weeks gestation
B. Between 18 and 24 weeks gestation
C. Between 16 and 28 weeks gestation
D. Between 16 and 24 weeks gestation
E. Between 12 and 28 weeks gestation

Q14: In which population is vaginal progesterone recommended as a management option to reduce the risk of preterm birth?

A. Asymptomatic women pregnant with a singleton without a history of preterm birth noted to have a shortened cervical length less than 25 mm before 24 weeks gestation
B. Asymptomatic women pregnant with a singleton without a history of preterm birth noted to have a shortened cervical length less than 20 mm before 24 weeks gestation
C. Asymptomatic women pregnant with twins without a history of preterm birth noted to have a shortened cervical length less than 25 mm before 24 weeks gestation
D. A and C
E. All the above

Answers

Q1: E, Q2: A, Q3: E, Q4: B, Q5: D, Q6: D, Q7: A, Q8: C, Q9: D, Q10: D, Q11: A, Q12: D, Q13: D, Q14: B.

Resources

1. Gabbe SG, Niebyl JR, Simpson JL, Landon MB, Galan HL, Jauniaux ERM, Driscoll DA. Obstetrics: normal and problem pregnancies. Chapter 28. 6th ed. Philadelphia, PA: Elsevier; 2012.
2. American College of Obstetricians and Gynecologists. Practice bulletin no. 130: prediction and prevention of preterm birth. Obstet Gynecol. 2012;120:964–73.

Chapter 23
Antiphospholipid Syndrome

Antiphospholipid antibody syndrome (APS) is associated with both venous and arterial thromboses. In pregnancy, APS accounts for 14% of thromboembolic events. Diagnostic criteria include thrombosis or obstetrical comications with at least one laboratory abnormality. Despite prophylaxis, there is still a 5% risk for thromboembolism during pregnancy [1].

Recommended resource—ACOG Practice Bulletin 132: Antiphospholipid Syndrome [2].

Q1: Patients with antiphospholipid syndrome (APS) are at risk for all of the following EXCEPT?

A. Arterial thrombosis
B. Stroke
C. Autoimmune thrombocytopenia
D. Fetal loss
E. All of the above

Q2: What lab criteria are required in diagnosing APS?

A. All three antiphospholipid antibodies must be positive once
B. Two out of three antiphospholipid antibodies must be positive on more than one occasion 6 weeks apart
C. One antiphospholipid antibody must be positive on more than one occasion 12 weeks apart

K.C. Arnold, C.J. Flint, *Obstetrics Essentials*,
DOI 10.1007/978-3-319-57675-6_23,

D. A and C
E. Any of the above

Q3: Which of the following is TRUE regarding lupus anticoagulant?
A. It is an anticoagulant
B. Testing involves screening and then a second confirmatory test
C. Results are reported as low, medium, or high levels
D. It can be tested while the patient is treated with anticoagulation
E. All of the above

Q4: Which of the following is TRUE regarding anticardiolipin antibodies and anit-B2 glycoprotein I?
A. Only IgG should be tested
B. Testing involves screening and then a second confirmatory test
C. A positive result is greater than the 99th percentile for normal population
D. IgA can be tested in patients that test negative when clinical suspicion is high
E. All of the above

Q5: Patients with APS have an increased risk for which of the following disorders involving pregnancy and hypertension?
A. Severe preterm preeclampsia
B. Pregnancy-induced hypertension
C. Severe pregnancy induced hypertension
D. A and C
E. All of the above

Q6: Which of the following pregnancy loss scenarios are concerning for APS?
A. Losses greater than 10 weeks
B. Sporadic embryonic loss
C. Recurrent embryonic loss

D. A and C
E. All of the above

Q7: What is the risk of thrombosis in pregnancy or postpartum in women who have APS?
A. Less than 1%
B. 10%
C. 25%
D. 50%
E. None of the above

Q8: Your 30-year-old G3P0030 has just been diagnosed with APS. She states that she was previously diagnosed with ITP. How do you counsel her?
A. Autoimmune thrombocytopenia occurs in up to 50% of patients with APS
B. A simple blood test will distinguish if she had ITP as well as APS
C. Treatment does not differ
D. A and B
E. A and C

Q9: All of the following patients meet clinical criteria for APS testing EXCEPT?
A. A 29-year-old with a DVT who is 36 weeks pregnant
B. A 60-year-old with retinal arterial thrombosis
C. An 18-year-old with three missed abortion at 6 weeks
D. A 30-year-old with a history of severe preeclampsia requiring delivery at 35 weeks gestation
E. All of the above meet criteria for testing

Q10: A 30-year-old G4P0030 presents for a new obstetrical visit at 10 weeks gestation and asks if you recommend anticoagulation. She has never had a thrombotic event. You counsel here that:
A. Clinical surveillance is recommended
B. Prophylactic anticoagulation until 6 weeks postpartum

C. Aspirin is recommended
D. A and C
E. All of the above are reasonable

Q11: A 35-year-old G1P0 at 22 weeks gestation with a history of a DVT with subsequent diagnosis of APS. Which of the following is TRUE regarding your recommendation?
A. Prophylactic anticoagulation through 12 weeks postpartum is recommended
B. Aspirin is strongly recommended
C. After delivery anticoagulation can be continued with Coumadin
D. She should use SCDs while asleep
E. All of the above are true

Q12: What do you recommend for patients with APS in terms of antenatal testing?
A. A detailed anatomic survey at 20 weeks gestation
B. Growth ultrasounds every 4 weeks
C. Biophysical profiles every week in the third trimester
D. Data support all of the above
E. Expert opinion supports all of the above

Answers

Q1: E, Q2: C, Q3: B, Q4: C, Q5: E, Q6: D, Q7: B, Q8: E, Q9: D, Q10: E, Q11: C, Q12: E.

Resources

1. Gabbe SG, Niebyl JR, Simpson JL, Landon MB, Galan HL, Jauniaux ERM, Driscoll DA. Obstetrics: normal and problem pregnancies. Chapter 43. 6th ed. Philadelphia, PA: Elsevier; 2012.
2. American College of Obstetricians and Gynecologists. Practice bulletin no. 132: antiphospholipid syndrome. Obstet Gynecol. 2012;120:1514–21.

Chapter 24
Fetal Growth Restriction

Fetuses who are growth restricted are at a high risk for perinatal mortality, with rates 6–10 times greater than normally grown fetuses. Specific patterns of growth restriction include asymmetric and symmetric which generally reflect the timing and duration of the underlying etiology. Possible underlying conditions include constitutionally small fetuses, abnormal fetuses (aneuploidy, infection, syndromes), and placental insufficiency [1].

Recommended resource—ACOG Practice Bulletin 134: Fetal Growth Restriction [2].

Q1: Which of the following is TRUE regarding the commonly used terms "small for gestational age (SGA)" and "intrauterine growth restriction" (IUGR)?

A. SGA refers to a fetus in utero
B. IUGR is defined as a fetus with an estimated fetal weight of less than the fifth percentile for gestational age
C. The terms are interchangeable
D. SGA refers to a newborn whose birth weight is less than the 10% for gestational age

K.C. Arnold, C.J. Flint, *Obstetrics Essentials*,
DOI 10.1007/978-3-319-57675-6_24,

Q2: Which of the following maternal disorders have been associated with IUGR or SGA?

A. Hypertension
B. Hereditary thrombophilias
C. Antiphospholipid syndrome
D. A and C
E. All of the above

Q3: All of the following have been associated with IUGR and SGA EXCEPT:

A. Tobacco use during pregnancy
B. Extremely poor protein intake in the third trimester
C. Multiple gestation
D. Intrauterine infection
E. All the above are true

Q4: Fetal growth restriction has been associated with both chromosomal abnormalities and structural malformations.

A. TRUE
B. FALSE

Q5: The most common pathology associated with fetal growth restriction is the finding of a single umbilical artery.

A. TRUE
B. FALSE

Q6: Examples of the morbidity and mortality associated with fetal growth restriction include all of the following EXCEPT?

A. Increased risk of stillbirth
B. Cognitive delay in childhood
C. Hypoglycemia
D. Seizures
E. All the above are true

Q7: Fundal height measurements are most useful at what gestational age?
A. 20–40 weeks
B. 20–36 weeks
C. 24–38 weeks
D. 28–42 weeks

Q8: What is the next BEST step when a growth-restricted fetus is diagnosed by ultrasound?
A. Repeat the study in a week due to the low sensitivity of ultrasound
B. Perform Doppler blood flow studies of the umbilical artery
C. Give steroids for fetal lung maturity and move toward delivery
D. Order weekly biophysical profiles for the fetus for the remainder of the pregnancy

Q9: What is the risk of recurrence of an SGA birth?
A. 10%
B. 20%
C. 30%
D. 40%

Q10: Which of the following strategies have been proven to be effective in preventing fetal growth restriction?
A. Daily aspirin
B. Dietary supplementation
C. Bed rest
D. Nutritional counseling
E. None of the above

Q11: Use of umbilical artery Doppler velocimetry is associated with improved outcomes in fetuses with fetal growth restriction.
A. TRUE
B. FALSE

Q12: In which of the following scenarios is delaying delivery until 38 0/7–39 6/7 weeks recommended?

A. A 24-year-old G1P0 diagnosed with IUGR and oligohydramnios
B. A 32-year-old G2P1001 diagnosed with IUGR and reverse end-diastolic flow on umbilical artery studies
C. A 18-year-old G1P0 diagnosed with IUGR and severe hypertension
D. A 28-year-old G3P2002 with a history of an SGA fetus diagnosed with IUGR and an inherited thrombophilia

Q13: Ultrasonography is the best method for evaluating a growth-restricted fetus and growth assessments should be performed every 2 weeks.

A. TRUE
B. FALSE

Q14: Which of the following is true regarding the effects of teratogen exposure on IUGR?

A. The effect is dependent on the timing, duration, exposure, and dosage of the drug
B. Drugs commonly associated with IUGR include cyclophosphamide, valproic acid, warfarin, and lisinopril
C. Individual genetic predisposition for drug metabolism can mediate the effect of a teratogen
D. A and B
E. A and C

Q15: All of the following infections are associated with IUGR EXCEPT:

A. HSV
B. CMV
C. Rubella
D. Malaria
E. Varicella

Answers

Q1: D, Q2: D, Q3: B, Q4: A, Q5: B, Q6: E, Q7: C, Q8: B, Q9: B, Q10: E, Q11: A, Q12: D, Q13: B, Q14: E. Q15: A.

Resources

1. Gabbe SG, Niebyl JR, Simpson JL, Landon MB, Galan HL, Jauniaux ERM, Driscoll DA. Obstetrics: normal and problem pregnancies. Chapter 31. 6th ed. Philadelphia, PA: Elsevier; 2012.
2. American College of Obstetricians and Gynecologists. Practice Bulletin No. 134: Fetal growth restriction. Obstet Gynecol. 2013;121:1122–33.

Chapter 25
Gestational Diabetes

The incidence of gestational diabetes is increasing. Adequate treatment of gestational diabetes reduces the associated poor outcomes. Nutritional and dietary counseling are first-line treatment options. However, if glucose levels are not adequately controlled, then oral hypoglycemic therapy or insulin therapy should be initiated. After pregnancy, all women with gestational diabetes should be screened for overt diabetes and should receive early screening for gestational diabetes in future pregnancies [1].

Recommended resources—ACOG Practice Bulletin 137: Gestational Diabetes [2].

Q1: Women with pregnancies complicated by gestational diabetes are at increased risk for hypertensive disorders of pregnancy, cesarean section, macrosomia, and:

A. Neonatal hyperglycemia
B. Hyperbilirubinemia
C. Fetal hypoinsulinemia
D. All of the above
E. None of the above

K.C. Arnold, C.J. Flint, *Obstetrics Essentials*,
DOI 10.1007/978-3-319-57675-6_25,

Q2: Gestational diabetes is defined by:
A. Carbohydrate intolerance with onset or recognition during pregnancy
B. Carbohydrate intolerance at 20 or more weeks gestation
C. Glucose intolerance with onset or recognition during pregnancy
D. Glucose intolerance at 20 or more weeks gestation
E. None of the above

Q3: Which of the following patients should have early screening for gestational diabetes?
A. A woman with a BMI if 28
B. A woman with gestational diabetes during her past pregnancy who passed her postpartum glucose screen
C. A woman with gestational diabetes during her past pregnancy who did not have a postpartum glucose screen
D. A and C
E. B and C

Q4: Which of the following describes the correct method of diagnosis of gestational diabetes?
A. Screening should be performed at 24–30 weeks gestation
B. A 1 h, 50 g oral glucose test followed by a 3 h, 100 g glucose test
C. A one-step approach with a 2 h, 75 g oral glucose test
D. A and B
E. All of the above are acceptable

Q5: What are the diagnostic criteria for gestational diabetes using Carpenter and Coustan in mg/dL?
A. 100, 180, 150, 130
B. 95, 160, 155, 140
C. 100, 180, 150, 130
D. 95, 180, 155, 140

Q6: What cutoff is recommended per ACOG for the 1 h, 50 g glucose challenge?

A. 130
B. 135
C. 140
D. 130 for women who are high risk, 140 for women who are low risk
E. Individual practitioner should select a single consistent cutoff

Q7: Treatment for gestational diabetes is associated with a decrease in which of the following EXCEPT:

A. Hypertensive disorders
B. Shoulder dystocia
C. Cesarean section
D. Neonatal hypoglycemia
E. All of the above were decreased

Q8: Your patient was recently diagnosed with gestational diabetes. She asks you what you recommend in terms of management of gestational diabetes for the rest of her pregnancy. You counsel her:

A. To eat three meals a day and limit snacks
B. To check her glucose 3 times a day, 1 or 2 h postprandial
C. To initiate a moderate exercise program
D. A and C
E. All of the above

Q9: Patients with gestational diabetes should ideally have a caloric allotment of:

A. Carbohydrates 40%, protein 20%, fat 40%
B. Carbohydrates 60%, protein 20%, fat 20%
C. Carbohydrates 40%, protein 40%, fat 20%
D. Carbohydrates 60%, protein 30%, fat 10%
E. ACOG does not have a formal recommendation

Q10: Which of the following is TRUE regarding the initiation of pharmacologic treatment of gestational diabetes?

A. There is consensus regarding thresholds for starting medical therapy
B. Insulin and oral medications are equivalent in efficacy
C. Insulin and oral medications can be appropriate first-line therapy
D. Traditionally, insulin is standard therapy and is started if fasting or postprandials are persistently elevated
E. All of the above

Q11: Which of the following is TRUE regarding dosage of insulin?

A. Typical starting dosage is 0.7–1.0 units/day given in divided doses
B. Insulin lispro has a peak action of 1–2 h and therefore may be helpful in postprandial glucose control
C. Insulin glargine has a peak action of 12 h
D. Insulin crosses the placenta
E. All of the above

Q12: Which of the following is TRUE regarding the usage of glyburide and metformin in gestational diabetes?

A. They are both FDA approved for this indication and can be considered for glycemic control in gestational diabetes
B. Metformin increases insulin secretion and insulin sensitivity of peripheral tissues
C. Glyburide should not be used in patients with a sulfa allergy
D. Glyburide inhibits hepatic gluconeogenesis and glucose absorption
E. All of the above are true

Q13: A 37-year-old with polycystic ovarian syndrome is referred to you. She reports taking metformin, but denies a history of diabetes. How do you counsel her?

A. Metformin should be stopped now as it was only helpful in achieving pregnancy
B. Metformin should be continued until the end of the first trimester
C. Metformin should be continued throughout the entire pregnancy given her diagnosis of polycystic ovarian syndrome
D. Metformin should be continued and patient can defer screening for gestational diabetes

Q14: Which of the following is FALSE regarding treatment options for gestational diabetes?

A. Glyburide, metformin, and insulin area all acceptable first-line treatments
B. Glyburide may be superior to metformin in that less women require the addition of insulin
C. Glyburide is known to cross the placenta, as opposed to insulin, which does not
D. Insulin can be added to both metformin and glyburide if needed
E. All of the above are true

Q15: When is antenatal surveillance recommended?

A. In women with pregestational diabetes
B. In all women with gestational diabetes
C. In women with gestational diabetes with poor glycemic control
D. At the discretion of the provider in women with well-controlled gestational diabetes
E. A and C

Q16: When does ACOG recommend delivery of pregestational diabetics who are well controlled?

A. 37th
B. 38th week
C. 39th week
D. 40th week
E. There are insufficient data to make a recom mendation

Q17: Your 33-year-old G4P3003 with gestational diabetes controlled with insulin is concerned because her friend mentioned she may need a cesarean section if her baby gets too big. Which of the following is TRUE?

A. Fetal growth will be assessed by clinical exam or by ultrasound to identify macrosomia
B. Fifty-eight cesarean sections for an estimated fetal weight of 4500 g to prevent a single case of permanent brachial plexus palsy
C. Given the risks and benefits, women with gestational diabetes should be offered a cesarean section if the estimated fetal weight is 4500 g or more
D. A and B
E. A and C

Q18: Your 30-year-old patient presents for her postpartum checkup. Her pregnancy was complicated by gestational diabetes. All of the following are true EXCEPT:

A. She will need to be screened at this visit for diabetes or impaired fasting glucose
B. Fasting plasma glucose is less sensitive; hence, the 2 h glucose test is recommended
C. If she is found to have a normal screen, she should have her glycemic status assessed every 3 years
D. All of the above are true

Answers

Q1: B, Q2: A, Q3: E, Q4: B, Q5: D, Q6: E, Q7: E, Q8: C, Q9: A, Q10: E, Q11: B, Q12: C, Q13: B, Q14: E, Q15: E, Q16: C, Q17: E, Q18: D.

Resources

1. Gabbe SG, Niebyl JR, Simpson JL, Landon MB, Galan HL, Jauniaux ERM, Driscoll DA. Obstetrics: normal and problem pregnancies. Chapter 39. 6th ed. Philadelphia, PA: Elsevier; 2012.
2. American College of Obstetricians and Gynecologists. Practice bulletin no. 137: gestational diabetes mellitus. Obstet Gynecol. 2013;122:406–16.

Chapter 26
Inherited Thrombophilias in Pregnancy

Inherited thrombophilias are associated with arterial and venous clots, as well as fetal loss. Risk for thromboembolic events with these conditions is increased significantly in the setting of a personal history or a family history of a venous thrombosis. Inherited thrombophilias are classified as low or high risk for thrombotic events during pregnancy [1].

Recommended resources—ACOG Practice Bulletin 138: Inherited Thrombophilias in Pregnancy [2].

Q1: Pregnancy is characterized by increased thrombotic potential. Which of the following factors contribute to this known state?
A. Decreased fibrinolysis
B. Increased insulin resistance and hyperlipidemia
C. Compression of the aorta by the pregnant uterus
D. A and B
E. All of the above

Q2: Venous thromboembolism is a leading cause of maternal mortality in the United States.
A. TRUE
B. FALSE

K.C. Arnold, C.J. Flint, *Obstetrics Essentials*,
DOI 10.1007/978-3-319-57675-6_26,

Q3: Which inherited thrombophilia accounts for the greatest percentage, as high as 40%, of thromboembolism in pregnancy?

A. Antithrombin deficiency
B. Factor V Leiden heterozygote
C. Protein C deficiency
D. Prothrombin gene homozygote

Q4: Which of the following confers the greatest risk for thromboembolism?

A. A 32-year-old pregnant patient who is a heterozygote for Factor V Leiden and has a personal history of thromboembolism
B. A 32-year-old pregnant patient with protein C deficiency
C. A 32-year-old pregnant patient who is a homozygote for Factor V Leiden and has a sister with a history of thromboembolism
D. A and C have the same risk

Q5: Which of the following is TRUE regarding prothrombin G20210A mutations?

A. Is a point mutation that results in decreased circulating prothrombin levels
B. Has a synergistic hypercoagulable effect when also present with Factor V Leiden mutations
C. Having a personal history of thromboembolism increases the risk for thromboembolism in carriers during pregnancy
D. B and C
E. All of the above are true

Q6: Screening for which thrombophilia is less reliable during pregnancy?

A. Protein C deficiency
B. Protein S deficiency
C. Factor V Leiden mutation
D. Prothrombin G20210A mutation
E. Antithrombin deficiency

Q7: Which of the following is FALSE regarding methylenetetrahydrofolate reductase (MTHFR) mutations?

A. Pregnant patients should not be screened for MTHFR mutations
B. Homozygosity for MTHFR mutations is the most common cause of hyperhomocysteinemia
C. MTHFR mutations do not increase the risk for thromboembolism in nonpregnant women
D. MTHFR mutations increase the risk for thromboembolism in pregnant women
E. A and C

Q8: Which thrombophilia infers the greatest risk for thromboembolism in pregnancy regardless of history?

A. Antithrombin deficiency
B. Protein C deficiency
C. Protein S deficiency
D. Factor V Leiden homozygote
E. None of the above

Q9: Inherited thrombophilias are associated with which of the following?

A. Fetal loss
B. Preeclampsia
C. Placenta abruption
D. All the above
E. None of the above

Q10: In which of the following patient(s) would it be appropriate to screen for an inherited thrombophilia at their first obstetrical visit?

A. A 32-year-old G2P1001 with a first cousin with a known antithrombin deficiency
B. A 29-year-old G1P0 with a history of a DVT following a pelvic fracture sustained in a motor vehicle accident
C. A 42-year-old G6P5005 with bulging varicose veins on exam

D. A 23-year-old G2P1001 whose brother is known to be a homozygote for Factor V Leiden
E. All the above
F. B and D

Q11: Ideally, the BEST time to screen a patient for an inherited thrombophilia is:
A. At least 4 weeks from the acute thrombotic event
B. While the patient is not pregnant
C. While the patient is on anticoagulation
D. A and B
E. All the above

Q12: Unfractionated heparin is the preferred agent for prophylaxis in pregnancy.
A. TRUE
B. FALSE

Q13: When is the risk of venous thromboembolism the greatest during pregnancy?
A. First trimester
B. Before 20 weeks gestation
C. Third trimester
D. After 30 weeks gestation
E. The risk is the same throughout

Q14: Postpartum anticoagulation may be indicated for low-risk thrombophilias in certain situations even if not recommended antepartum.
A. True, if they have additional risk factors including obesity or prolonged mobility.
B. True, if they have a history of a first-degree relative with a thrombotic episode before age 50 years
C. False, if antepartum prophylaxis is not indicated than neither is postpartum prophylaxis
D. False, anticoagulation is indicated for all low-risk thrombophilias both antepartum and postpartum
E. A and B

Q15: A 33-year-old G1P0 is one-day postpartum and necessitates prophylactic anticoagulation. She is also breastfeeding and asks which medication is safest to use. You counsel her:

A. Only low-molecular-weight heparin is safe to use in women breastfeeding
B. Low-molecular-weight heparin and unfractionated heparin are safe to use in women breastfeeding
C. Low-molecular-weight heparin, unfractionated heparin, and warfarin are all safe to use in women breastfeeding
D. Unfortunately, none of the anticoagulant medications are safe in women who are breastfeeding so she will have to bottle-feed instead

Q16–20: For the following thrombophilias, indicated whether it is high risk or low risk.

Q16: Factor V Leiden heterozygote

A. Low risk
B. High risk

Q17: Protein C deficiency

A. Low risk
B. High risk

Q18: Double heterozygote for prothrombin G20210A and Factor V Leiden

A. Low risk
B. High risk

Q19: Factor V Leiden homozygote

A. Low risk
B. High risk

Q20: Protein S deficiency

A. Low risk
B. High risk

Q21: The risk of procedure-related bleeding is limited with administration of regional anesthesia after how many hours after the last dose of low-molecular-weight heparin?

A. 4 h after prophylactic dosing; 8 h after therapeutic dosing
B. 6 h after prophylactic dosing; 12 h after therapeutic dosing
C. 12 h after prophylactic dosing; 24 h after therapeutic dosing
D. 18 h after prophylactic dosing; 36 h after therapeutic dosing

Q22: How soon after a cesarean section can unfractionated heparin or low-molecular-weight heparin be restarted?

A. 4–6 h
B. 6–12 h
C. 12–16 h
D. 20–24 h

Q23: Which of the following is TRUE regarding inherited thrombophilias and contraception?

A. The risk of venous thromboembolism is not appreciably increased in Factor V Leiden heterozygotes using estrogen-containing oral contraceptives
B. As long as patients are counseled regarding the risks of thromboembolism, it is reasonable to prescribe estrogen-containing contraceptives to patients with low-risk thrombophilias
C. Due to the increased risk of venous thromboembolism in patients with low-risk inherited thrombophilias, progestin-only pills or implants should the only prescribed hormonal contraceptives
D. A and B
E. None of the above

Answers

Q1: D, Q2: A, Q3: B, Q4: C, Q5: D, Q6: B, Q7: D, Q8: A, Q9: E, Q10: F, Q11: B, Q12: B, Q13: B, Q14: E, Q15: C, Q16: A, Q17: A, Q18: B, Q19: B, Q20: A, Q21: C, Q22: B, Q23: C.

Resources

1. Gabbe SG, Niebyl JR, Simpson JL, Landon MB, Galan HL, Jauniaux ERM, Driscoll DA. Obstetrics: normal and problem pregnancies. Chapter 43. 6th ed. Philadelphia, PA: Elsevier; 2012.
2. American College of Obstetricians and Gynecologists. Practice bulletin no. 138: inherited thrombophilias in pregnancy. Obstet Gynecol. 2013;122:706–17.

Chapter 27
Cerclage for the Management of Cervical Insufficiency

Cervical insufficiency is commonly described as painless cervical dilation with subsequent delivery. Cerclages may be placed in three distinct settings: history-indicated, ultrasound-indicated, and physical examination-indicated. Cerclages are most commonly placed vaginally, however, abdominal cerclages may be needed if a vaginal approach is not possible or if the patient has a history of failed vaginal cerclage [1].

Recommended resource—ACOG Practice Bulletin 142: Cerclage for the Management of Cervical Insufficiency [2].

Q1: How is cervical insufficiency diagnosed?

A. Painless cervical dilation at any time during pregnancy
B. Shortened cervical length in the second trimester
C. History of a second trimester delivery after painless dilation
D. Balloon elastin test
E. B and C

Q2: Which of the following are risk factors for cervical insufficiency?

A. Cold knife cone
B. In utero exposure to DES
C. Müllerian anomalies

K.C. Arnold, C.J. Flint, *Obstetrics Essentials*,
DOI 10.1007/978-3-319-57675-6_27,

D. A and B
E. All of the above

Q3: Which of the following are effective treatments for cervical insufficiency?
A. Bed rest
B. Pelvic rest
C. Activity restriction
D. None of the above
E. All of the above

Q4: Choose the most correct description of the three different types of cerclage:
A. Transabdominal is reserved for patients who have failed other types of cerclages; Shirodkar involves placing a single suture around the cervix; McDonald involves placing a double suture around the cervix
B. Transabdominal may be a first choice option in Müllerian anomalies; Shirodkar involves dissection of the vesicocervical mucosa; McDonald involves placing a single suture around the cervix
C. Transabdominal is reserved for patients who have failed other types of cerclages; Shirodkar involves dissection of the vesicocervical mucosa; McDonald involves placing a double suture around the cervix
D. None of the above are correct

Q5: Which of the following is TRUE regarding a transabdominal cerclage:
A. Can be placed in any trimester; must be removed at time of delivery
B. Can be placed in any trimester; can be left in place between pregnancies
C. Requires delivery by cesarean section
D. A and C
E. B and C

Q6: A 25-year-old G2P0101 presents with a cervical length of 23 mm at 23 weeks gestation. What type of cerclage would you offer her?

A. History indicated
B. Physical exam indicated
C. Ultrasound indicated
D. Do not offer cerclage
E. Do not offer cerclage but would offer her vaginal progesterone therapy

Q7: A 36-year-old G4P3003 is found to be 2 cm dilated at 20 weeks gestation. She denies complaints. What type of cerclage would you offer her?

A. History indicated
B. Physical exam indicated
C. Ultrasound indicated
D. Do not offer cerclage
E. Do not offer cerclage but would offer her vaginal progesterone therapy

Q8: A 28-year-old G2P0101 at 13 weeks gestation presents for routine obstetric care. What type of cerclage would you offer her?

A. History indicated
B. Physical exam indicated
C. Ultrasound indicated
D. Do not offer cerclage
E. Do not offer cerclage but would offer her vaginal progesterone therapy

Q9: A 30-year-old G2P1001 at 13 weeks gestation who had a previous term delivery after cerclage placement presents for a routine obstetric visit. What type of cerclage would you offer her?

A. History indicated
B. Physical exam indicated
C. Ultrasound indicated
D. Do not offer cerclage
E. Do not offer cerclage but would offer her vaginal progesterone therapy

Q10: An 18-year-old G2P1001 at 23 weeks gestation is found to have a cervical length of 15 mm. Her cervix is found to be closed on vaginal exam. What type of cerclage would you offer her?

A. Rescue cerclage
B. Physical exam indicated
C. Ultrasound indicated
D. Do not offer cerclage
E. Do not offer cerclage but would offer her vaginal progesterone therapy

Q11: A 20-year-old G2P0101 presents for a new obstetric visit at 13 weeks gestation and would like to discuss the risks and benefits of having a cerclage placed now versus undergoing ultrasound monitoring. How do you counsel her?

A. Ultrasound surveillance involves monitoring cervical length starting now until 30 weeks gestational age
B. It is safer to have one placed now because 90% of women with a history of preterm delivery develop cervical effacement and will need rescue cerclage placement
C. By monitoring your cervical length, there is a 50% chance we could avoid needing to place a cerclage
D. If cerclage is placed, it would need to be removed on your due date
E. A and C

Q12: Which of the following are recommended by ACOG during cerclage placement?

A. Antibiotics are shown to decrease inflammation
B. Prophylactic tocolysis improves efficacy
C. Monitoring of cervical lengths after cerclage placement to assure efficacy
D. B and C
E. None of the above

Q13: In which of the following situations would cerclage removal be recommended?
A. A 32-year-old at 37 weeks gestation with no complaints at her routine office visit
B. A 25-year-old G2P0101 at 34 weeks gestation who complains of cramping
C. A 37-year-old G5P0400 at 25 weeks gestation with vaginal bleeding and painful contractions
D. A and C
E. All of the above

Q14: Cerclage should always be removed at the time of preterm premature rupture of membranes.
A. TRUE
B. FALSE

Answers

Q1: C, Q2: E, Q3: D, Q4: B, Q5: C, Q6: C, Q7: B, Q8: D, Q9: A, Q10: E, Q11: C, Q12: E, Q13: D, Q14: B.

Resources

1. Gabbe SG, Niebyl JR, Simpson JL, Landon MB, Galan HL, Jauniaux ERM, Driscoll DA. Obstetrics: normal and problem pregnancies. Chapter 27. 6th ed. Philadelphia, PA: Elsevier; 2012.
2. American College of Obstetricians and Gynecologists. Practice bulletin no. 142: cerclage for the management of cervical insufficiency. Obstet Gynecol. 2014;123:372–9.

Chapter 28
Antepartum Fetal Surveillance

Antepartum fetal surveillance aims to decrease perinatal morbidity and mortality; however, unnecessary iatrogenic preterm delivery should be avoided as well. Antenatal testing may include contraction stress tests, nonstress tests, biophysical profiles, and modified biophysical profiles. Decreased fetal movement by maternal report is appealing as an inexpensive, simple screening method, but evidence is mixed regarding its utility [1].

Recommended resources—ACOG Practice Bulletin 145: Antepartum Fetal Surveillance [2].

Q1: What is the ultimate goal of fetal surveillance?

A. To detect academia
B. To detect hypoxemia
C. To assess fetal well-being in pregnancies complicated by preexisting maternal conditions and conditions which have developed
D. To prevent fetal death

Q2: Tests of fetal well-being can predict which of the following:

A. Oligohydramnios caused by decreased renal perfusion
B. Umbilical cord accidents

K.C. Arnold, C.J. Flint, *Obstetrics Essentials*,
DOI 10.1007/978-3-319-57675-6_28,

C. Duration of the acid base disturbance
D. Severity of the acid base disturbance

Q3: Which of the following is TRUE regarding fetal kick counts?
A. Decreases in fetal movement are seldom correlated with clinical outcomes
B. The optimal number of movements and duration for counting is evidence based
C. One method includes counting fetal movement for 1 h every day
D. It is considered a form of antepartum fetal surveillance

Q4: A 40-year-old G1P0 presents to triage with a term gestation. Her baby is known to have intrauterine growth restriction. The team decides to perform a contraction stress test. Which of the following describes the correct method of performing the test?
A. Contractions may be spontaneous, produced by oxytocin, or by nipple stimulation
B. An adequate test must include at least two contractions for 30 sections each in a 10-min period
C. This test relies on the premise that fetal oxygenation is worsened by contractions; hence, internal monitoring should be used to measure Montevideo units
D. A and B
E. All of the above

Q5: Your intern asks you how to interpret the results of a contraction stress test. You answer:
A. A negative test means that there are no variable or late contractions
B. A positive test indicates the presence of late decelerations after every contraction
C. An equivocal test means that the decelerations occur if contractions are longer than 90 s or more frequent than every 2 min

D. A and C
E. All of the above

Q6: How is a nonstress test conducted?
A. The patient is placed in the semi-Fowler position
B. The test should be conducted for 20 min, but may last as long as 40 min
C. Vibroacoustic stimulation safely reduces the frequency of nonreactive tests
D. Accelerations are defined as 15 beats per minute above the baseline for 15 s for term pregnancies
E. All of the above are true

Q7: Which of the following is the cutoff for when 10 by 10 accelerations appear to sufficiently predict fetal well-being?
A. 28 weeks or less
B. 30 weeks or less
C. 32 weeks or less
D. 34 weeks or less
E. Exact week is not known

Q8: Which of the following is FALSE regarding the components of a biophysical profile?
A. Amniotic fluid volume as defined by measurement of four pockets
B. Fetal breathing movements defined as one or more of 30 s
C. Fetal movement including three or more body or limb movements
D. Fetal tone defined as one or more episodes of extension and then flexion
E. A nonstress test can be omitted if other components are normal

Q9: Which of the following defines a modified biophysical profile?
A. Amniotic fluid assessment and nonstress test
B. Fetal breathing and fetal movement

C. Fetal tone and amniotic fluid assessment
D. Any of the above, but only valid in the third trimester

Q10: A 31-year-old G4P3003 presents to your office for umbilical artery Doppler velocimetry. She asks why this is being done. What do you tell her?
A. It is used to assess vascular resistance, but correlates poorly with perinatal mortality
B. Abnormal flow is defined as absent or reversed end-diastolic flow
C. It can be used in the fetus with growth restriction or cardiac anomalies
D. B and C
E. All of the above are true

Q11: The negative predictive value is above 99% for a stillbirth occurring within 1 week of a normal test result of all of the following EXCEPT:
A. Contraction stress test
B. Biophysical profile
C. Nonstress test
D. Modified biophysical stress test
E. All of the above have a 99% negative predictive value

Q12: Which of the following are indications for antepartum fetal surveillance?
A. Hemoglobinopathies
B. Recurrent pregnancy loss
C. Hypothyroidism
D. Dichorionic diamniotic twin gestation
E. All of the above

Q13: Antepartum fetal surveillance should begin:
A. When delivery would be considered for perinatal benefit
B. For most at-risk patients, 32/0 weeks gestation

C. For most at-risk patients, 34/0 weeks gestation
D. A and B
E. A and C

Q14: Your patient presents to clinic complaining of decreased fetal movement at 35 weeks gestation. Her pregnancy is otherwise uncomplicated. A biophysical profile is performed, and the result is 8/10. The patient reports return of fetal movement. When should subsequent fetal testing be performed?
A. Weekly until delivery
B. In 1 week and then no further testing required if reassuring
C. No further testing is indicated
D. All of the above are reasonable options

For the following scenarios choose:
A. Immediate delivery
B. Repeat biophysical profile in 24 h or extended monitoring

Q15: A type 1 diabetic patient at 31 weeks gestation in diabetic ketoacidosis with a biophysical profile of 4/10:
A. Immediate delivery
B. Repeat biophysical profile in 24 h or extended monitoring

Q16: A healthy woman at 36 weeks gestation with a biophysical profile of 6/10.
A. Immediate delivery
B. Repeat biophysical profile in 24 h or extended monitoring

Q17: A healthy woman at 33 weeks gestation with a biophysical profile of 4/10.
A. Immediate delivery
B. Repeat biophysical profile in 24 h or extended monitoring

Q18: A healthy woman at 31 weeks gestation with a biophysical profile of 4/10.

A. Immediate delivery
B. Repeat biophysical profile in 24 h or extended monitoring

Q19: A healthy woman with a fetus with intrauterine growth restriction at 38 weeks gestation who is found to have presence of diastolic flow with an elevated S/D ratio:

A. Immediate delivery
B. Repeat biophysical profile in 24 h or extended monitoring

Q20: A woman at 38 weeks with a new finding of oligohydramnios.

A. Immediate delivery
B. Repeat biophysical profile in 24 h or extended monitoring

Q21: Which method of amniotic fluid measurement is associated with a reduction in unnecessary interventions without an increase in adverse perinatal outcomes?

A. Measurement of a 2 cm by 2 cm pocket
B. Measurement of a single vertical pocked of 2 cm, not containing umbilical cord
C. An amniotic fluid index of 5 cm or less
D. All of the above are equivalent and decision made be based on provider's preference

Answers

Q1: D, Q2: A, Q3: D, Q4: A, Q5: D, Q6: E, Q7: C, Q8: A, Q9: A, Q10: B, Q11: E, Q12: A, Q13: D, Q14: C, Q15: B, Q16: B, Q17: A, Q18: B, Q19: A, Q20: A, Q21: B.

Resources

1. Gabbe SG, Niebyl JR, Simpson JL, Landon MB, Galan HL, Jauniaux ERM, Driscoll DA. Obstetrics: normal and problem pregnancies. Chapter 12. 6th ed. Philadelphia, PA: Elsevier; 2012.
2. American College of Obstetricians and Gynecologists. Practice bulletin no. 145: antepartum fetal surveillance. Obstet Gynecol. 2014;124:182–92.

Chapter 29
Management of Late-Term and Postterm Pregnancies

The incidence of postterm pregnancies is reported to be between 5% and 6%. Risk factors include primigravity, previous history of a postterm pregnancy, male fetus, and maternal obesity. Infants delivered postterm are at risk for neonatal convulsions, meconium aspiration syndrome, and low Apgar scores. Stillbirth is also increased; hence antenatal surveillance is recommended [1].

Recommended resource—ACOG Practice Bulletin 146: Management of Late-Term and Postterm Pregnancies [2].

Q1: Late-term pregnancy refers to a pregnancy between:
- A. 40 0/7 weeks and 42 0/7 weeks
- B. 40 6/7 weeks and 41 6/7 weeks
- C. 41 0/7 weeks and 42 6/7 weeks
- D. 41 0/7 weeks and 41 6/7 weeks

Q2: A 42-year-old G2P1001 presents to OB triage with intrauterine gestation at 42/2 weeks gestation. When discussing the morbidities associated with her gestational age, you refer to her pregnancy as:
- A. Term
- B. Late term
- C. Postterm
- D. Advanced term

K.C. Arnold, C.J. Flint, *Obstetrics Essentials*,
DOI 10.1007/978-3-319-57675-6_29,

Q3: A 29-year-old G1P0 with intrauterine pregnancy at 42 weeks presents to your office for her last OB visit. She has an induction scheduled at the end of the week. She is carrying a female fetus and has a BMI of 21. In conversation she mentions that her mother also carried her 2 weeks beyond her due date. What risk factors does this patient have for a postterm pregnancy?

A. Maternal weight and sex of fetus
B. Nulliparity and maternal weight
C. Sex of fetus and genetic predisposition
D. Nulliparity and genetic predisposition

Q4: The risks associated with postterm pregnancy include all the following EXCEPT:

A. Macrosomia
B. Oligohydramnios
C. Neonatal convulsions
D. 5 min Apgar less than 4
E. All of the above are risks

Q5: There is an increased risk of cesarean delivery in late-term and postterm pregnancies.

A. TRUE
B. FALSE

Q6: Membrane sweeping should not be performed in women who are Group B strep positive.

A. TRUE
B. FALSE

Q7: Which of the following has been shown to reduce the risk of late-term and postterm pregnancies?

A. Confirmation of menstrual dating with ultrasonography
B. Membrane sweeping
C. Walking and frequent intercourse
D. A and B
E. All of the above

Q8: A 27-year-old G2P1001 with intrauterine gestation at 40 weeks presents for her OB visit. She is scheduled for induction in 12 days. She asks if there are any special precautions that need to be taken starting at her next visit in 1 week. You counsel her:

A. Yes, antenatal testing should be instituted, though the frequency is provider dependent due to insufficient data
B. Yes, ultrasound measurement of amniotic fluid should be considered with nonstress test or biophysical profile
C. Yes, antenatal testing should be started due to the increased risk of stillbirth in postterm pregnancies
D. B and C
E. All of the above

Q9: Which definition of oligohydramnios may reduce unnecessary interventions without compromising perinatal outcomes?

A. Amniotic fluid index of 5 cm or less
B. Maximum vertical pocket of 2 cm or less
C. Maximum vertical pocket of 3 cm or less
D. Amniotic fluid index of 7 cm or less

Q10: Which of the following is FALSE in regard to oligohydramnios in postterm pregnancies?

A. Associated with an increased risk of fetal demise
B. Is an indication for delivery
C. Increased risk of fetal heart rate abnormalities
D. All of the above are true

Q11: Expectant management in late-term and postterm pregnancies is associated with a decreased risk of cesarean delivery.

A. TRUE
B. FALSE

Q12: A 27-year-old G2P1001 with intrauterine gestation at 37 weeks presents for OB visit. She has a past obstetrical history significant for primary cesarean delivery at term due to non-reassuring fetal heart tones. She desires trial of labor after cesarean. Her cervix is currently closed and her pregnancy is otherwise uncomplicated. She asks you about your policy on expectant management versus induction of labor if she goes past her estimated due date. You counsel her:

A. If she does not go into labor spontaneously before her estimated due date, she should have a repeat cesarean section due to the increased risk of uterine rupture
B. Her chances of having a successful vaginal birth after cesarean delivery decrease beyond 41 weeks gestational age
C. The use of Pitocin during an induction is associated with a greater risk of uterine rupture in late-term pregnancies compared to early-term pregnancies
D. Induction of labor is contraindicated in patients who have had a prior cesarean delivery

Answers

Q1: D, Q2: C, Q3: D, Q4: E, Q5: A, Q6: B, Q7: D, Q8: E, Q9: B, Q10: D, Q11: B, Q12: B.

Resources

1. Gabbe SG, Niebyl JR, Simpson JL, Landon MB, Galan HL, Jauniaux ERM, Driscoll DA. Obstetrics: normal and problem pregnancies. Chapter 34. 6th ed. Philadelphia, PA: Elsevier; 2012.
2. American College of Obstetricians and Gynecologists. Practice bulletin no. 146: management of late-term and postterm pregnancies. Obstet Gynecol. 2014;124:390–6.

Chapter 30
Thyroid Disease in Pregnancy

Pregnancy results in increased thyroxine-binding globulin and increased thyroid-stimulating hormone receptor activation due to human chorionic gonadotropin. This results in increased secretion of thyroid hormones. In hyperthyroidism patients, propylthiouracil and methimazole are the drugs of choice depending on fetal gestational age. More than half of patients with hypothyroidism will need to increase the dose of their replacement during pregnancy. Thyroid storm is rare but life-threatening and should be managed in an intensive care unit [1].

Recommended resources—ACOG Practice Bulletin 148: Thyroid Disease in Pregnancy [2].

Q1: Which of the following is TRUE regarding thyroid changes in pregnancy?
- A. Maternal thyroid size increases 30% by the third trimester
- B. TSH increases in early pregnancy because of stimulation by BhCG
- C. Thyroid-binding globulin decreases throughout pregnancy
- D. All of the above are false
- E. All of the above are true

K.C. Arnold, C.J. Flint, *Obstetrics Essentials*,
DOI 10.1007/978-3-319-57675-6_30,

Q2: A 26-year-old presents to your office at 14 weeks gestation. Her lab values reveal an increased TSH and a decreased free T4. Which of the following is the correct diagnosis?

A. Overt hyperthyroidism
B. Subclinical hyperthyroidism
C. Overt hypothyroidism
D. Subclinical hypothyroidism
E. Additional antibody testing is required for a diagnosis

Q3: At what gestation does the fetal thyroid begin to synthesize its own thyroid hormone?

A. 8 weeks gestation
B. 12 weeks gestation
C. 20 weeks gestation
D. 24 weeks gestation
E. At birth

Q4: In which of the following cases is the fetus at the highest risk for fetal thyrotoxicosis?

A. A woman with Graves' disease being treated with methimazole
B. A woman with Graves' disease who was previously treated with a thyroidectomy
C. A woman with a suppressed TSH but normal free T4 who is on no medications
D. All of the above have equal risk for adverse outcomes

Q5: Which of the following adverse effects is associated with inadequately treated maternal hyperthyroidism?

A. Severe preeclampsia
B. Fetal hypothyroidism
C. Fetal hyperthyroidism
D. A and C
E. All of the above

Q6: In which of the following scenarios would umbilical cord blood sampling be reasonable if disease could not be excluded based on clinical or ultrasound findings?

A. Any mother with Graves' disease should be offered umbilical cord sampling
B. Mothers with uncontrolled Graves' disease
C. Fetal growth restriction and hydrops
D. Fetal macrosomia and tachycardia
E. Patients with any of the above should be offered umbilical cord sampling to assess fetal thyroid status

Q7: Which of the following substances are LEAST likely to cross the placenta?

A. Thyroid antibodies in Graves' disease
B. Maternal free T4
C. Thioamide medications
D. Thyroid inhibitory antibodies

Q8: A 30-year-old pregnant patient has an elevated TSH and a low free T4. Which of the following are TRUE?

A. If she does not start treatment, she will be at risk for preeclampsia, preterm birth, and abruption
B. Regardless of treatment, her fetus is at risk for low birth rate and for impaired neuropsychologic development
C. The most likely cause for her symptoms is Hashimoto's thyroiditis
D. The most likely cause for her symptoms is Graves' disease
E. A and C

Q9: Which of the following is TRUE in a pregnant woman with an elevated TSH but a normal free T4?

A. Treatment will not improve her pregnancy outcomes
B. Left untreated, she will likely develop overt hypothyroidism

C. Universal prenatal screening for this condition is recommended
D. B and C
E. All of the above

Q10: Which of the following pregnant women should have a thyroid laboratory evaluation?
A. A woman with a mildly enlarged thyroid
B. A woman with thyroid nodules
C. A woman with a family history of thyroid disorders
D. A woman with a BMI of 40
E. All of the above

Q11: Which of the following reflects the upper limit of normal for TSH in the first trimester?
A. 2.0 mlU/L
B. 2.5 mIU/L
C. 3.0 mIU/L
D. There is no consensus

Q12: A 30-year-old patient complains of sweating, weight loss, heat intolerance, and insomnia. Her TSH is found to be suppressed and her free T4 is normal. Which of the following is TRUE?
A. A free T3 should be obtained
B. She currently meets criteria for subclinical hyperthyroidism
C. She should be tested for antithyroid peroxidase and antithyroglobulin antibodies
D. A and B
E. All of the above

Q13: Which of the following is TRUE regarding the treatment of overt hyperthyroidism in pregnancy?
A. Labs should be checked every trimester and doses adjusted accordingly
B. Doses should be adjusted to keep TSH at the upper limit of normal or just above
C. Patients should be given precautions regarding symptoms of agranulocytosis

D. Propylthiouracil should be used in the first and second trimester, and then the patient should be transitioned to methimazole
E. A and C

Q14: Which of the following statements are TRUE regarding thioamides in the treatment of overt hyperthyroidism of pregnancy?
A. Propylthiouracil is associated with aplasia cutis
B. Propylthiouracil inhibits the conversion of T3 to T4
C. Methimazole is associated with choanal atresia
D. Methimazole is associated with maternal hepatotoxicity
E. All of the above are true

Q15: An 18-year-old G1P0 presents to your office and is found to have a new diagnosis of overt hypothyroidism. She asks you what your treatment plan is and you tell her:
A. She'll start at a dose of approximately 100 mcg of T4 replacement per day
B. Her TSH will be checked every 2 weeks until it is within normal limits
C. After initiation of treatment, if her TSH remains high, her dose will be increased by 25–50 mcg
D. A and B
E. A and C

Q16: All of the following regarding classic thyroid storm are true, EXCEPT:
A. Thyroid storm is a hypermetabolic state
B. Symptoms include fever, central nervous dysfunction, cardiac dysrhythmia
C. It has an insidious onset leading to multiorgan decompensation
D. It is a life-threatening condition
E. Treatment should not be delayed until laboratory confirmation

Q17: A patient presents to urgent care with cardiomyopathy and is diagnosed with thyrotoxic heat failure. She is transferred to the ICU, and her husband asks why this happened and what will happen to his wife. You counsel him that:

A. Her condition is due to an elevated TSH which caused heart failure and pulmonary hypertension.
B. Her condition is unfortunately not reversible
C. She has a rare form of thyroid storm
D. Decompensation generally has an additional underlying cause such as sepsis or anemia
E. All of the above are true

Q18: When treating thyroid storm, all of the following medications should be administered, EXCEPT:

A. Propylthiouracil
B. Methimazole
C. Lugol's solution
D. Dexamethasone
E. Propranolol

Q19: A 27-year-old G3P2002 presents to your office distraught because the thyroid ultrasound you ordered showed a nodule which is suspicious for malignancy. Which of the following are true?

A. Fine needle aspiration is the next step in diagnosis
B. Thyroid cancer is generally an extremely aggressive cancer
C. Radioiodine scanning should be utilized to aid in diagnosis
D. Surgery should always be postponed until postpartum if needed

Q20: Your patient presents to her postpartum visit and you suspect postpartum thyroiditis. After confirming the diagnosis with labs, how will you treat her?

A. Methimazole, then T4 replacement
B. Beta blockers, then T4 replacement

C. Propylthiouracil, then T4 replacement
D. T4 replacement, then propylthiouracil
E. T4 replacement, then methimazole

Q21: Your patient with postpartum thyroiditis would like to know how long her condition will last. You tell her:
A. The hyperthyroid phase generally lasts 6–12 months
B. The hypothyroid phase generally lasts 6–12 months
C. One half of patients develop overt hypothyroidism
D. All of the above are true

Answers

Q1: A, Q2: C, Q3: B, Q4: B, Q5: E, Q6: C, Q7: D, Q8: E, Q9: A, Q10: B, Q11: B, Q12: D, Q13: C, Q14: C, Q15: E, Q16: C, Q17: D, Q18: B, Q19: A, Q20: B, Q21: B.

Resources

1. Gabbe SG, Niebyl JR, Simpson JL, Landon MB, Galan HL, Jauniaux ERM, Driscoll DA. Obstetrics: normal and problem pregnancies. Chapter 40. 6th ed. Philadelphia, PA: Elsevier; 2012.
2. American College of Obstetricians and Gynecologists. Practice bulletin no. 148: thyroid disease in pregnancy. Obstet Gynecol. 2015;125:996–1005.

Chapter 31
Cytomegalovirus, Parvovirus B19, Varicella Zoster, and Toxoplasmosis in Pregnancy

Cytomegalovirus is a common childhood illness and in utero infection often causes hearing loss. Parvovirus can cause Fifth's disease and eventually hydrops fetalis by preferentially infecting rapidly dividing cells. Varicella, commonly known as chickenpox, is highly contagious and can cause congenital varicella syndrome if the mother is exposed prior to 13 weeks gestation. Toxoplasmosis is acquired through eating infected meat or cat feces with 40% of mothers acutely infected during pregnancy giving birth to babies with congenital toxoplasmosis [1].

Recommended resources—ACOG Practice Bulletin 151: Cytomegalovirus, Parvovirus B19, Varicella Zoster, and Toxoplasmosis in Pregnancy [2].

Q1: Cytomegalovirus (CMV) is a double-stranded DNA virus that is transmitted through:

A. Consumption of undercooked meat
B. Respiratory secretions
C. Sexual contact
D. Hand-to-mouth contact

Q2: Adults infected with primary CMV may experience:

A. No symptoms as many are asymptomatic with infection
B. Mononucleosis-like syndrome with fevers, chills, and myalgias
C. Reticular rash on the trunk

K.C. Arnold, C.J. Flint, *Obstetrics Essentials*,
DOI 10.1007/978-3-319-57675-6_31,

D. A and B
E. All of the above

Q3: Which of the following is FALSE in regard to secondary infection with CMV?
A. The incidence of secondary infection is higher than primary infection in pregnant women
B. Rate of vertical transmission after a secondary infection is much lower than after a primary infection
C. Unlikely to cause multiple sequelae in the fetus
D. Congenital hearing loss is the most common severe sequelae
E. All the above are true

Q4: A 33-year-old G1P0 is known to have contracted CMV, and vertical transmission to her fetus is strongly suspected. You counsel her regarding the potential clinical manifestations of congenital CMV telling her that her newborn may have:
A. Jaundice, petechiae, and thrombocytopenia
B. Chorioretinitis
C. Periventricular calcifications and ventriculomegaly
D. Microcephaly

Q5: Vertical transmission of CMV:
A. Has the same probability of occurring in all trimesters
B. Is more likely to occur in the third trimester
C. Is more likely to cause severe disease if occurs in the first trimester
D. A and C
E. B and C

Q6: Which of the following is FALSE regarding parvovirus B19?
A. Is a single-stranded DNA virus
B. Causes “fifth disease” in children
C. Serious manifestation is more likely to occur in patients with a hemoglobinopathy

D. Most common symptoms in adult include reticular rash on trunk and peripheral arthropathy
E. All of the above are true

Q7: A person infected with parvovirus B19 is no longer infectious to others once a rash has developed.
A. TRUE
B. FALSE

Q8: A 39-year-old G3P2002 with 18 weeks gestation presents to your clinic reporting exposure to parvovirus B19 with subsequent development of rash and arthritis. Serology studies confirm acute infection revealing:
A. Positive IgM antibodies and IgG antibodies
B. Positive IgM antibodies alone
C. Positive IgG antibodies alone
D. A and B

Q9: You inform the above patient that the risk of her male fetus having severe effects if vertical transmission occurs is more likely due to:
A. The severity of her symptoms
B. Her gestational age
C. Sex of her fetus
D. All of the above

Q10: This same patient has now progressed to 27 weeks gestation, and there is no ultrasound evidence of parvovirus B19 infection in her fetus. You tell her:
A. Until the fetus is born, she cannot be assured that her fetus will not suffer severe effects
B. Since more than 8 weeks has passed since her infection, it is unlikely that severe manifestations such as hydrops will occur
C. Repeat serology is necessary to confirm maternal infection
D. Serology will need to be drawn on fetus once it is born to determine newborn sequelae

Q11: Which of the following is TRUE regarding transmission of parvovirus B19?

A. Transmitted through respiratory secretions and hand-to-mouth contact
B. Risk of exposure and subsequent transmission is higher in a child care setting than in household setting
C. Prevalence of seropositivity increases with age
D. A and C
E. All the above

Q12: Parvovirus B19 is cytotoxic to:

A. Immunoglobulin precursors
B. Neuronal precursors
C. Erythroid precursors
D. Hepatocyte precursors
E. All the above

Q13: Varicella zoster is a highly contagious virus that has a period of infectivity lasting:

A. 24 h before a rash appears until the first vesicles form
B. 24 h before a rash appears until the vesicles crust over
C. 48 h before a rash appears until the first vesicles form
D. 48 h before a rash appears until the vesicles crust over

Q14: A 29-year-old G2P1001 with intrauterine pregnancy at 31 weeks gestation develops symptoms of acute varicella zoster infection including rash and vesicle formation. You counsel her that she is at risk of developing ________ which is a significant risk factor for maternal mortality.

A. Pneumonia
B. Coagulopathy
C. SIRS
D. Myocarditis

Q15: The risk of a fetus developing congenital varicella syndrome is high.

A. TRUE
B. FALSE

Q16: A 25-year-old G1P0 is noted to develop a maculopapular rash and vesicles 24 h after vaginally delivering a term infant. You counsel her:

A. There is no need for concern since her infant has already been delivered
B. Her infant is at risk of developing neonatal varicella zoster virus infection which has a high neonatal death rate
C. Her infant may have been exposed to varicella zoster, but the robust neonatal immune system will likely prevent infection from developing
D. As long as the patient is placed in isolation from her infant until her vesicles resolve, the infant should be safe from developing infection

Q17: Toxoplasmosis is caused by:

A. A double-stranded DNA virus
B. A single-stranded RNA virus
C. An intracellular parasite
D. A gram-negative bacterium

Q18: Congenital transmission of toxoplasmosis is most likely to occur during the ______ trimester and most likely to cause severe disease if transmitted in the _____trimester.

A. First; first
B. Second; first
C. Third; third
D. Third; first

Q19: Acute maternal infection with CMV can be diagnosed by:

A. Seroconversion from negative to positive anti-CMV IgG
B. Greater than twofold increase in anti-CMV IgG titers

C. Presence of anti-CMV IgM antibodies
D. A and B
E. All the above

Q20: Amniocentesis with positive culture for CMV is predictive of severe congenital infection.
A. TRUE
B. FALSE

Q21: A 22-year-old G1P0 with intrauterine pregnancy at 24 weeks gestation has confirmed fetal cytomegalovirus infection. The next best steps include:
A. Administration of ganciclovir
B. Passive immunization with CMV-specific hyperimmune globulin
C. Serial ultrasound surveillance
D. A and C
E. B and C

Q22: For which of the following infectious diseases should women undergo routine serologic screening prior to or during pregnancy?
A. Cytomegalovirus
B. Parvovirus B19
C. Toxoplasmosis
D. All of the above
E. None of the above

Q23: A 30-year-old G2P0101 with intrauterine gestation at 31 weeks presents to your office with concerns that she has been exposed to a child at work who has parvovirus. You immediately obtain serologic screening. A few days later, the lab results return and your patient is IgM negative but IgG positive. You call her and inform her:
A. She should be closely monitored for potential fetal infection
B. She should undergo repeat serologic testing in four weeks

C. She is not at risk of transplacental transmission
D. A and B

Q24: How is parvovirus fetal infection diagnosed?
A. PCR analysis of fractionated fetal blood obtained from maternal blood samples
B. PCR analysis of amniotic fluid
C. Culture of amniotic fluid
D. By ultrasonography revealing hydrops fetalis

Q25: Fetal parvovirus infection is diagnosed. What specific ultrasound measurement will be important in monitoring for signs of developing sequelae?
A. Femur length
B. Biparietal diameter
C. Umbilical artery systolic to diastolic ratio
D. Middle cerebral artery Doppler assessment

Q26: Administration of varicella zoster immune globulin (VZIG) should be considered in the following situation(s):
A. To an infant when maternal infection develops 36 h following delivery
B. To a nonimmune pregnant mother who has been exposed to someone with active varicella zoster infection within the past 5 days
C. To a pregnant mother who has personal history of varicella zoster infection as a child who has been exposed to someone with active varicella zoster within the past 2 days
D. A and B
E. All the above

Q27: Oral acyclovir has been proven effective in reducing maternal symptoms and preventing fetal effects of congenital varicella syndrome if started within 24 h of developing a varicella zoster-associated rash.
A. TRUE
B. FALSE

Q28: How long should pregnancy be delayed after administration of the last varicella vaccine dose?
A. 1 month
B. 2 months
C. 3 months
D. No delay is necessary

Questions 29–30 pertain to the same patient:

Q29: A 31-year-old G3P2002 with intrauterine gestation at 16 weeks has recently confirmed acute toxoplasmosis infection. Spiramycin is immediately prescribed to the mother. You explain to your patient that the medication:
A. Reduces transplacental parasitic transfer
B. Does not readily cross the placenta
C. Cannot prevent fetal infection
D. A and B
E. All the above

Q30: Which of the following are appropriate recommendations for pregnant patients to prevent toxoplasmosis infection?
A. Avoid consuming undercooked meat or dairy products
B. Avoid working in the soil without gloves
C. Avoid handling cat litter
D. A and C
E. All the above

Answers

Q1: C, Q2: D, Q3: E, Q4: A, Q5: E, Q6: E, Q7: A, Q8: D, Q9: B, Q10: B, Q11: D, Q12: C, Q13: D, Q14: A, Q15: B, Q16: B, Q17: C, Q18: D, Q19: A, Q20: B, Q21: C, Q22: E, Q23: C, Q24: B, Q25: D, Q26: D, Q27: B, Q28: A, Q29: E, Q30: E.

Resources

1. Gabbe SG, Niebyl JR, Simpson JL, Landon MB, Galan HL, Jauniaux ERM, Driscoll DA. Obstetrics: normal and problem pregnancies. Chapter 50. 6th ed. Philadelphia, PA: Elsevier; 2012.
2. American College of Obstetricians and Gynecologists. Practice bulletin no. 151: cytomegalovirus, parvovirus B19, varicella zoster, and toxoplasmosis in pregnancy. Obstet Gynecol. 2015;125:1510–25.

Chapter 32
Nausea and Vomiting of Pregnancy

Nausea and vomiting are frequent complaints during pregnancy. Symptoms can range from mildly bothersome to severely debilitating, even requiring hospitalization. Management should include dietary counseling as well as medications. Hyperemesis gravidarum is rare, but should be suspected if patients lose more than 5% of the body weight [1].

Recommended resource—ACOG Practice Bulletin 153: Nausea and Vomiting of Pregnancy [2].

Q1: In general, which of the following is TRUE regarding nausea and vomiting of pregnancy?

A. It is overtreated and patients should be reassured that 75% of pregnancy women experience nausea
B. Early treatment is recommended to prevent hospitalizations
C. Assessment tools to categorize degree of nausea in a patient can help distinguish who needs treatment
D. It is caused by excessive life stress

K.C. Arnold, C.J. Flint, *Obstetrics Essentials*,
DOI 10.1007/978-3-319-57675-6_32,

Q2: Hyperemesis gravidarum:

A. Is defined by a strict set of criteria involving specific lab abnormalities
B. Has an incidence of approximately 0.1% of pregnancies
C. Is a clinical diagnosis
D. Fifth most common cause of hospitalization during pregnancy

Q3: All of the following criteria are most commonly cited in the diagnosis of hyperemesis gravidarum, EXCEPT?

A. Other possible causes have been ruled out
B. Documented weight loss
C. Volume of emesis
D. Ketonuria
E. Electrolyte abnormalities

Q4: Which of the following would suggest a diagnosis other than nausea/vomiting of pregnancy?

A. Symptoms starting before 9 weeks gestation
B. Headache
C. Mild epigastric pain
D. A and B
E. B and C

Q5: A 23-year-old presents to your office as a transfer of care at 12 weeks gestation stating that another practitioner diagnosed her with hyperemesis gravidarum. You review her labs and note a suppressed TSH. She requests that you start treatment as it may help with her nausea and vomiting. Which of the following are appropriate?

A. Thyroid exam with initiation of treatment only if a goiter is present
B. Initiation of treatment for symptomatic hyperthyroidism
C. No initiation of treatment given she has an established diagnosis which accounts for her suppressed TSH
D. None of the above are correct

Q6: Which of the following should you discuss with your patient regarding possible causes for nausea and vomiting during pregnancy?

A. Estrogen and human chorionic gonadotropin levels
B. Psychological predisposition
C. Smoking
D. A and C
E. All of the above

Q7: Which of the following supports the theory that hCG and estrogen can cause nausea and vomiting?

A. Lower levels of hormones caused by multiple gestations and molar pregnancies generally cause less nausea and vomiting
B. Smokers have increased levels of these hormones and are more likely to have nausea and vomiting
C. Women who experienced nausea and vomiting with combined oral contraceptive pills are more likely to have nausea and vomiting during pregnancy
D. A and C
E. All of the above

Q8: Which of the following does NOT increase the risk for nausea and vomiting of pregnancy?

A. Increased placental mass
B. Motion sickness
C. Family history of nausea and vomiting of pregnancy
D. Obesity
E. All of the above increase the risk of nausea and vomiting of pregnancy

Q9: Which of the following is a severe maternal effect related to nausea and vomiting of pregnancy?

A. Esophageal rupture
B. Splenic avulsion
C. Psychosocial morbidity
D. A and B
E. All of the above

Q10: A 36-year-old G1P0 presents for a routine obstetric. She is followed for hyperemesis gravidarum and is worried about what effect this will have on her baby. How do you counsel her?

A. It often portends well for pregnancy outcome, may be associated with low birth weight, gives a lower risk of miscarriage, and is unlikely associated with malformations
B. Its impact on the fetus is unknown overall. It may be associated with low birth weight, but it is unlikely associated with malformations
C. The risk for miscarriage is decreased, the risk for low birth weight infants is significantly increased, and long-term health of children appears to be unaffected
D. It often portends well for pregnancy outcomes. Although it is associated with low birth weight, it is also associated with a lower risk of miscarriage and is unlikely associated with malformations. Long-term health of children is unaffected

Q11: All of the following have been shown in studies to decrease nausea and vomiting in pregnancy, EXCEPT:

A. Small frequent meals
B. Multivitamins at the time of conception
C. Ginger pills
D. All of the above have been proven to decrease nausea and vomiting

Q12: Which of the following is TRUE regarding the use of pyridoxine combined with doxylamine for the treatment of nausea and vomiting of pregnancy?

A. It is shown to decrease nausea and vomiting of pregnancy compared to placebo
B. It should be used as a second-line therapy
C. Fetal effects are unlikely; however, there is not enough data yet to know
D. It should be taken as soon as nausea begins for greatest decrease in symptoms

Q13: A 20-year-old G1P0 pregnant patient presents complaining of nausea and vomiting. She asks you to discuss the risks and benefits of ondansetron treatment. Which of the following is FALSE?

A. Ondansetron is more effective at decreasing nausea and vomiting than pyridoxine and doxylamine combined
B. High doses should be avoided to decrease the risk of torsades de pointes
C. It has been shown to cause a significant increase in birth defects
D. Continuous infusion pumps are associated with complications in approximately 1/3 of patients
E. All of the above are true

Q14: Which of the following is a side effect of ondansetron?

A. Headache
B. Diarrhea
C. Hyperkalemia
D. Hypocalcemia
E. All of the above

Q15: Your patient asks about the possibility of using methylprednisolone to decrease her nausea and vomiting of pregnancy. You tell her that it is effective and:

A. It should only be used in the third trimester do decrease the risk of anomalies
B. If no improvement is seen after 3 days of use, the dose should be increased
C. It is associated with fetal cardiac defects
D. It should only be used in refractory patients as a last resort treatment
E. All of the above

Q16: Which of the following medications are contraindicated for patients taking ondansetron?

A. Diuretics
B. Metronidazole
C. HIV protease inhibitors

D. Oxycodone
E. All of the above

Q17: Which of the following lab value is NOT consistent with a diagnosis of hyperemesis gravidarum?
A. Amylase ten times normal
B. Ketonuria
C. Increased liver function tests in the 100 s
D. Elevated serum bilirubin of 3
E. Hypochloremic metabolic alkalosis

Q18: All of the following are options to consider in the differential for nausea and vomiting of pregnancy, EXCEPT:
A. Acute pancreatitis
B. Chronic hepatitis
C. Helicobacter pylori
D. Gastric ulcer

Q19: To rehydrate a woman with hyperemesis gravidarum, what IV fluids should you give her?
A. First dextrose, then vitamins including thiamine
B. First thiamine, then vitamins and dextrose
C. First thiamine and dextrose, then vitamins and dextrose
D. First vitamins, then dextrose and thiamine

Q20: A pregnant patient has tried medical management, and despite this, she is unable to maintain her weight. She begins to ask about other ways of getting nutrition. How do you counsel her?
A. Enteral nutrition is associated with sepsis and thromboembolic events
B. Enteral nutrition is not well tolerated during pregnancy
C. Enteral nutrition is indicated in her case
D. Parenteral nutrition is the preferred method
E. C and B

Q21: You receive a phone call as triage physician regarding a woman at 22 weeks gestation. She reports that she has tried scheduled doxylamine and pyridoxine; however, she has been unable to keep food down without vomiting for the last 5 days. She is able to tolerate liquids. She asks you if she needs to be admitted to the hospital. How do you respond?

A. Yes, because you have tried medicine and still cannot tolerate food
B. No, because you can still tolerate liquids
C. No, but I can prescribe additional antiemetics to assist you
D. Yes, because if we admit you we may be able to prevent long-term hospitalization E. B and C

Answers

Q1: B, Q2: C, Q3: C, Q4: B, Q5: A, Q6: A, Q7: C, Q8: D, Q9: E, Q10: A, Q11: A, Q12: A, Q13: C, Q14: A, Q15: D, Q16: E, Q17: A, Q18: B, Q19: B, Q20: C, Q21: E.

Resources

1. Gabbe SG, Niebyl JR, Simpson JL, Landon MB, Galan HL, Jauniaux ERM, Driscoll DA. Obstetrics: normal and problem pregnancies. Chapter 7. 6th ed. Philadelphia, PA: Elsevier; 2012.
2. American College of Obstetricians and Gynecologists. Practice bulletin no. 153: Nausea and vomiting of pregnancy. Obstet Gynecol. 2015;126:e12–24.

Chapter 33
Operative Vaginal Delivery

Operative vaginal delivery includes the use of the vacuum extractor or forceps. Vacuum deliveries have an increased fetal risk for cephalohematoma, subgaleal, and retinal hemorrhages, while forceps have an increased fetal risk for scalp and facial injuries. The two methods should not be used sequentially on the same patient as this creates unacceptable risk [1].

Recommended resource—ACOG Practice Bulletin 154: Operative Vaginal Delivery [2].

Q1: Between 1992 and 2013, the rate of cesarean sections ________ and rate of operative vaginal deliveries ________.

A. Increased; decreased
B. Increased; increased
C. Decreased; decreased
D. Decreased; increased

Q2: Choice to use forceps or vacuum extractor depends on the indication for operative delivery.

A. TRUE
B. FALSE

K.C. Arnold, C.J. Flint, *Obstetrics Essentials*,
DOI 10.1007/978-3-319-57675-6_33,

Q3: Successfully performing an operative vaginal delivery has many potential benefits in comparison to performing a cesarean section such as:

A. Preventing the increased morbidity associated with repeat cesarean sections
B. Decreased cost
C. Reducing or preventing the potential exposure of intrapartum insults to the fetus
D. All the above

Q4: Which of the following is NOT a necessary component of the clinicians' assessment prior to performing an operative vaginal delivery?

A. Estimation of fetal weight
B. Adequacy of maternal effort with pushing
C. Clinical adequacy of maternal pelvis
D. Identification of fetal station and position

Q5: A 34-year-old G1P0 at 36 weeks gestational age presents to your office for a routine OB visit. During this visit, you discuss the potential circumstances and associated risks that accompany an operative vaginal delivery. While comparing the two different instruments available to perform an operative delivery, you inform her that if an operative vaginal delivery is indicated:

A. She would be more likely to achieve a vaginal birth with use of a vacuum extractor
B. She would be more likely to sustain a third or fourth degree laceration with forceps
C. Her infant would be more likely to develop a cephalohematoma with use of a forceps extractor
D. She would be more likely to have anal sphincter dysfunction 5 years after delivery with use of forceps
E. All of the above

Q6: The best technique for use of vacuum extraction includes:

A. Placing the cup 2 cm posterior to anterior fontanelle
B. Centering the cup over the lambdoid suture
C. Placing the cup 2 cm anterior to the posterior fontanelle
D. Centering the cup over the coronal suture

Q7: Episiotomies are no longer routinely performed with operative vaginal deliveries because:

A. Of the association between midline episiotomies and increased risk of injury to the anal sphincter
B. Of poor healing and increased likelihood of dyspareunia with use of mediolateral episiotomies
C. Of the increased risk of perineal infection with either type of episiotomy
D. A and B
E. All of the above

Q8: Which type of incontinence was reported to be more prevalent at 6 weeks postpartum than before delivery in patients who had an operative vaginal delivery without anal sphincter laceration?

A. Urinary incontinence
B. Anal incontinence of flatus and liquids
C. Anal incontinence of solids
D. None of the above

Q9: Which type of incontinence was reported to be more prevalent at 1 year postpartum than before delivery in patients who had an operative vaginal delivery without anal sphincter laceration?

A. Urinary incontinence
B. Anal incontinence of flatus and liquids
C. Anal incontinence of solids
D. None of the above

Q10: Studies have shown that the rates of newborn intracranial hemorrhage are similar between infants delivered by forceps, vacuum, and cesarean section during labor.

A. TRUE
B. FALSE

For the following types of infant injuries, please indicate which type of delivery is more associated with their occurrence in comparison to delivery by cesarean section:

Q11: Facial nerve palsy:

A. Vacuum extractor
B. Forceps
C. A and B

Q12: Brachial nerve palsy:

A. Vacuum extractor
B. Forceps
C. A and B

Q13: A 34-year-old patient presents for her 6-week postpartum visit. She underwent an operative vaginal delivery due to non-reassuring fetal status, and examination of the newborn afterward revealed no obvious defects. Today in your clinic, she asks you about the likelihood of her baby having long-term effects stemming from her mode of delivery. You tell her:

A. Her child may have slightly impaired scholastic performance
B. Her child may have delayed speech
C. The long-term outcomes of operative vaginal delivery are not well understood
D. Her mode of delivery will not have long-term effects on her child

Q14: Which of the following statements regarding operative vaginal delivery and fetal macrosomia are TRUE?

A. Macrosomic infants delivered by operative vaginal delivery had an overall higher injury rate compared to those in a lower birth weight group
B. The risk of persistent injury in infants does not differ between operative vaginal delivery and spontaneous vaginal delivery in birth weights greater than 4000 g
C. Use of operative vaginal delivery in a macrosomic infant is not contradicted
D. A and C
E. All of the above

Q15: In which of the following scenarios would an operative vaginal delivery not be contraindicated?

A. 22-year-old G3P2002 at term with a fetus suspected of having osteogenesis imperfecta
B. 24-year-old G4P3003 with a term gestation has reached complete dilation and is at +1 station. Fetus is noted to be in occiput posterior position with Category III fetal heart tracing
C. 27-year-old G2P1001 with term gestation has reached complete dilation though head is not engaged in the pelvis. Category III fetal heart tracing noted
D. 21-year-old G1P0 at term with known autosomal-dominant bleeding disorder

Q16: Which of the follow factors has been associated with an increased rate of failed operative vaginal delivery?

A. Increased birth weight
B. Primagravda
C. Increased duration of second stage of labor
D. Occiput posterior position
E. A and C

Q17: Operative vaginal delivery should not be attempted if provider feels chances of success are low.
A. TRUE
B. FALSE

Q18: It is reasonable to attempt both forceps and vacuum extraction on the same patient to avoid cesarean delivery.
A. TRUE
B. FALSE

Q19: Operative vaginal delivery with vacuum should be abandoned after three vacuum detachments even if descent is noted with each pull.
A. TRUE
B. FALSE

Q20: There is evidence of increased neonatal morbidity associated with failed operative vaginal delivery followed by cesarean section in comparison to cesarean section or operative delivery alone.
A. TRUE
B. FALSE

Q21: With vacuum extractor use, cephalohematomas are more likely to occur as the duration of vacuum application increases. Given this finding, you:
A. Release vacuum pressure between contractions to improve outcomes
B. Alert pediatricians of vacuum application as soon as decision is made to perform an operative delivery
C. Apply rocking motion and torque with each pull to decrease time to delivery
D. A and B
E. All the above

Q22: Potential indications for operative vaginal delivery include all of the following, EXCEPT:
A. Multigravida who has been pushing for greater than 2 h without delivery of fetus
B. Fetal monitoring reveals repetitive early decelerations with each contraction
C. Primigravida with cardiac condition which prevents her from being able to valsalva safely
D. All of the above are appropriate indications for operative vaginal delivery

Answers

Q1: A, Q2: B, Q3: D, Q4: B, Q5: B, Q6: C, Q7: D, Q8: C, Q9: D, Q10: A, Q11: B, Q12: C, Q13: D, Q14: E, Q15: B, Q16: E, Q17: A, Q18: B, Q19: B, Q20: A, Q21: B, Q22: B.

Resources

1. Gabbe SG, Niebyl JR, Simpson JL, Landon MB, Galan HL, Jauniaux ERM, Driscoll DA. Obstetrics: normal and problem pregnancies. Chapter 15. 6th ed. Philadelphia, PA: Elsevier; 2012.
2. American College of Obstetricians and Gynecologists. Practice bulletin no. 154: operative vaginal delivery. Obstet Gynecol. 2015;126:e56–65.

Chapter 34
Obesity in Pregnancy

Obesity is defined as a BMI of greater than 30 kg/m^2. Its prevalence continues to increase in the United States which is salient for obstetric providers given its association with complications such as hypertensive disorders and increased risk for cesarean delivery. Obesity is described in terms of class I, II, or III [1].

Recommended resources—ACOG Practice Bulletin 156: Obesity in Pregnancy [2].

Questions 1–6 all refer to the same patient:

Q1: A 25-year-old G2P1001 comes to your office for her first prenatal visit. Her BMI is 41. What class of obesity is she?

A. Class I
B. Class II
C. Class III
D. Class IV

Q2: Based on her obesity, she has an increased risk of all of the following, EXCEPT:

A. Spontaneous abortion
B. Fetal gastroschisis
C. Fetal neural tube defects
D. Fetal limb reduction
E. Her risk for all of the above is increased

K.C. Arnold, C.J. Flint, *Obstetrics Essentials*,
DOI 10.1007/978-3-319-57675-6_34,

Q3: Her first delivery was a cesarean section and she asks you about the possibility of a trial of labor after cesarean section. How do you counsel her on her risks compared to a non-obese woman?

A. Her risk of maternal morbidity is increased
B. She has an equal chance of having a successful vaginal delivery
C. Her risk of neonatal injury is increased
D. A and C
E. All of the above

Q4: Which of the following is TRUE regarding her risk of stillbirth?

A. Antepartum surveillance has been shown to improve outcomes
B. The risk for stillbirth increases with each class of obesity
C. Her risk of stillbirth decreases at term; thus she should be induced due to her obesity
D. Obese women are 30% more likely to experience stillbirth than non-obese women
E. All of the above are true

Q5: Which of the following are potential consequences for her baby?

A. Fetal macrosomia
B. Impaired fetal growth
C. Childhood obesity
D. A and C
E. All of the above

Q6: Postpartum she is at increased risk for which of the following?

A. Postpartum depression
B. Mastitis
C. Retained products of conception
D. A and B

Q7: A 35-year-old woman with a BMI of 52 presents to your office for preconceptual counseling. What do you recommend for weight loss?

A. Anorectics
B. Weight loss surgery
C. Behavioral interventions
D. B and C
E. All of the above

Q8: The same patient expresses concern that no matter how much she loses prior to pregnancy, her outcomes will be the same. You counsel her a weight loss of ____% will improve her metabolic health.

A. 3%
B. 5%
C. 10%
D. The percentage is unknown

Q9: She returns to your clinic pregnant and asks which interventions are most useful in avoiding excessive gestational weight gain. Which of the following appears to be most effective?

A. Dietary control
B. Exercise
C. None of the above

Q10: In a randomized controlled trial, interventions were able to reduce the risk of gestational weight gain by 20%. Which outcomes were also improved?

A. Decreased cesarean section rates
B. Decreased risk of preterm delivery
C. Decreased risk of macrosomia in obese women
D. Decreased risk of macrosomia in overweight women
E. All of the above

Q11: Risk for various outcomes should be assessed by calculating the patient's BMI at each trimester.
A. TRUE
B. FALSE

Q12: How many pounds should an overweight patient gain during her pregnancy?
A. 10–20 pounds
B. 15–25 pounds
C. 20–30 pounds
D. 30–40 pounds

Q13: A 19-year-old has just learned she is pregnant. At her new obstetric visit, you counsel her on the increased risk for complications based on her BMI of 37. She asks if she should lose weight. How do you counsel her?
A. Yes, but no more than 5 pounds a trimester
B. No, because it can lead to vitamin deficiencies
C. Yes, but only during the first trimester
D. No, because it increases the risk of a small-for-gestational-age infant

Q14: Detection of fetal anomalies by standard ultrasonography is ___ for women with a normal BMI and ____ for women with class III obesity.
A. 49%; 22%
B. 76%; 45%
C. 76%; 22%
D. 66%; 22%

Q15: Which of the following is TRUE regarding the first trimester screening in obese women?
A. The detection rate for trisomy 18 is decreased by analyte screening
B. It is equally as effective in women who are obese as those who are not

C. The detection of neural tube defects is decreased with analyte screening
D. Nuchal fold measurements are not affected by obesity
E. All the above are true

Q16: Your patient complains of daytime sleepiness and you suspect she may have obstructive sleep apnea. If she does, which of the following does she have an increased risk of?
A. Preeclampsia
B. In hospital mortality
C. Cardiomyopathy
D. A and B
E. All of the above

Q17: Which of the following are indications to screen for gestational diabetes at the first prenatal visit?
A. A BMI of 25 or above
B. A history of gestational diabetes
C. Chronic hypertension
D. A and B
E. All of the above

Q18: Your 25-year-old patient will undergo a primary cesarean section. She weighs 100 kg. What dose of cefazolin should she receive?
A. 1 gram
B. 2 grams
C. 3 grams
D. 4 grams

Q19: In planning for her surgery, you remember:
A. The best incision for primary cesarean sections in obese women is a vertical midline
B. Drains should be left in place if there is 4 cm or more of subcutaneous tissue

C. The subcutaneous tissue should be closed if it is greater than 2 cm
D. A and B
E. A and C

Q20: Which of the following increase the risk for venous thromboembolism?
A. Preeclampsia
B. Fetal growth restriction
C. Infection
D. All of the above

Q21: You elect to start prophylactic low-molecular-weight heparin on your patient. Her BMI is 52. What dose should you use?
A. 40 mg once a day
B. 40 mg twice a day
C. 60 mg once a day
D. 60 mg twice a day
E. 0.5 mg/kg twice a day

Answers

Q1: C, Q2: B, Q3: D, Q4: B, Q5: E, Q6: A, Q7: D, Q8: B, Q9: A, Q10: C, Q11: B, Q12: B, Q13: D, Q14: D, Q15: D, Q16: E, Q17: B, Q18: B, Q19: C, Q20: D, Q21: E.

Resources

1. Gabbe SG, Niebyl JR, Simpson JL, Landon MB, Galan HL, Jauniaux ERM, Driscoll DA. Obstetrics: normal and problem pregnancies. Chapter 7. 6th ed. Philadelphia, PA: Elsevier; 2012.
2. American College of Obstetricians and Gynecologists. Practice bulletin no. 156: obesity in pregnancy. Obstet Gynecol. 2015;126:e112–26.

Chapter 35
External Cephalic Version

In patient with a breech fetus at term, counseling for external cephalic version should be performed if appropriate. Success of external cephalic version is reported to be between 60% and 75%. The use of both regional anesthesia and tocolysis increases success rates [1].

Recommended resource—ACOG Practice Bulletin 161: External Cephalic Version [2].

Q1: What percentage of term fetuses are breech?
A. 1–2%
B. 3–4%
C. 5–6%
D. 7–8%

Q2: Patients are ideal candidates for external cephalic version (ECV) starting at:
A. 35/0 weeks
B. 36/0 weeks
C. 37/0 weeks
D. 38/0 weeks
E. 39/0 weeks

K.C. Arnold, C.J. Flint, *Obstetrics Essentials*,
DOI 10.1007/978-3-319-57675-6_35,

Q3: Ideal timing for ECV is based on all of the following, EXCEPT:

A. The fetus is unlikely to spontaneously turn to vertex after this gestation
B. After a successful version, the fetus is unlikely to spontaneously turn to breech at this gestation
C. If complications necessitate delivery, there is low fetal morbidity at given gestation
D. All of the above are true

Q4: A 26-year-old G3P2002 at 36/0 weeks gestation presents to your office for routine prenatal care. On ultrasound her fetus is breech. She has had one previous term cesarean section and one successful VBAC and strongly desires a vaginal delivery. How should you counsel her?

A. ECV is known to be higher risk in patients with previous cesarean section
B. ECV is thought to be safe only if attempted prior to the start of labor
C. Small studies show no increased rate in adverse events in ECV in patients with previous cesarean section
D. ECV success rates are lower in patients with prior cesarean section

Q5: Attempted ECV is associated with:

A. Lower risk of cesarean section
B. Low Apgar score
C. Low umbilical cord blood pH
D. B and C
E. All of the above

Q6: All of the following occur at rates of less than 1% of ECVs, EXCEPT:

A. Fetal heart rate decelerations
B. Abruption
C. Rupture of membranes
D. Umbilical cord prolapse
E. All of the above occurred in less than 1% of cases

Q7: Which of the following is most consistently associated with increased rate of success for ECV?
A. Nulliparous patient
B. Low fetal station
C. Normal amniotic fluid index
D. Parous patient

Q8: The use of terbutaline was shown in a randomized controlled trial to ____ of ECV. ACOG states that the evidence _______ the use of tocolytics in ECV.
A. Increase the success; is inconclusive regarding
B. Increase the success; is in support of
C. Have no effect on the success; is inconclusive regarding
D. Have no effect on the success; does not support

Q9: Regarding regional anesthesia during ECV attempts, which is true?
A. Data supports its utility in increasing success
B. Data are inconclusive
C. Data does not support its use

Q10: Choose the correct sequence for performing an ECV:
A. Informed consent; elevate breech fetal part; attempt forward roll; NST
B. NST; informed consent; attempt forward roll; elevate breech fetal part; NST
C. NST; informed consent; elevate breech fetal part; attempt forward roll
D. NST; informed consent; elevate breech fetal part; attempt forward roll; NST

Q11: You attempt an ECV on your patient, which, however, is unsuccessful. Which of the following are acceptable options?
A. Schedule a cesarean section at 39 weeks gestation with plans to confirm breech prior to the surgery
B. Schedule a retrial of ECV prior to delivery planning

C. Monitor through 41 weeks gestation for spontaneous version with plans to deliver by a cesarean section if still breech
D. A and C
E. All of the above

Q12: Which of the following patients would NOT be a candidate for an ECV?
A. 29-year-old G2P1001 at 37/3 weeks gestation with a previous classical cesarean section
B. 37-year-old G1P0 with a BMI of 40 at 38 weeks gestation
C. 23-year-old G2P1001 at 40/3 weeks gestation presenting with contractions and I kept found to be 3 cm dilated
D. A and C
E. None of the above would be candidates

Q13: Which is true regarding monitoring fetal heart tones during an attempted ECV?
A. It is only indicated if the attempt lasts more than 5 min
B. Ultrasound monitoring of fetal heart tones intermittently is recommended
C. Continually monitoring fetal heart tones using a Doppler is recommended
D. There is no recommendation to guide fetal monitoring during the procedure

Q14: Which of the following Rh-negative patients should receive anti-D immune globulin immediately after the ECV attempt?
A. A woman who undergoes a failed ECV at 39 weeks gestation and will undergo a primary cesarean section tomorrow
B. A woman who undergoes a successful ECV at 37 weeks gestation and will return at 39 weeks gestation for induction

C. A woman who undergoes a failed ECV at 38 weeks gestation and will return at 39 weeks gestation for her cesarean section
D. B and C
E. All of the above

Answers

Q1: B, Q2: C, Q3: D, Q4: C, Q5: A, Q6: A, Q7: D, Q8: B, Q9: B, Q10: D, Q11: E, Q12: A, Q13: B, Q14: D.

Resources

1. Gabbe SG, Niebyl JR, Simpson JL, Landon MB, Galan HL, Jauniaux ERM, Driscoll DA. Obstetrics: normal and problem pregnancies. Chapter 18. 6th ed. Philadelphia, PA: Elsevier; 2012.
2. American College of Obstetricians and Gynecologists. Practice bulletin no. 161: external cephalic version. Obstet Gynecol. 2016;127:e54–61.

Chapter 36
Prenatal Diagnostic Testing for Genetic Disorders

Antenatal diagnosis of genetic disorders requires the acquisition of fetal or placental tissue. Invasive procedures are indicated if a fetus is at increased risk for a genetic condition. Risk factors include advanced maternal age, known parental genetic conditions, abnormal aneuploidy screening, soft markers for aneuploidy on ultrasound, and fetal growth restriction [1].

Recommended resource—ACOG Practice Bulletin 162: Prenatal Diagnostic Testing for Genetic Disorders [2].

Q1: How frequently does a live birth involve some type of chromosomal abnormality that results in an abnormal fetal or neonatal phenotype?

A. 1 in 50 live births
B. 1 in 100 live births
C. 1 in 150 live births
D. 1 in 200 live births

Q2: Which of the following statements regarding chromosomes is FALSE?

A. Chromosome irregularities are more common early in pregnancy
B. The most common abnormality of chromosome number is aneuploidy

K.C. Arnold, C.J. Flint, *Obstetrics Essentials*,
DOI 10.1007/978-3-319-57675-6_36,

C. Balanced translocations are often associated with a normal phenotype
D. Epigenetics means an abnormal number of chromosomes are not present in all cell lines

Q3: Isolated structural birth defects are more common than chromosomal abnormalities.
A. TRUE
B. FALSE

Q4: Which of the following is TRUE regarding isolated structural birth defects?
A. Occur less within an affected family than in the general population
B. Diagnosis is rarely made by ultrasound or other imaging techniques
C. Usually determined by multiple genes in combination with environmental factors
D. Diagnosed using specific DNA methods

Q5: The primary function of mitochondria is in anaerobic metabolism.
A. TRUE
B. FALSE

Q6: During which phase of mitosis is karyotype analysis performed?
A. Interphase
B. Metaphase
C. Anaphase
D. Telophase

Q7: Karyotype analysis is an adequate method to detect:
A. Genetic abnormalities obtained from stillbirth specimens
B. Small gene rearrangements
C. Mosaicism
D. Aneuploidies
E. All of the above

Q8: Which of the following should be considered a screening test?

A. FISH analysis
B. Microarray analysis
C. Karyotype analysis
D. None of the above

Q9: Why can results from FISH analysis be obtained within 2 days compared to the 7–14 days needed to complete karyotype analysis?

A. FISH analysis is cheaper and more accessible
B. FISH can be performed on uncultured cells
C. FISH analysis uses probes for specific chromosomes and chromosomal regions
D. None of the above

Q10: What two abnormalities can be detected by karyotype analysis but not chromosomal microarray analysis?

A. Unbalanced translocations and monosomy
B. Balanced translocations and monosomy
C. Unbalanced translations and triploidies
D. Balanced translocations and triploidies

Q11: What is the preferred method to analyze cells from cases of fetal death or stillbirth?

A. FISH
B. Karyotype analysis
C. Chromosomal microarray analysis
D. No single method is preferred

Q12: Which of the following statements is FALSE regarding chromosomal microarray analysis?

A. Should not be the primary diagnostic test offered for a fetal structural anomaly detected by ultrasound
B. Low-level mosaicism may not be identified
C. Best suited to detect copy number variants in the fetus
D. Results can be obtained within 3–7 days

Q13: Which of the following statements is FALSE about preimplantation genetic diagnosis?
A. Refers to the testing of an embryo for a specific genetic disorder prior to implantation
B. Can be performed on polar bodies from the oocyte and zygote
C. Can be performed using molecular or cytogenetic techniques
D. It is not recommended that results be confirmed with CVS or amniocentesis

For the following statements (Q14–Q20), choose which one BEST applies:

Q14: Should be performed between 10 and 13 weeks gestational age.
A. CVS
B. Amniocentesis
C. Neither

Q15: Obtains sample of the placental villi without entering the amniotic sac.
A. CVS
B. Amniocentesis
C. Neither

Q16: When performed at the appropriate gestational age, has a higher risk of limb reduction defects:
A. CVS
B. Amniocentesis
C. Neither

Q17: Associated with a 2% procedure-related pregnancy loss rate.
A. CVS
B. Amniocentesis
C. Neither

Q18: Viable cells obtained by this process require shorter processing time of 5–7 days compared to 7–14 days.
A. CVS
B. Amniocentesis
C. Neither

Q19: Most frequently performed between 15 and 20 weeks gestational age.
A. CVS
B. Amniocentesis
C. Neither

Q20: The perinatal outcomes following spontaneous preterm rupture of membranes are equivalent to the outcomes for membrane rupture after amniocentesis at a similar gestational age.
A. TRUE
B. FALSE

Q21: Early amniocentesis is associated with all of the following, EXCEPT:
A. Increased risk of membrane rupture
B. Increased incidence of club foot
C. Increased risk of culture failure
D. All of the above are true

Q22: A 37-year-old woman presents to your office for her new OB visit. When discussing her specific risk of genetic disorders, it would be most accurate to explain to her:
A. If she has a prior history of having a child with an autosomal trisomy, her risk of recurrence is not increased above her risk based on age
B. Risk of aneuploidy increases with maternal age; however this correlation is not seen with structural chromosomal abnormalities

C. Paternal age is inconsequential in the discussion of risk of genetic disorders
D. That discussing her screening options for genetic disorders should be deferred until the next visit

Q23: A 24-year-old women presents for her Level I ultrasound at which time her fetus is noted to have a major structural abnormality that is not strongly suggestive of a particular aneuploidy. What is the BEST next step?
A. CVS with karyotype analysis with or without FISH should be offered
B. Amniocentesis with karyotype analysis with or without FISH should be offered
C. CVS with chromosomal microarray should be offered
D. Amniocentesis with chromosomal microarray should be offered

Q24: A 32-year-old woman has a QUAD screen which results with an increased risk of trisomy 13. When you call her to discuss the results, what testing in particular should be offered?
A. CVS with karyotype analysis with or without FISH
B. Amniocentesis with karyotype analysis with or without FISH
C. CVS with chromosomal microarray
D. Amniocentesis with chromosomal microarray

Q25: Which of the following statements is FALSE in regard to counseling patients about prenatal diagnostic testing for genetic disorders who have blood-borne infections?
A. Women who are positive for hepatitis B e antigen have a lower risk of vertical transmission with amniocentesis

B. Risk of vertical transmission of hepatitis B with amniocentesis is related to viral load
C. Risk of vertical transmission of HIV with amniocentesis is related to viral load
D. Risk of vertical transmission is higher in patients with multiple infections, i.e., HIV and hepatitis C

Answers

Q1: C, Q2: D, Q3: A, Q4: C, Q5: B, Q6: B, Q7: D, Q8: A, Q9: B, Q10: D, Q11: C, Q12: A, Q13: D, Q14: A, Q15: A, Q16: C, Q17: C, Q18: A, Q19: B, Q20: B, Q21: D, Q22: B, Q23: D, Q24: B, Q25: A.

Resources

1. Gabbe SG, Niebyl JR, Simpson JL, Landon MB, Galan HL, Jauniaux ERM, Driscoll DA. Obstetrics: normal and problem pregnancies. Chapter 11. 6th ed. Philadelphia, PA: Elsevier; 2012.
2. American College of Obstetricians and Gynecologists. Practice bulletin no. 162: prenatal diagnostic testing for genetic disorders. Obstet Gynecol. 2016;127(5):e108–22.

Chapter 37
Screening for Fetal Aneuploidy

The goal of screening is to identify fetuses at increased risk of having a genetic disorder. Screening for aneuploidy can be accomplished using different modalities at specific gestational ages. Examples include first trimester screen, second trimester screen, integrated screen, and sequential screen. Screening should be offered to all women as part of comprehensive prenatal care [1].

Recommended resource—ACOG Practice Bulletin 163: Screening for Fetal Aneuploidy [2].

Q1: Which of the following statement is FALSE regarding Down syndrome?

A. The severity of the syndrome can be predicted prenatally
B. It is the most common autosomal aneuploidy
C. It occurs at a rate of 1/800 live births
D. It is usually due to nondisjunction
E. Detection rates are roughly equivalent between first trimester screen and quad screen

K.C. Arnold, C.J. Flint, *Obstetrics Essentials*,
DOI 10.1007/978-3-319-57675-6_37,

Q2: Which of the following women should be offered screening for aneuploidy at the first prenatal visit?

A. A 36-year-old G1P0 at 6 weeks gestational age by LMP
B. A 36-year-old G3P2002 at 16 weeks gestational age with history of a baby with Down syndrome
C. A 25-year-old G1P0 at 19 weeks gestational age who has a normal Level 1 ultrasound
D. A and B
E. All of the above

Q3: The triple screen has been largely replaced by the quad screen because of its lower sensitivity for which of the following?

A. Open fetal defects
B. Down syndrome
C. Trisomy 13
D. Neural tube defects
E. None of the above

A patient is trying to decide between the first trimester screen and the quad screen. Choose the best test for the patient in the following scenarios:

A. FTS
B. Quad screen

Q4: A 27-year-old G1P0 with pregnancy at 11 weeks gestational age

Q5: A 38-year-old at her new OB appointment whose doctor does not have a professional ultrasonographer on staff

Q6: A 37-year-old who is especially concerned about her risk of neural tube defects

Q7: A 32-year-old who would consider termination if her fetus is diagnosed with an aneuploidy

Q8: Which of the following are components of a first trimester screen?
A. PAPP-A
B. Inhibin A
C. B-hCG
D. A and C
E. B and C

Q9: In which of the following is it possible for a patient be told she has low risk for aneuploidy without completion of a quad screen?
A. Integrated
B. Contingent
C. Sequential
D. A and B
E. A and C

Q10: Which of the following tests provide no information regarding risk stratification until the second trimester?
A. Integrated
B. Contingent
C. Sequential
D. A and B
E. A and C

Q11: A 19-year-old G1P0 has completed a normal first trimester screen. She now presents to her 16-week appointment with concerns regarding neural tube defects because she has a friend who had a baby with spina bifida. What test would you offer her?
A. AFP
B. Quad screen
C. Sequential screen
D. Detailed anatomy scan
E. None of the above

Q12: A 39-year-old G6P1311 presents to your clinic for a new OB visit at 8 weeks gestation. She reports that during her last pregnancy, she had a positive FTS and then had a cell-free fetal DNA test that showed a fetus with Down syndrome. She did not pursue diagnostic testing and the baby was born with 46XX chromosomes. She conveys how much stress the false-positive cell-free fetal DNA testing caused her and requests counseling regarding what tests she should undergo for this pregnancy. As her provider your next best step is to:

A. Counsel her regarding her options for screening for aneuploidy and order said tests
B. Refer her to a genetic counselor
C. Refer to a genetic counselor prior to ordering any testing
D. None of the above

Q13: Which of the following syndromes is most commonly missed by ultrasound screening alone?

A. Patau syndrome
B. Edwards syndrome
C. Down syndrome

Q14: Which of the following is associated with the lowest risk of aneuploidy?

A. Thickened nuchal fold
B. Echogenic bowel
C. Renal pelvis dilation
D. Echogenic intracardiac focus
E. They are all equally associated with aneuploidy

Q15: For which of the following isolated findings are follow-up ultrasounds recommended?

A. Echogenic bowel
B. Renal pelvis dilation
C. Echogenic intracardiac focus
D. A and B
E. A and C

Q16: Which of the following statements is FALSE regarding cell-free fetal DNA?
A. Cells are derived from fetal skin
B. It can be tested from 10 weeks gestation to term
C. It can identify Rh-negative babies in Rh-positive moms
D. It has the highest detection rate for Down syndrome

Q17: A 37-year-old G3P2002 comes to your office for a return OB visit. You had previously counseled her on screening for aneuploidy and she elected for cell-free fetal DNA. The result is "no reportable result." How do you counsel her?
A. Given no result, repeat free-cell DNA or diagnostic testing is recommended
B. From baseline, her risk for aneuploidy is decreased
C. From baseline, her risk for aneuploidy is increased
D. A and B
E. A and C

Q18: Which of the following places the screening tests in correct order from lowest rate of detection for Down syndrome to highest rate of detection?
A. Ultrasound, cell-free fetal DNA, serum screening
B. Cell-free fetal DNA, ultrasound, serum screening
C. Serum screening, cell-free fetal DNA, ultrasound
D. Ultrasound, serum screening, cell-free fetal DNA

Q19: Your 23-year-old patient was previously very nervous as her nuchal translucency measurement was 4 mm. She then underwent an amniocentesis revealing a normal XY fetus. In regard to her current risk for abnormalities, you counsel her that:
A. Her fetus has a decreased risk for genetic syndromes
B. Her risk for adverse outcome is comparable to having a nuchal translucency of 6 mm
C. A fetal ECHO should be performed
D. None of the above

Q20: Your patient comes to her return OB appointment and is very concerned following the finding of a cystic hygroma on her first trimester ultrasound. How do you counsel her?

A. Her risk for aneuploidy is approximately 50%
B. Her risk for structural malformation in the absence of aneuploidy is 50%
C. Her chance for a healthy live-born term infant is approximately 50%
D. A and B
E. A and C

Q21: Which of the following is NOT associated with an increased risk for aneuploidy?

A. Choroid plexus cyst
B. Shortened femur length
C. Pyelectasis
D. Echogenic bowel
E. Ventriculomegaly

Q22: Regarding cell-free fetal DNA testing, which of the following statements is FALSE?

A. It can detect Down syndrome at a rate of 93%
B. It is more effective at detecting trisomy 18 than trisomy 13
C. It has not been proven to detect microdeletions
D. All of the above are true

Q23: Two pregnant patients, a 23-year-old and a 47-year-old, present to their NOB visit requesting cell-free DNA because they both desire to know the sex of their fetus as early as possible. Both have unremarkable past OB histories. Both have cell-free fetal DNA results that are positive for T18. Which of the following is TRUE?

A. The 23-year-old is more likely to have a T18 fetus
B. The 47-year-old is more likely to have a T18 fetus
C. They are equally both likely to have a T18 fetus

Q24: A 32-year-old patient has a positive first trimester screen. Which of the following are acceptable options for follow-up assessment?

A. Cell-free fetal DNA
B. CVS
C. Amniocentesis
D. Any of the above

Q25: Which of the following are NOT associated with IUGR, preeclampsia, and fetal death in the absence of structural abnormalities?

A. Elevated AFP
B. Elevated inhibin A
C. Elevated unconjugated estriol
D. Elevated b-hCG

Q26: Which of the following has an increased risk for aneuploidy above that of the mother's age-adjusted risk?

A. A dizygotic twin
B. A monozygotic twin
C. Both
D. Neither

Q27: Nuchal translucency is:

A. If discordant in monochorionic gestations, may be a marker for twin-twin transfusion syndrome
B. A reliable way to evaluate twins and higher order multifetal gestations independently
C. Useful if cutoffs are adjusted for twins and higher order gestations
D. A and B
E. All of the above

Answers

Q1: A, Q2: E, Q3: B, Q4: A, Q5: B, Q6: B, Q7: A, Q8: D, Q9: B, Q10: A, Q11: A, Q12: A, Q13: C, Q14: D, Q15: D, Q16: A, Q17: E, Q18: D, Q19: C, Q20: D, Q21: A, Q22: B, Q23: B, Q24: D, Q25: C, Q26: D, Q27: D.

Resources

1. Gabbe SG, Niebyl JR, Simpson JL, Landon MB, Galan HL, Jauniaux ERM, Driscoll DA. Obstetrics: normal and problem pregnancies. Chapter 10. 6th ed. Philadelphia, PA: Elsevier; 2012.
2. American College of Obstetricians and Gynecologists. Practice bulletin no. 163: screening for fetal aneuploidy. Obstet Gynecol. 2016;127(5):e123–37.

Chapter 38
Prevention and Management of Obstetric Lacerations at Vaginal Delivery

After all vaginal deliveries, a thorough exam should be performed to evaluate for lacerations. In classifying lacerations, it is important to note if the perineal body, external anal sphincter, or rectal mucosa are involved. Episiotomy may be useful in specific situations; however, routine use is not indicated [1].

Recommended resource—ACOG Practice Bulletin 165: Prevention and Management of Obstetric Lacerations at Vaginal Delivery [2].

Q1: Which of the following is NOT part of the perineal body?
- A. Deep muscle of the perineal membrane
- B. Transverse perineal muscle
- C. Bulbocavernosus muscle
- D. External anal sphincter
- E. The perineal body includes all of the above

Q2: The internal anal sphincter is under autonomic control and provides 80% of the resting pressure of the anal canal.
- A. True
- B. False

K.C. Arnold, C.J. Flint, *Obstetrics Essentials*,
DOI 10.1007/978-3-319-57675-6_38,

Q3: Which of the following is a characteristic of a medio-lateral episiotomy?

A. It starts within 10 mm of midline
B. It is angled at least 30 degrees
C. It is aimed toward the ischial tuberosity
D. It is more common in the United States
E. It is associated with increased rates of pelvic organ prolapse

Q4: Episiotomy is associated with:

A. Increased risk of anal incontinence if there is extension into the anal sphincter complex
B. Increased risk of anal incontinence regardless of extension
C. No increased risk of anal incontinence
D. Decreased risk of anal incontinence
E. Increased risk or stress urinary incontinence

Q5: Which of the following would give the highest risk for an obstetric anal sphincter injury?

A. Midline episiotomy combined with forceps
B. Vacuum-assisted delivery
C. Increased fetal birth weight
D. Persistent occiput posterior position
E. Duration of the second stage of labor

Q6: Which of the following is associated with increased risk for an obstetric anal sphincter injury?

A. Maternal age
B. Maternal BMI
C. Duration of the second stage of labor
D. Epidural anesthesia
E. Occiput transverse

Q7: Third- and fourth-degree lacerations are quality care measures

A. True
B. False

Q8: Perineal massage has been shown to:

A. Decrease perineal trauma that required suture repair when done at 34 weeks gestation and further
B. Decrease third- and fourth-degree lacerations when done during the second stage of labor
C. Increase the rate of women with intact perineum after delivery
D. A and B
E. All of the above

Q9: Delayed pushing has been shown to:

A. Decrease third- and fourth-degree lacerations
B. Decrease operative deliveries
C. Decrease the risk of lacerations requiring repair
D. Decrease rates of episiotomy
E. None of the above

Q10: Episiotomy is indicated in which of the following situations?

A. Routine use is advocated
B. Shoulder dystocia
C. Vacuum-assisted vaginal delivery
D. Restricted use is recommended
E. B and C

Q11: Mediolateral episiotomy is associated with a ____ in third- and fourth-degree lacerations and an _____ likelihood of perineal pain.

A. Increase, increased
B. Decrease, increased
C. Increase, decreased
D. Decrease, decreased

Q12: The intern calls/requests assistance in evaluation of a laceration following delivery. On exam, a hemostatic laceration on the labia that distorts the anatomy and a hemostatic first-degree laceration are noted. How should you proceed?

A. Repair the labial laceration to make it heal faster, and repair the first degree as sexual activity will be able to be resumed sooner
B. Do not repair either; there has been no evidence to support repair of lacerations that are hemostatic
C. Repair the labial laceration to restore anatomy, and repair the first degree as recommended by ACOG
D. Repair the labial laceration to restore anatomy, and defer repair on the first degree as it is hemostatic

Q13: How is an occult OASIS defined?
A. Laceration of the anal sphincter that is only palpated on a rectal exam, but is unable to be visualized
B. A laceration that is visualized without needing to perform a rectal exam
C. A laceration that involves the perineal skin and the rectal mucosa, but spares much of the perineal body
D. A laceration that has no clinical findings, but is identified on endoanal ultrasonography
E. None of the above

Q14: Endoanal ultrasonography has a high:
A. False-positive rate
B. False-negative rate
C. Positive predictive value
D. Negative predictive value

Q15: Following a vaginal delivery, a hemostatic first-degree laceration is noted. Which of the following are reasonable options?
A. Adhesive glue
B. Standard suture
C. No repair
D. A and B
E. All of the above

Q16: Which of the following are important considerations in choosing a suture to repair a second degree?

A. Absorbable synthetic suture may require a postpartum visit for suture removal
B. Closure of the perineal skin with adhesive glue results in decreased repair time, but increased pain
C. Interrupted sutures are recommended as they achieve improved hemostasis
D. Choice of suture can impact dyspareunia at 3 months to a year
E. None of the above

Q17: Which of the following describes the correct repair of a cervical laceration?

A. A 3-0 polyglactin suture should be placed above the apex of the laceration. Running suture should then be continued incorporating half the thickness of the cervix
B. A 2-0 polyglactin suture should be placed above the apex of the laceration. Running locking suture should then be continued incorporating full thickness of the cervix
C. A 3-0 polyglactin suture should be placed at the apex of the laceration. Running suture should then be continued incorporating half the thickness of the cervix
D. A 2-0 polyglactin suture should be placed at the apex of the laceration. Running suture should then be continued incorporating half the thickness of the cervix
E. None of the above

Q18: All of the following are important considerations in repairing the external anal sphincter EXCEPT:

A. Care should be taken to suture just the muscle, not the fascial sheath
B. End-to-end repair is most appropriate for 3a and 3b sphincter injuries

C. Allis clamps may be necessary to grasp the edges of the sphincter
D. 2-0 or 3-0 suture is recommended
E. For full thickness external anal sphincter lacerations, either end-to-end or overlap repair is reasonable

Q19: The recommendation that a single dose of antibiotics should be given for repair of an OASIS is based on what evidence?
A. Cohort investigation
B. Randomized controlled trial
C. Retrospective case series
E. Expert opinion

Q20: Following repair of an OASIS, a patient should be counseled regarding the ______ risk of wound infection.
A. 3%
B. 5%
C. 10%
D. 15%
E. 20%

Q21: Obstetric lacerations are the most common cause of rectovaginal fistulas in the United States.
A. True
B. False

Q22: Which of the following may decrease patient pain following OASIS repair?
A. Topical anesthetics
B. Local cooling treatments
C. Rectal suppositories
D. A and B
E. All of the above

Q23: A patient presents to clinic to establish prenatal care. She reports a history of a fourth-degree laceration with her previous delivery and requests a cesarean delivery with this pregnancy. What aspect of her history would justify this?

A. Reported anal incontinence
B. Reported need for repeat laceration repair
C. Reported psychological trauma from event
D. A and B
E. Any of the above could be indications for a cesarean delivery

Answers

Q1: D, Q2: A, Q3: C, Q4: B, Q5: A, Q6: D, Q7: B, Q8: D, Q9: E, Q10: D, Q11: B, Q12: D, Q13: D, Q14: A, Q15: E, Q16: A, Q17: B, Q18: A, Q19: A, Q20: E, Q21: B, Q22: E, Q23: E.

Resources

1. Gabbe SG, Niebyl JR, Simpson JL, Landon MB, Galan HL, Jauniaux ERM, Driscoll DA. Obstetrics: normal and problem pregnancies. 6th ed. Philadelphia: Elsevier; 2012.
2. American College of Obstetricians and Gynecologists. Practice bulletin no. 165: prevention and management of obstetric lacerations at vaginal delivery. Obstet Gynecol. 2016;128:e1–15.

Chapter 39
Thrombocytopenia in Pregnancy

Thrombocytopenia in pregnancy is a common complication. Common causes include gestational thrombocytopenia, severe preeclampsia, HELLP syndrome, and disseminated intravascular coagulation. Rare causes include TTP, HUS, rheumatologic conditions, and HIV. Treatment varies by cause; however, it can include steroids, IVIG, platelet transfusions, plasma exchange, and delivery [1].

Recommended resource—ACOG Practice Bulletin 166: Thrombocytopenia in Pregnancy [2].

Q1: Thrombocytopenia affects approximately what percentage of pregnancies?
- A. 1–5%
- B. 6–15%
- C. 16–25%
- D. 26–35%

Q2: Which of the following is NOT a common manifestation of thrombocytopenia?
- A. Bleeding into mucous membranes
- B. Ecchymosis
- C. Bleeding into joints
- D. Menometrorrhagia

K.C. Arnold, C.J. Flint, *Obstetrics Essentials*,
DOI 10.1007/978-3-319-57675-6_39,

Q3: Which of the following is FALSE regarding thrombocytopenia and platelet counts?

A. The normal range of platelet count in nonpregnant individuals is approximately 150–400/μL
B. Excessive bleeding associated with trauma or surgery is uncommon unless the patient's platelet count is less than 50,000/μL
C. Thrombocytopenia is often caused by increased platelet destruction during pregnancy
D. The mean platelet count in pregnant women is higher than in nonpregnant individuals

Q4: Clinically significant spontaneous bleeding is usually limited to patients with platelet counts less than ______.

A. 50,000/μL
B. 30,000/μL
C. 20,000/μL
D. 10,000/μL
E. Is often not predicted by platelet counts due to variable function

Q5: What is the most common cause of thrombocytopenia during pregnancy?

A. Immune thrombocytopenia purpura (ITP)
B. Gestational thrombocytopenia
C. Pregnancy-induced hypertension (PIH)
D. Pseudothrombocytopenia

Q6: Which of the following would make a diagnosis of gestational thrombocytopenia less likely?

A. A platelet count of 60,000/μL
B. Thrombocytopenia incidentally detected during routine prenatal testing
C. No history of thrombocytopenia prior to pregnancy
D. Platelet count normalizes in the postpartum period
E. All of the above are consistent with gestational thrombocytopenia

Q7: A 33-year-old G2P1001 with intrauterine pregnancy at 38 weeks gestational age presents to labor and delivery in active labor. Review of her antenatal records reveals a diagnosis of gestational thrombocytopenia which was made at 35 weeks. The patient's platelet count is 80,000/μL prior to delivery. The risk of bleeding complications in this fetus compared to a fetus delivered by a patient without gestational thrombocytopenia is:

A. 50% greater
B. 20% greater
C. The same
D. 20% less

Q8: Which of the following is TRUE regarding preeclampsia and thrombocytopenia?

A. Thrombocytopenia may be the first clinical sign of preeclampsia
B. In the setting of new-onset hypertension, it can be a diagnostic indicator of preeclampsia if platelet count is less than 120,000/μL
C. Clinical hemorrhage is common
D. A and B
E. All of the above

Q9: Fetal-neonatal alloimmune thrombocytopenia affects women and fetuses.

A. TRUE
B. FALSE

Q10: A 33-year-old G2P1001 at 31 weeks gestational age presents for routine obstetrical visit. Her pregnancy has been complicated by maternal immune thrombocytopenia purpura (ITP). Her most recent platelet count was 90,000/μL. She asks you how her diagnosis will affect her fetus. You counsel her:

A. Maternal antibodies do not cross the placenta, protecting her fetus from the risk of thrombocytopenia

B. There is no relationship between maternal platelet count at time of delivery and infant platelet count at birth
C. Up to one half of infants born to mothers with ITP will develop platelet counts less than 150,000/μL
D. The risk of severe hemorrhagic complications in newborns is high in neonates born to mothers with ITP
E. None of the above

Q11: Chronic immune thrombocytopenia is classified by a duration of symptoms:
A. Greater than 6 months
B. Greater than 8 months
C. Greater than 10 months
D. Greater than 12 months
E. Greater than three episodes requiring hospitalization

Q12: All the following are examples of secondary causes of immune thrombocytopenia EXCEPT:
A. Systemic lupus erythematosus
B. Disseminated intravascular coagulation
C. Infection with human immunodeficiency virus
D. Drug-induced thrombocytopenia
E. Preeclampsia

Q13: Fetal-neonatal alloimmune thrombocytopenia shares many similarities with hemolytic (Rh) disease of the newborn. What is a key difference between the two disorders?
A. One is mediated by maternal alloimmunization, while the other is mediated by paternal alloimmunization
B. One involves placental transfer of antibodies, while the other involves placental transfer of antigens

C. One can affect the first pregnancy, while the other typically affects subsequent pregnancies
D. All of the above
E. None of the above

Q14: Which of the following is FALSE in regard to fetal intracranial hemorrhage due to fetal-neonatal alloimmune thrombocytopenia?
A. Can occur in utero
B. Is the most serious complication of the disorder
C. Can occur in up to 50% of infants with platelet counts less than 50,000/μL
D. None of the above

Q15: Gestational thrombocytopenia and immune thrombocytopenia purpura (ITP) can be differentiated by antiplatelet antibody testing.
A. TRUE
B. FALSE

Q16: In a patient diagnosed with gestational thrombocytopenia, how often should a provider check the platelet count antepartum?
A. Weekly starting at 34 weeks gestational age
B. Every other week starting at 34 weeks gestational age
C. Weekly starting at 37 weeks gestational age
D. Once at term

Q17: In general, it is recommended that a platelet transfusion be employed in patients undergoing cesarean delivery to increase the count above ____________ prior to surgery.
A. 10,000/μL
B. 30,000/μL
C. 50,000/μL
D. 70,000/μL

Q18: What treatment modality is an option for the management of patients with ITP if first-line treatment fails?

A. Platelet transfusion
B. Intravenous steroids
C. Intravenous immunoglobulins
D. Splenectomy

Q19: Delivery via cesarean section is safer for the fetus in patients with maternal ITP.

A. TRUE
B. FALSE

Q20: What defines a "high-risk" pregnancy for intracranial hemorrhage?

A. Fetal platelet count less than 30,000/μL at 30 weeks of gestation
B. History of a sibling with a perinatal intracranial hemorrhage
C. Fetal platelet count less than 20,000/μL at 20 weeks of gestation
D. B and C
E. All of the above

Q21: How should a pregnancy at "high risk" for fetal intracranial hemorrhage be managed?

A. Combination of maternal intravenous immunoglobulin and intravenous prednisone should be given
B. Direct fetal administration of intravenous immunoglobulin
C. Cesarean section should be performed if fetal platelet count is less than 50,000/μL at time of delivery
D. A and C
E. All of the above

Q22: If platelet count is stable, it is reasonable to provide epidural or spinal anesthesia if maternal platelet count is equal to or above ________

A. 60,000/μL
B. 70,000/μL
C. 80,000/μL
D. 90,000/μL
E. 100,000/μL

Q23: Thrombocytopenia in pregnancy is defined as:

A. 100,000/μL
B. 120,000/μL
C. 130,000/μL
D. 140,000/μL
E. 150,000/μL

Answers

Q1: B, Q2: C, Q3: D, Q4: D, Q5: B, Q6: A, Q7: C, Q8: A, Q9: B, Q10: B, Q11: D, Q12: B, Q13: C, Q14: C, Q15: B, Q16: A, Q17: C, Q18: D, Q19: B, Q20: D, Q21: D, Q22: C, Q23: E.

Resources

1. Gabbe SG, Niebyl JR, Simpson JL, Landon MB, Galan HL, Jauniaux ERM, Driscoll DA. Obstetrics: normal and problem pregnancies, Chapter 42. 6th ed. Philadelphia: Elsevier; 2012.
2. American College of Obstetricians and Gynecologists. Practice bulletin no. 166: thrombocytopenia in pregnancy. Obstet Gynecol. 2016;128:e43–53.

Chapter 40
Twin, Triplet, and Higher-Order Multifetal Pregnancies

Multifetal gestations have increased significantly in the past 30 years, mostly due to the increase in fertility treatments. Diagnosis can be made as early as 5 weeks gestation. Determination of both chorionicity and zygosity is most accurate early in pregnancy. Maternal and fetal complications are elevated in multifetal gestations, and such patients should receive specialized prenatal care [1].

Recommended resource—ACOG Practice Bulletin 169: Twin, Triplet, and Higher-Order Multifetal Pregnancies [2].

Q1: What is the most common complication encountered in multifetal gestations?
- A. Neonatal death
- B. Stillbirth
- C. Preeclampsia
- D. Spontaneous preterm birth

Q2: Multifetal gestations are associated with all the following, EXCEPT:
- A. Increased prevalence of cerebral palsy
- B. Higher costs
- C. Increase in short-term morbidity neonatal morbidity
- D. Increase in long-term infant morbidity
- E. All of the above are true

K.C. Arnold, C.J. Flint, *Obstetrics Essentials*,
DOI 10.1007/978-3-319-57675-6_40,

Q3: Excluding ART use, the likelihood of a multifetal gestation increases with maternal age.
A. TRUE
B. FALSE

Q4: Which of the following ART techniques may have the most significant effect on the increase of multifetal pregnancies?
A. In vitro fertilization
B. Ovulation induction with clomiphene
C. Controlled ovarian hyperstimulation with gonadotropins
D. A and C
E. All of the above

Q5: A woman presents to your office with quadruplets and requests information about multifetal reduction. How would you counsel her?
A. She would have a decreased risk of IUGR and decreased risk of cesarean section, but an increased risk of preterm delivery
B. She would have an increased risk of IUGR, decreased risk of cesarean section, and no change in her risk of preterm delivery
C. She would have a decreased risk of IUGR, decreased risk of cesarean section, and a decreased risk of preterm delivery
D. She would have an increased risk of IUGR, decreased risk of cesarean section, and an increased risk of preeclampsia

Q6: Further review of this patient's records reveals that she has one monochorionic pair. What would you recommend in terms of reduction?
A. Reduction of one of the non-monochorionic fetuses
B. Reduction of one of the monochorionic fetuses
C. Reduction of both monochorionic fetuses
D. Recommend against reduction given the increased risks associated with it

Q7: Another woman with triplets voices interest in selective fetal termination. How would you counsel her on the difference?

A. Selective fetal termination refers to reduction based on desired sex of live-born children
B. Selective fetal termination refers to reduction of an abnormal fetus
C. Selective fetal termination is associated with higher risks compared to multifetal reduction
D. B and C
E. All of the above

Q8: How can dichorionicity be established?

A. Sex discordance
B. Two placentas
C. IVF with documentation of two embryos transferred
D. Twin peak sign
E. A, B, and D
F. All of the above

Q9: Given risk for preterm delivery, all women with multifetal gestations should be screened using the following method:

A. Serial cervical lengths
B. Cervical length at growth US
C. Fetal fibronectin at visits between 24 and 34 weeks gestational age
D. All of the above
E. B and C
F. None of the above

Q10: Which of the following interventions have been shown to prolong pregnancy in women with multifetal gestations without a history of cervical insufficiency?

A. Bed rest
B. Prophylactic cerclage
C. Prophylactic tocolysis
D. Vaginal progesterone in setting of a shortened cervix
E. Prophylactic pessary
F. None of the above

Q11: How should preterm labor with multifetal gestations be managed?

A. Hold tocolysis regardless of gestational age, give betamethasone if 23–34 weeks gestation, and hold magnesium sulfate for neuroprotection
B. Give tocolysis for steroid benefit, give betamethasone if 23–34 weeks gestation, and hold magnesium sulfate for neuroprotection
C. Give tocolysis for steroid benefit, give betamethasone if 23–34 weeks gestation, and give magnesium sulfate for neuroprotection up to 32 weeks gestation
D. Give magnesium for tocolysis and for neuroprotection up to 32 weeks gestation, and give betamethasone if between 23 and 34 weeks gestation

Match the following tests with the current knowledge of their use in multiple gestations:

A. Not as sensitive because average of values can mask abnormal values
B. Can be technically challenging, but is equally as sensitive in singletons and multiples
C. Insufficient evidence to recommend its use
D. Can be performed for definitive diagnosis, higher risk of sampling error
E. Can be performed for definitive diagnosis, lower risk of sampling error

Q12: CVS

Q13: Nuchal translucency

Q14: Amniocentesis

Q15: Cell-free fetal DNA

Q16: Serum screening

Q17: How is discordance calculated?
A. (Larger twin – smaller twin) × 100/smaller twin
B. (Larger twin – smaller twin) × 100/larger twin

For questions 18–22—True or False:

Q18: Twins are considered discordant when there is a 25% difference in fetal weight between larger and smaller fetus.

Q19: Twins with isolated growth discordance are at no increased risk for morbidity or mortality.

Q20: IUGR twins have equivalent outcomes to singleton IUGR babies once gestational age is controlled for.

Q21: Dichorionic-diamniotic twin gestations should undergo growth ultrasounds every 46 weeks.

Q22: Dichorionic-diamniotic twin gestations should undergo antenatal testing starting at 32 weeks gestational age.

Q23: Which of the following is FALSE regarding twin-twin transfusion syndrome?
A. Ultrasounds should be performed to monitor for twin-twin transfusion syndrome starting at 20 weeks gestational age
B. Twin-twin transfusion syndrome occurs in 10–15% of monochorionic-diamniotic twin gestations
C. Twin-twin transfusion syndrome is generally diagnosed in the second trimester
D. Twin-twin transfusion syndrome results from AV anastomoses in the placenta

Q24: Which of the following is the correct sequence for the progression of twin-twin transfusion?

A. Absent bladder in the donor, abnormal Doppler ultrasonography, oligohydramnios/polyhydramnios, hydrops, and death
B. Oligohydramnios/polyhydramnios, absent bladder in the donor, abnormal Doppler ultrasonography, hydrops, and death
C. Oligohydramnios/polyhydramnios, abnormal Doppler ultrasonography, absent bladder in the donor, and death
D Absent bladder in the donor, oligohydramnios/polyhydramnios, abnormal Doppler ultrasonography, hydrops, and death
E. Oligohydramnios/polyhydramnios, absent bladder in the donor, abnormal Doppler ultrasonography, and death

Q25–27: In uncomplicated pregnancies, choose the latest recommended gestational age to deliver at: A, 34 weeks; B, 35 weeks; C, 36 weeks; D, 37 weeks; E, 38 weeks; F, 39 weeks.

Q25: Dichorionic-diamniotic twin gestations.

Q26: Monochorionic-diamniotic twin gestations.

Q27: Monochorionic-monochorionic twin gestations.

Q28: Which of the following factors are necessary to attempt a vaginal delivery in dichorionic-diamniotic twin gestations?

A. No prior cesarean sections
B. Gestational age at 32 weeks or greater
C. Presenting twin is vertex
D. A and C
E. B and C
F. All of the above

Q29: If all criteria are met, planned vaginal delivery compared to planned cesarean section in dichorionic-diamniotic twin gestations is associated with:

A. Increased risk of fetal death
B. Increased risk of serious neonatal morbidity
C. Increased risk of cerebral palsy
D. B and C
E. None of the above

Answers

Q1: D, Q2: E, Q3: A, Q4: D, Q5: C, Q6: C, Q7: D, Q8: E, Q9: F, Q10: F, Q11: C, Q12: D, Q13: B, Q14: E, Q15: C, Q16: A, Q17: B, Q18: False, Q19: True, Q20: False, Q21: True, Q22: False, Q23: A, Q24: B, Q25: E, Q26: D, Q27: A, Q28: E, Q29: E.

Resources

1. Gabbe SG, Niebyl JR, Simpson JL, Landon MB, Galan HL, Jauniaux ERM, Driscoll DA. Obstetrics: normal and problem pregnancies. Chapter 30. 6th ed.. Philadelphia, Elsevier. 2012.
2. American College of Obstetricians and Gynecologists. Practice bulletin No. 169: multifetal gestations: twin, triplet, and higher-order multifetal pregnancies. Obstet Gynecol. 2016;128:e131–46.

Chapter 41
Critical Care in Pregnancy

Pregnancy causes expansion of blood volume which, while adaptive, can also cause a delay in the recognition of significant hemorrhage. The critically ill pregnant patient requires thorough knowledge of physiologic changes that are normal during pregnancy. Logistics of their care may require a multidisciplinary approach [1].

Recommended resource—ACOG Practice Bulletin 170: Critical Care in Pregnancy [2].

Q1: What percent of pregnant women require critical care services in the United States each year?
A. Less than 1%
B. 1–3%
C. 3–5%
D. Up to 10%

Q2: As a practicing physician, it can be difficult to maintain competency in skills necessary for critical care. All of the following are examples of ways to develop or maintain these important skills EXCEPT:
A. Practicing intubation under the direct supervision of an anesthesiologist
B. Participating in a sepsis simulation

K.C. Arnold, C.J. Flint, *Obstetrics Essentials*,
DOI 10.1007/978-3-319-57675-6_41,

C. Completing an online course reviewing the interpretation of electrocardiograms
D. All of the above are examples of ways to maintain critical care skills

Q3: Which of the following is FALSE in regard to a closed ICU?
A. Only critical care attendings or house staff can write orders
B. Considered a type of high-intensity ICU
C. Associated with lower ICU mortality and decreased length of stay
D. Allows any physician to write orders as long as there is an on-site critical care physician to provide consultation

Q4: A critically ill OB patient is being transferred to another hospital due to the availability of ICU services. Which of the following are true?
A. Patient needs to have secure IV access prior to transfer
B. Minimal maternal monitoring during transfer includes pulse oximetry, electrocardiography, and frequent assessment of vital signs
C. Minimal fetal assessment during transfer includes continuous external fetal monitoring
D. A and B
E. All of the above

Q5: The most common causes for ICU admission for obstetric patients are hemorrhage and sepsis.
A. TRUE
B. FALSE

Q6: Key differences in laboratory values during pregnancy include all the following EXCEPT:
A. Decreased blood pressure
B. Increased serum creatinine levels

C. Increased heart rate
D. Increased D-dimer levels
E. All of the above are true

Q7: About 75% of obstetric patients admitted to the ICU are postpartum.
A. TRUE
B. FALSE

Q8: Delivery in the ICU is associated with:
A. Increased likelihood of operative vaginal delivery
B. Lack of space to accommodate key pediatric equipment and providers
C. Decreased risk of nosocomial infection with drug-resistant organisms
D. A and B
E. All of the above

Q9: A 28-year-old G1P0 with pregnancy at 32 weeks gestation is admitted to the ICU for airway management due to acute sepsis related to suspected pneumonia. The ICU critical care physician is concerned about how the medications and additional workup needed for this patient will affect the fetus. You advise:
A. Necessary medications should not be withheld
B. Only non-contrast imaging studies should be ordered
C. Corticosteroids for fetal lung maturity are contraindicated in the setting of sepsis
D. A and C
E. All of the above

Q10: After how long should a cesarean section be considered for maternal and fetal benefit when a pregnant woman has cardiopulmonary arrest in the third trimester?
A. 2 min
B. 3 min
C. 4 min
D. 5 min

Q11: Which of the following is TRUE regarding management of sepsis in an OB patient?

A. It is critical for blood cultures to be drawn prior to the administration of antibiotics

B. It is reasonable to wait to start antibiotics until transfer to ICU has been completed

C. Broad-spectrum antibiotics should be started within 1 h of diagnosis of severe sepsis or septic shock

D. Fetal resuscitation in utero is difficult; thus cesarean section should strongly be considered with fetal heart tone abnormalities

Q12: Which of the following are interventions that can be accomplished when a pregnant patient is being transported and fetal heart tones become non-reassuring?

A. Alert the receiving institution of possible need for delivery

B. Return to transferring facility for delivery planning if it is closer

C. Emergency cesarean delivery for Category III fetal heart rate tracings

D. All of the above

Q13: A 19-year-old G0 at 30 weeks gestational age is admitted to the ICU after a car accident. Her fetus is intermittently Category II, however predominantly Category I. Which of the following need to be determined as soon as possible?

A. Where delivery will occur

B. Preferred mode of delivery

C. Which family members will be present

D. A and B

E. All of the above

Answers

Q1: B, Q2: D, Q3: D, Q4: D, Q5: B, Q6: B, Q7: A, Q8: D, Q9: A, Q10: C, Q11: C, Q12: A, Q13: D.

Resources

1. Gabbe SG, Niebyl JR, Simpson JL, Landon MB, Galan HL, Jauniaux ERM, Driscoll DA. Obstetrics: normal and problem pregnancies, Chapter 24. 6th ed.. Philadelphia, Elsevier. 2012.
2. American College of Obstetricians and Gynecologists. Practice bulletin no. 170: critical care in pregnancy. Obstet Gynecol. 2016;128:e147–54.

Chapter 42
Management of Preterm Labor

Preterm birth occurs in 9.6% of pregnancies worldwide with gestational age being most strongly correlated with fetal outcomes. Goals in the treatment of preterm labor include transfer to an appropriate hospital and administration of the following medications if indicated: antibiotics, steroids for fetal lung maturity, tocolysis, and magnesium sulfate for neuroprotection. Intrapartum care is often complicated due to multiple comorbidities. Indications for cesarean delivery are similar to those at term [1].

Recommended resource—ACOG Practice Bulletin 171: Management of Preterm Labor [2].

Q1: What is the average cost per premature infant in the Unites States according to the Institute of Medicine?
A. $20,000
B. $26,000
C. $40,000
D. $51,000

Q2: Preterm birth is defined as delivery between what gestational ages?
A. 20/0 and 38/6 weeks gestational age
B. 20/0 and 36/6 weeks gestational age
C. 24/0 and 38/6 weeks gestational age
D. 24/0 and 36/6 weeks gestational age

K.C. Arnold, C.J. Flint, *Obstetrics Essentials*,
DOI 10.1007/978-3-319-57675-6_42,

Q3: According to ACOG, preterm labor is defined by which of the following in a 23-year-old G3P2002 at 33/0 weeks gestational age?

A. Symptomatic regular contractions and dilation of more than 1 cm
B. Regular contractions with a cervical dilation of 2/50/–3 stable over 3 h and 2 cervical exams
C. Regular contractions with a cervical dilation of 1/80/–2 stable over 3 h and 2 cervical exams
D. A and B
E. All of the above

Q4: A 35-year-old at 28 weeks gestational age is admitted with preterm labor. She is very concerned and asks how certain you are that she will delivery prematurely. What percent of women with the diagnosis of preterm labor give birth within 7 days of initial presentation?

A. 75%
B. 50%
C. 25%
D. 10%

Q5: What is the percent likelihood that after her hospitalization she will deliver at term?

A. 75%
B. 50%
C. 25%
D. 10%

Q6: A 30-year-old G3P0202 at 30 weeks gestational age calls your office. She reports becoming increasingly nervous as she gave birth at 32 weeks in her previous pregnancy. She asks if she should go on bed rest and abstain from sexual activities. How should you counsel her?

A. Tell her to go on bed rest but that she may continue sexual activity

B. Tell her there is no need to go on bed rest but that she should abstain from sexual activity
C. Inform her that neither has been proven to be effective
D. Advise her that neither can hurt and with her history she should play it safe

Q7: Tocolytics should be considered in which of the following situations?
A. A 37-year-old G5P0040 presents at 32 weeks gestational age with moderate contractions; cervical exam is 2/50/−2. She is not ruptured
B. A 37-year-old G5P0040 presents to triage at 26 weeks gestation. She is found to be ruptured. The first dose of betamethasone is administered. The patient has mild contractions; her abdomen is soft, nontender to palpation; and she has no leukocytosis. She requests tocolysis until steroid benefit has been reached
C. An 18-year-old G1P0 at 18 weeks gestation who has just had an appendectomy
D. All of the above
E. None of the above

Q8: A 30-year-old G2P0101 at 32 weeks gestation in your office. She is your patient and also your co-worker. She reports contractions throughout the day that interfere with her ability to focus on her job and requests nifedipine for symptomatic relief to use as needed.
A. You tell her that the use of chronic tocolytics does not prevent preterm delivery
B. You empathize with her symptoms and give her a prescription for nifedipine prn
C. Tell her that there is no indication to give her nifedipine and do not write a prescription

D. A and B
E. A and C

Q9: At what gestational ages should steroid administration be considered?
A. 23/0 to 36/6 weeks gestational age
B. 24/0 to 33/6 weeks gestational age
C. 23/0 to 33/6 weeks gestational age
D. 24/0 to 36/6 weeks gestational age

Q10: A patient presents to triage at 29 weeks gestational age and is found to be in preterm labor. Betamethasone is administered and a tocolytic is started. Eleven hours later, she has progressed to 8/100/−1. A medical student asks if we can administer the second dose of steroids 12 h after the first. What is your response?
A. There is no proven benefit hence second dose will not be given early despite probable imminent delivery
B. Yes, it is called accelerated dosing. Please notify nursing and I'll place the order

Q11: Which of the following is true regarding magnesium given for neuroprotection?
A. It should be given if birth is anticipated before 30 weeks gestational age
B. It also has the dual function of prolonging pregnancy
C. It reduces respiratory distress syndrome in neonates
D. It reduces the risk and severity of cerebral palsy in neonates
E. B and D

Q12: In which of the following situations may tocolytic therapy be useful?

A. During transport to another hospital
B. During administration of magnesium for neuro-protection and steroids for fetal lung maturity
C. To decrease contractions so the fetus can be delivered at a more favorable age
D. A and B
E. B and C

Q13: Which of the following are contraindications to tocolysis?

A. Non-reassuring fetal status
B. Mild preeclampsia
C. Insulin-dependent diabetes
D. Maternal drug use
E. All of the above

Q14–17: Match the tocolytic class or agent to its associated characteristics:

A. Maternal side effect: gastritis, platelet dysfunction. Fetal adverse effect: oligohydramnios
B. Maternal side effect: flushing, elevation of transaminases. Contraindications: preload-dependent maternal cardiac lesions
C. Maternal side effect: diaphoresis, respiratory depression, suppresses heart rate. Fetal adverse effect: deonatal depression
D. Maternal side effect: palpitations, shortness of breath, pulmonary edema. Fetal adverse effect: tachycardia. Contraindication: poorly controlled diabetes

Q14: Calcium channel blocker.

Q15: Nonsteroidal anti-inflammatory drugs.

Q16: Beta-adrenergic receptor agonists.

Q17: Magnesium sulfate.

Q18: In women with multiple gestations who are in preterm labor, which of the following are indicated?

A. Tocolysis
B. Antenatal steroids
C. Magnesium sulfate
D. B and C
E. All of the above

Q19: Which of the following patients would be a candidate for rescue dose steroid administration?

A. A patient initially given a course of steroids at 23/4 weeks gestation who represents to labor and delivery with continued concern for preterm labor at 27 weeks gestational age
B. A patient initially given a course of steroids at 24/0 weeks gestation who then begins to show signs of imminent delivery at 25/0 weeks gestation
C. A patient initially given a course of steroids at 29/0 weeks gestation who represents with concerns of labor at 34/2 weeks gestation
D. A and B
E. All the above

Answers

Q1: D, Q2: B, Q3: D, Q4: D, Q5: B, Q6: C, Q7: D, Q8: E, Q9: A, Q10: A, Q11: D, Q12: D, Q13: A, Q14: B, Q15: A, Q16: D, Q17: C, Q18: D, Q19: D.

Resources

1. Gabbe SG, Niebyl JR, Simpson JL, Landon MB, Galan HL, Jauniaux ERM, Driscoll DA. Obstetrics: normal and problem pregnancies, chapter 28. 6th ed. Philadelphia: Elsevier; 2012.
2. American College of Obstetricians and Gynecologists. Practice bulletin no. 171: management of preterm labor. Obstet Gynecol. 2016;128:e155–64.

Chapter 43
Premature Rupture of Membranes

Preterm rupture of membranes is defined as rupture of membranes prior to the start of labor. It is more common in African American patients. Rupture of membranes increases the risk of perinatal infection and umbilical cord compression. Diagnosis is generally confirmed by either visualization of amniotic fluid from the cervical os, a vaginal pH of more than 6.0, or ferning on microscopic exam. Management is highly variable depending on gestational age and the clinical setting [1].

Recommended resource—ACOG Practice Bulletin 172: Premature Rupture of Membranes [2].

Q1: Preterm premature rupture of membranes (preterm PROM) complicates ____% of pregnancies.
- A. 1%
- B. 3%
- C. 9%
- D. 12%

Q2: Preterm PROM is defined as the rupture of membranes before the onset of labor prior to:
- A. 40 weeks gestational age
- B. 39 weeks gestational age
- C. 37 weeks gestational age
- D. 34 weeks gestational age

K.C. Arnold, C.J. Flint, *Obstetrics Essentials*,
DOI 10.1007/978-3-319-57675-6_43,

Q3: Which of the following has been shown to be associated with preterm PROM?
A. Intraamniotic infection
B. Prior history of preterm PROM
C. Shortened cervical length
D. A and B
E. All of the above

Q4: What is the most significant maternal consequence of term PROM?
A. Intrauterine infection
B. Abruption with hemorrhage
C. Labor dystocia
D. Impaired fetal lung maturity

Q5: Which of the following is *TRUE* regarding preterm PROM?
A. Delivery will occur within 1 week in 50% of patients regardless of management
B. Latency after membrane rupture is directly correlated with gestational age at time of membrane rupture
C. Incidence of infection is higher at earlier gestational age
D. B and C
E. A and C

Q6: What is the most common complication of prematurity for the fetus?
A. Sepsis
B. Necrotizing enterocolitis
C. Intraventricular hemorrhage
D. Respiratory distress

Q7: Which of the following fetal complications is more likely to be seen with preterm PROM pregnancies than preterm deliveries due to other causes?
A. Intraventricular hemorrhage
B. White matter damage

C. Necrotizing enterocolitis
D. Respiratory distress

Q8: Which of the following is *FALSE* regarding fetal pulmonary hypoplasia?
A. Associated with a high risk of mortality
B. Less common after 23–24 weeks gestation
C. Early gestational age at membrane rupture and low residual amniotic fluid volume are primary determinants
D. All of the above are true

Q9: Digital examinations are discouraged in preterm PROM patients unless absolutely necessary due to:
A. Increased risk of infection
B. Add little information to sterile speculum exam
C. Increased risk of bleeding
D. A and B
E. All of the above

Q10: Which of the following can cause a false-negative test result for membrane rupture?
A. Prolonged rupture
B. Blood or semen
C. Bacterial vaginosis
D. Continued leakage of fluid

Q11: Fetal fibronectin is a specific test for ruptured membranes.
A. TRUE
B. FALSE

Q12: In regard to labor induction in term patients with PROM, which of the following is *TRUE*?
A. Induction with prostaglandins has been shown to be more effective than induction with Pitocin
B. Induction with Pitocin has been shown to be more effective than induction with prostaglandins

C. Induction with prostaglandins is associated with a higher risk of chorioamnionitis
D. Induction with Pitocin versus prostaglandins has been shown to have equal risks for chorioamnionitis
E. A and C

Q13: A 36-year-old G1P0 at 40 weeks gestation presents to the hospital loss of fluid starting 2 h ago and is confirmed to have rupture of membranes. Sterile vaginal exam is closed/thick/high. The patient reports cramping. Review of patient chart reveals a recent GBS-negative status. Fetus is cephalic and Category I. The next BEST steps include:
A. Induction of labor
B. Induction of labor and administration of prophylactic antibiotics
C. Expectant management
D. Expectant management and administration of prophylactic antibiotics
E. Induction of labor and cesarean section for failed induction if still in latent phase 10–14 h later

Q14: Which of the following has NOT been shown to be useful in the monitoring of patients with preterm PROM?
A. Maternal temperature assessments
B. Ultrasound monitoring of fetal growth
C. Periodic fetal heart rate monitoring
D. Serial monitoring of maternal leukocyte count
E. None of the above

Q15: Which of the following is true in the setting of preterm PROM?
A. Prophylactic tocolysis is associated with a longer latency period
B. Prophylactic tocolysis increases risk of chorioamnionitis

C. Prophylactic tocolysis is not recommended in preterm PROM
D. A and B
E. All of the above

Q16: Administration of magnesium for neuroprotection should be considered in preterm PROM patients:
A. At less than 28 weeks gestational age
B. At less than 30 weeks gestational age
C. At less than 32 weeks gestational age
D. At less than 34 weeks gestational age

Q17: Which of the following statement(s) are *TRUE* regarding preterm PROM and antibiotic administration?
A. Can prolong pregnancy and reduce maternal and neonatal infections
B. Regimen includes 7-day course of IV erythromycin and ampicillin combined with oral erythromycin and amoxicillin-clavulanic acid
C. Should be administered in pregnancies less than 34 weeks gestation
D. A and C
E. All of the above

Q18: Due to lack of adequate evidence regarding the management of patients with preterm PROM and cerclage, no recommendation can be made as to whether or not cerclage should be removed following preterm PROM.
A. TRUE
B. FALSE

Q19: What is the risk of vertical transmission at the time of delivery with primary and recurrent HSV, respectively?
A. 30–50%; 3%
B. 50–70%; 6%
C. 20–40%; 3%
D. 30–50%; 6%

Q20: A single course of corticosteroids can be considered in women as early as _____ weeks gestation in the setting of preterm PROM.

A. 20 weeks gestation
B. 21 weeks gestation
C. 22 weeks gestation
D. 23 weeks gestation
E. 24 weeks gestation

Q21: A 33-year-old G3P2002 with intrauterine pregnancy at 21 weeks gestation presents to the emergency department with confirmed rupture of membranes. She is afebrile without evidence of infection. Fetal heart tones auscultated.

A. Immediate delivery should be offered
B. Outpatient surveillance should be offered
C. Latency antibiotic administration can be considered
D. A and C
E. All of the above are true

Q22: Patients with a previous history of preterm PROM with subsequent preterm birth are known to have an increased risk of recurrent preterm PROM and preterm delivery. Which of the following intervention(s) may be helpful to prevent recurrence?

A. Progesterone supplementation starting at 16 weeks to 24 weeks gestation
B. Daily administration of ASA 81 mg with confirmation of fetal heart tones
C. Prophylactic cerclage placement
D. Progesterone supplementation starting with conception up to 10 weeks gestation
E. A and B
F. A, B, and C

Answers

Q1: B, Q2: C, Q3: E, Q4: A, Q5: E, Q6: D, Q7: B, Q8: D, Q9: D, Q10: A, Q11: B, Q12: C, Q13: A, Q14: D, Q15: D, Q16: C, Q17: D, Q18: A, Q19: A, Q20: D, Q21: E, Q22: A.

Resources

1. Gabbe SG, Niebyl JR, Simpson JL, Landon MB, Galan HL, Jauniaux ERM, Driscoll DA. Obstetrics: normal and problem pregnancies, chapter 29. 6th ed. Philadelphia: Elsevier; 2012.
2. American College of Obstetricians and Gynecologists. Practice bulletin no. 172: premature rupture of membranes. Obstet Gynecol. 2016;128:e165–77.

Chapter 44
Macrosomia

Macrosomia is defined as a birth weight over 4000–4500 g and is associated with an increased risk for shoulder dystocia. Women with overt or gestational diabetes are more likely to have macrosomic fetuses because maternal hyperglycemia results in infant hyperinsulinemia causing accelerated growth [1].

Recommended resource—ACOG Practice Bulletin 173: Macrosomia [2].

Q1: Infants born to diabetic mothers have higher rates of shoulder dystocia, clavicular fracture, and brachial plexus injury.

A. True, regardless of birth weight
B. True, if the birth weight is above 4500 g
C. True, if the birth weight is above 5000 g
D. False

Q2: A 29-year-old G1P0 at 40 weeks gestation is admitted in active labor. She has gestational diabetes with an estimated fetal weight of 4600 g. What is the reported risk of shoulder dystocia in this patient?

A. 5–10%
B. 10–20%
C. 20–30%
D. 20–50%
E. 50–60%

K.C. Arnold, C.J. Flint, *Obstetrics Essentials*,
DOI 10.1007/978-3-319-57675-6_44,

Q3: Most shoulder dystocias occur with delivery of a:
A. Normal weight fetus
B. Macrosomic fetus with a diabetic mother
C. Macrosomic fetus with an untreated diabetic mother
D. Macrosomic fetus with a nondiabetic mother
E. B and C

Q4: Which of the following is NOT a risk factor for fetal macrosomia?
A. Positive 50 g glucose screen with normal 3-h glucose tolerance test
B. Advanced maternal age
C. Excessive gestational weight gain
D. Postterm pregnancy
E. Nulliparity

Q5: The macrosomic fetus of a diabetic mother would likely have ____ compared to the macrosomic fetus of a nondiabetic mother?
A. Lesser upper-extremity skinfold measurement
B. Larger head to abdominal circumference
C. Greater total body fat
D. A and C
E. All of the above

Q6: Which of the following is superior for prediction of macrosomia?
A. Ultrasound in the third trimester
B. Clinical palpation maneuvers
C. Multiparous mothers' estimate
D. A and C
E. None of the above has been proven superior

Q7: A 27-year-old G2P1001 has a fundal height concerning for macrosomia. She has an increased risk for all of the following complications EXCEPT:
A. Postpartum hemorrhage
B. Third- and fourth-degree lacerations
C. Cesarean delivery

D. Labor abnormalities
E. Risk is increased for all of the above

Q8: Which of the following is TRUE regarding brachial plexus injuries associated with macrosomia?
A. Cesarean section prevents brachial plexus injuries
B. 65% are resolved at 1 year of age
C. If there was no shoulder dystocia, the diagnosis of brachial plexus injury is likely false
D. Damage to C5 and C6 can produce Erb-Duchenne paralysis
E. None of the above

Q9: Which of the following is TRUE regarding the ability of ultrasound to predict macrosomia?
A. The estimated fetal weight would need to exceed 4800 to have more than a 50% chance of being macrosomic
B. Hadlock's formula is most accurate in estimating fetal weight in the macrosomic fetus
C. The utility of ultrasound for obtaining fetal weight is operator and equipment dependent
D. Abdominal circumference is most predictive of macrosomia
E. None of the above

Q10: A 41-year-old G1P0 without diabetes has an estimated fetal weight of 5000 g on the day of her induction. She asks about a cesarean section. How do you counsel her?
A. A cesarean delivery is required given risk of brachial plexus injury of 30%
B. A cesarean section should be considered given brachial plexus injury rate of 10%
C. A cesarean delivery should not be offered given emphasis on preventing the primary cesarean section
D. None of the above are true
E. All of the above are reasonable

Q11: Which of the following has been shown to decrease the risk of macrosomia?

A. Dietary regulation to prevent excess weight gain in nondiabetics
B. Daily exercise starting in the third trimester
C. Insulin therapy for diabetics
D. A and B
E. A and C

Q12: Which of the following is TRUE regarding the recommendations for cesarean delivery based on estimated fetal weight?

A. If the estimated fetal weight in a diabetic mother is above 4000 g, a cesarean delivery should be considered
B. If the estimated fetal weight in a diabetic mother is above 4500 g, a cesarean delivery is required
C. If the estimated fetal weight in a nondiabetic mother is above 4500 g, a cesarean delivery should be considered
D. If the estimated fetal weight in a nondiabetic mother is above 5000 g, a cesarean delivery should be considered
E. B and D

Q13: Given the risk for shoulder dystocia and brachial plexus injury, early induction should be considered if macrosomia is discovered at 37 weeks gestation.

A. Sometimes
B. Always
C. Never

Q14: The risk of shoulder dystocia is unaffected by assisted vaginal delivery.

A. TRUE
B. FALSE

Q15: Which of the following is TRUE regarding vaginal births after cesarean section for the macrosomic fetus?

A. Macrosomia is a contraindication
B. Success rates are less than 50%
C. All of the above
D. None of the above

Q16: Large for gestational age is defined as:
A. Birth weight at or above 4000 g
B. Birth weight at or above 5000 g
C. Birth weight at or above the 90th percentile
D. Birth weight at or above the 95th percentile
E. None of the above

Q17: A patient has an ultrasound with an estimated fetal weight of 4200 g. She should be informed that newborn weights of ____ and more are associated with increased stillbirth and neonatal mortality.
A. 3500 g
B. 4000 g
C. 4500 g
D. 5000 g
E. There are no data to support a cutoff

Q18: Approximately what percent of live-born infants in the United States have birth weights of more than 4500 g?
A. 1%
B. 2%
C. 5%
D. 8%
E. 10%

Q19: What is the sensitivity of fundal height measurement for detecting macrosomia?
A. 50% or less
B. 60%
C. 75%
D. 90%

Answers

Q1: A, Q2: D, Q3: A, Q4: E, Q5: C. Q6: E, Q7: E, Q8: D, Q9: A, Q10: B, Q11: C, Q12: D, Q13: C, Q14: B, Q15: D, Q16: C, Q17: D, Q18: A, Q19: A.

Resources

1. Gabbe SG, Niebyl JR, Simpson JL, Landon MB, Galan HL, Jauniaux ERM, Driscoll DA. Obstetrics: normal and problem pregnancies, chapter 39. 6th ed. Philadelphia: Elsevier; 2012.
2. American College of Obstetricians and Gynecologists. Practice bulletin no. 173: fetal macrosomia. Obstet Gynecol. 2016;128:e195–209.

Chapter 45
Ultrasound in Pregnancy

The use of ultrasound in pregnancy has increased immensely since it was first used during pregnancy in the 1960s. Elements of each type of ultrasound are clearly defined, and following these protocols with consistency is part of good clinical care. Diagnostic ultrasonography appears to be safe during pregnancy; however, ultrasound use for entertainment is discouraged [1].

Recommended resource— ACOG Practice Bulletin 175: Ultrasound in Pregnancy [2].

Q1: An obese patient presents to the ER and requires a viability scan for further evaluation. Which ultrasound settings would likely be most helpful?

A. High frequency as it provides better resolution and penetration
B. Low frequency as it provides worse resolution but better penetration
C. Low frequency as it provides better resolution but worse penetration
D. High frequency as it provides better resolution and penetration

K.C. Arnold, C.J. Flint, *Obstetrics Essentials*,
DOI 10.1007/978-3-319-57675-6_45,

Q2: Which of the following is NOT included in the standard obstetric ultrasound examination?
A. Fetal biometry
B. Anatomic survey
C. Cervix and adnexa
D. Placental position
E. All of the above are included

Q3: Which of the following is FALSE regarding a limited obstetric ultrasound examination?
A. Performed when a specific question requires investigation
B. Can be used to confirm fetal presentation
C. Can only be performed in the second or third trimester
D. Does not replace a standard examination
E. None of the above

Q4: First trimester ultrasound is performed before 12/0 weeks gestation, can be performed transabdominally or transvaginally, and should include an evaluation of the uterus and cervix.
A. TRUE
B. FALSE

Q5: Which of the following is most accurate when estimating gestational age?
A. Crown-rump length
B. Mean gestational sac diameter
C. Both are equivalent

Q6: Which of the following is diagnostic of a nonviable pregnancy?
A. A mean gestational sac of 20 mm or greater
B. Lack of cardiac motion with a 10 mm embryo
C. Lack of cardiac motion with a 5 mm embryo
D. A and C
E. All of the above

Q7: When measuring the biparietal diameter, which of the following is TRUE?

A. It should be measured at the level of the cerebellar hemispheres
B. Measurement should be taken from the inner edge of the proximal skull to the inner edge of the distal skull
C. It may be affected by fetal head shape in which case circumference may be more reliable
D. A and B
E. All of the above

Q8: Which of the following is TRUE regarding measurement of the femoral diaphysis?

A. It can be used for dating after 12 weeks gestation
B. It should include the femoral epiphysis
C. All of the above
D. None of the above

Q9: When measuring the abdominal circumference, all of the following should be in the transverse ultrasound view EXCEPT:

A. The umbilical vein
B. The portal sinus
C. The fetal stomach
D. The renal vessels

Q10: Estimated fetal weight by ultrasound can yield errors as high as:

A. 10%
B. 20%
C. 30%
D. 40%

Q11: Three-dimensional ultrasonography provides a clear clinical advantage in prenatal diagnosis.

A. TRUE
B. FALSE

Q12: Doppler has lower energy delivery and is therefore preferable to ultrasound in the first trimester.
A. TRUE
B. FALSE

Q13: The office has obtained a transvaginal ultrasound to use for patient care. How is microbial prevention accomplished when the same probe is used?
A. Single use disposable covers
B. High-level disinfection
C. Either A or B
D. Both A and B must be performed

Q14: A patient is considering paying for a nonmedical 3D ultrasound and asks your opinion. You counsel her that performing ultrasounds without a medical indication is:
A. Contrary to responsible medical practice
B. Known to cause fetal harm
C. Appropriate if only for keepsakes and patient is aware they are not for medical use
D. Outside the realm of ACOG recommendations and is a matter of personal preference

Q15: What is the latest gestational age a nuchal translucency should be performed at?
A. 12/0
B. 12/6
C. 13/0
D. 13/6
E. 14/0

Q16: An ultrasound is performed on a patient who is 10/5 weeks gestational age by LMP and the crown-rump length measures larger. At what difference would you change her estimated date of delivery?
A. More than 5 days
B. More than 6 days

C. More than 7 days
D. More than 10 days

Q17: Which single measurement is most predictive of gestational age during the second and third trimesters, respectively?
A. Femur length, head circumference
B. Head circumference, femur length
C. Biparietal diameter, femur length
D. Femur length, biparietal diameter
E. None is superior

Q18: Which of the following is FALSE in measuring amniotic fluid index (AFI)?
A. The width of the pocket must be 2 cm
B. ACOG favors using deepest vertical pocket to diagnose oligohydramnios
C. The transducer should be perpendicular to the floor
D. The maximum vertical pocket should be used in multiple pregnancies
E. None of the above

Q19: What percentage of fetuses with increased nuchal translucency will have a chromosomal abnormality?
A. 10%
B. 25%
C. 33%
D. 50%

Q20: How can ultrasound be used to assess for fetal anemia?
A. Diastolic velocity of the fetal middle cerebral artery
B. Systolic velocity of the fetal middle cerebral artery
C. Diastolic velocity of the umbilical artery
D. Systolic velocity of the umbilical artery
E. B and C

Q21: All of the following are recommended if IUGR is diagnosed EXCEPT:
A. Amniotic fluid assessment
B. Doppler blood flow of the umbilical artery
C. Assessment for structural abnormalities
D. Assessment for genetic abnormalities
E. All of the above are recommended

Q22: How frequently should monochorionic twins be monitored by ultrasound?
A. Every week starting at 20 weeks gestational age
B. Every 2 weeks starting at 16 weeks gestational age
C. Every 4 weeks starting at 20 weeks gestational age
D. Every week starting at 16 weeks gestational age

Answers

Q1: B, Q2: E, Q3: C, Q4: B, Q5: A, Q6: B, Q7: C, Q8: D, Q9: D, Q10: B, Q11: B, Q12: B, Q13: D, Q14: A, Q15: D, Q16: C, Q17: B, Q18: A, Q19: C, Q20: B, Q21: E, Q22: B.

Resources

1. Gabbe SG, Niebyl JR, Simpson JL, Landon MB, Galan HL, Jauniaux ERM, Driscoll DA. Obstetrics: normal and problem pregnancies. Chapter 9. 6th ed. Philadelphia: Elsevier; 2012.
2. American College of Obstetricians and Gynecologists. Practice bulletin no. 175: ultrasound in pregnancy. Obstet Gynecol. 2016;128:e241–56.

Part II
Questions Intermixed

Chapter 46
Questions Intermixed

Q1: It is suggested that a stillbirth includes fetal deaths that occur at ______ weeks gestation or greater or if gestational age is unknown, then in a fetus with a weight greater than or equal to _____ grams.

A. 20 weeks; 250 g
B. 20 weeks; 350 g
C. 24 weeks; 350 g
D. 24 weeks; 450 g

Q2: Fetal-neonatal alloimmune thrombocytopenia shares many similarities with hemolytic (Rh) disease of the newborn. What is a key difference between the two disorders?

A. One is mediated by maternal alloimmunization, while the other is mediated by paternal alloimmunization
B. One involves placental transfer of antibodies, while the other involves placental transfer of antigens
C. One can affect the first pregnancy, while the other typically affects subsequent pregnancies
D. All of the above
E. None of the above

K.C. Arnold, C.J. Flint, *Obstetrics Essentials*,
DOI 10.1007/978-3-319-57675-6_46

Q3: Infants born to diabetic mothers have higher rates of shoulder dystocia, clavicular fracture, and brachial plexus injury.

A. True, regardless of birth weight
B. True, if the birth weight is above 4500 g
C. True, if the birth weight is above 5000 g
D. False

Q4: A 29-year-old G1P0 at 40 weeks gestation is admitted in active labor. She has gestational diabetes with an estimated fetal weight of 4600 g. What is the reported risk of shoulder dystocia in this patient?

A. 5–10%
B. 10–20%
C. 20–30%
D. 20–50%
E. 50–60%

Q5: Which of the following is FALSE in regard to fetal intracranial hemorrhage due to fetal-neonatal alloimmune thrombocytopenia?

A. Can occur in utero
B. Is the most serious complication of the disorder
C. Can occur in up to 50% of infants with platelet counts less than 50,000/μL
D. None of the above

Q6: Late-term pregnancy refers to a pregnancy between:

A. 40 0/7 weeks and 42 0/7 weeks
B. 40 6/7 weeks and 41 6/7 weeks
C. 41 0/7 weeks and 42 6/7 weeks
D. 41 0/7 weeks and 41 6/7 weeks

Q7: Another woman with triplets voices interest in selective fetal termination. How would you counsel her on the difference between this and multifetal reduction?

A. Selective fetal termination refers to reduction based on desired sex of live-born children
B. Selective fetal termination refers to reduction of an abnormal fetus

C. Selective fetal termination is associated with higher risks compared to multifetal reduction
D. B and C
E. All of the above

Q8: How can dichorionicity be established?
A. Sex discordance
B. Two placentas
C. IVF with documentation of two embryos transferred
D. Twin peak sign
E. A, B, and D
F. All of the above

Q9: A 42-year-old G2P1001 presents to OB triage with intrauterine gestation at 42/2 weeks gestation. When discussing the morbidities associated with her gestational age, you refer to her pregnancy as:
A. Term
B. Late term
C. Postterm
D. Advanced term

Q10: Which of the following is FALSE regarding the management of diabetic ketoacidosis in pregnancy?
A. Start an insulin drip
B. Hydrate with 4–6 L of half normal saline in the first 12 h
C. Give 5% dextrose once glucose is below 250 mg/dL
D. If fetal heart tracing is Category II, continue to treat maternal condition and anticipate improvement in fetal status

Q11: When comparing electronic fetal monitoring (EFM) with intermittent auscultation of fetal heart tones, which of the following is TRUE?
A. Use of EFM decreases the risk of vacuum and forceps operative vaginal delivery
B. Use of EFM reduces perinatal mortality

C. Use of EFM reduces risk of neonatal seizures
D. Use of EFM reduces risk of cerebral palsy
E. All of the above are TRUE

Q12: You diagnose a patient at 30 weeks gestation with a new DVT. Which of the following are indications for initiating therapeutic anticoagulation as an inpatient?
A. Large clots
B. Patients who are past 35 weeks gestation
C. All patients should be hospitalized for initiation
D. A and B

Q13: When is monitoring labs recommended for pregnancy and anticoagulation?
A. Monitor platelet counts if using unfractionated or low-molecular-weight heparin
B. Xa should be monitored for prophylactic low-molecular-weight heparin dosing
C. Xa levels should be monitored for prophylactic unfractionated heparin dosing
D. aPTT should be monitored for therapeutic heparin dosing
E. All of the above

Q14: Misoprostol is a synthetic PGE2 analogue with published evidence to support its efficacy and safety when used appropriately.
A. True
B. False

Q15: The sensitivity of EFM for predicting cerebral palsy is high.
A. True
B. False

Q16: Thrombocytopenia affects approximately what percentage of pregnancies?
A. 1–5%
B. 6–15%

C. 16–25%
D. 26–35%

Q17: Which of the following is NOT a common manifestation of thrombocytopenia?
A. Bleeding into mucous membranes
B. Ecchymosis
C. Bleeding into joints
D. Menometrorrhagia

Q18: Variable decelerations are equally likely to occur among preterm deliveries and term deliveries.
A. True
B. False

Q19: What is the leading cause of perinatal mortality in pregnancies complicated by pregestational diabetes?
A. Congenital anomalies
B. Iatrogenic preterm deliveries
C. Spontaneous preterm deliveries
D. Diabetic ketoacidosis

Q20: Of all races, which group has the highest prevalence of anemia in pregnancy?
A. Mothers of advanced maternal age
B. Mothers of low income
C. Multiparous mothers
D. Teenaged mothers

Q21: Cytomegalovirus (CMV) is a double-stranded DNA virus that is transmitted through:
A. Consumption of undercooked meat
B. Respiratory secretions
C. Sexual contact
D. Hand-to-mouth contact

Q22: Adults infected with primary CMV may experience:
A. No symptoms as many are asymptomatic with infection
B. Mononucleosis-like syndrome with fevers, chills, and myalgias

C. Reticular rash on the trunk
D. A and B
E. All of the above

Q23: Iron deficiency anemia during pregnancy has been associated with all of the following EXCEPT:
A. Increased risk of perinatal mortality
B. Increased risk of structural abnormalities
C. Increased risk of low birth weight
D. Increased risk of preterm delivery

Q24: What is considered to be an elevated level of maternal serum alpha-fetoprotein (MSAFP) for a single gestation?
A. More than 1.5 times the normal median
B. More than 2.0 times the normal median
C. More than 2.5 times the normal median
D. More than 3.0 times the normal median

Q25: The risk of uterine rupture is greater when induction of labor is started on an unfavorable cervix versus a favorable cervix.
A. True
B. False

Q26: Studies have revealed that higher doses of oxytocin are associated with a dose-response effect with increasing risks of uterine rupture. Due to this, the following recommendation has been made:
A. The maximum Pitocin dosage for a patient attempting TOLAC is 32 mu/min
B. Unless location of previous uterine incision is clearly documented, Pitocin levels above 16 mu/min should not be used
C. There is not enough evidence to recommend an upper limit of oxytocin dosing in patients attempting TOLAC
D. In a patient with a history of two previous lower uterine segment incisions, Pitocin is clearly contraindicated

Q27: What is considered to be diagnostic for a fetal neural tube defect?

A. Elevated MSAFP and presence of acetylcholinesterase in amniotic fluid
B. Elevated MSAFP and elevated amniotic fluid AFP
C. Presence of acetylcholinesterase in amniotic fluid
D. Elevated amniotic fluid AFP and presence of acetylcholinesterase in amniotic fluid

Q28: What percent of gravid women undergo induction of labor in the United States?

A. 12%
B. 17%
C. 22%
D. 33%
E. 37%

Q29: All of the following are purposes of cervical ripening EXCEPT:

A. Cervical thinning
B. Decrease in time to painful contractions
C. Cervical dilation
D. Decrease in rate of failed induction
E. Decrease in induction to delivery time

Q30: Prior to the introduction of anti-D immune globulin, hemolytic disease of the fetus and newborn affected ______ pregnancies?

A. About 10% of pregnancies
B. About 20% of pregnancies
C. About 35% of pregnancies
D. About 45% of pregnancies

Q31: Which of the following is true regarding magnesium given for neuroprotection?

A. It should be given if birth is anticipated before 30 weeks gestational age
B. It also has the dual function of prolonging pregnancy

C. It reduces respiratory distress syndrome in neonates
D. It reduces the risk and severity of cerebral palsy in neonates
E. B and D

Q32: In which of the following situations may tocolytic therapy be useful?
A. During transport to another hospital
B. During administration of magnesium for neuro-protection and steroids for fetal lung maturity
C. To decrease contractions so the fetus can be delivered at a more favorable age
D. A and B
E. B and C

Q33: Which of the following are contraindications to tocolysis?
A. Non-reassuring fetal status
B. Mild preeclampsia
C. Insulin-dependent diabetes
D. Maternal drug use
E. All of the above

Q34: Transmission of this virus is generally through use of IV drugs or through blood products and is associated with B cell lymphomas, and its association with hepatocellular carcinoma is uncertain.
A. Hepatitis A
B. Hepatitis B
C. Hepatitis C
D. Hepatitis D
E. Hepatitis B and D

Q35: A 29-year-old G1P0 with intrauterine pregnancy at 42 weeks presents to your office for her last OB visit. She has an induction scheduled at the end of the week. She is carrying a female fetus and has a BMI of 21. In

conversation, she mentions that her mother also carried her 2 weeks beyond her due date. What risk factors does this patient have for a postterm pregnancy?
A. Maternal weight and sex of fetus
B. Nulliparity and maternal weight
C. Sex of fetus and genetic predisposition
D. Nulliparity and genetic predisposition

Q36: The risks associated with postterm pregnancy include all of the following EXCEPT:
A. Macrosomia
B. Oligohydramnios
C. Neonatal convulsions
D. 5 min Apgar less than 4
E. All of the above are risks

Q37: The prevalence of obesity has increased in reproductive aged women with the greatest proportion affecting Mexican Americans.
A. True
B. False

Q38: The negative predictive value is above 99% for a stillbirth occurring within 1 week of a normal test result of all of the following EXCEPT:
A. Contraction stress test
B. Biophysical profile
C. Nonstress test
D. Modified biophysical stress test
E. All of the above have above a 99% negative predictive value

Q39: What percent of pregnant women require critical care services in the United States each year?
A. Less than 1%
B. 1–3%
C. 3–5%
D. Up to 10%

Q40: As a practicing physician, it can be difficult to maintain competency in skills necessary for critical care. All of the following are examples of ways to develop or maintain these important skills EXCEPT:

A. Practicing intubation under the direct supervision of an anesthesiologist
B. Participating in a sepsis simulation
C. Completing an online course reviewing the interpretation of electrocardiograms
D. All of the above are examples of ways to maintain critical care skills

Q41: Which of the following is FALSE in regard to a closed ICU?

A. Only critical care attendings or house staff can write orders
B. Considered a type of high-intensity ICU
C. Associated with lower ICU mortality and decreased length of stay
D. Allows any physician to write orders as long as there is an on-site critical care physician to provide consultation

Q42: Which of the following are indications for antepartum fetal surveillance?

A. Hemoglobinopathies
B. Recurrent pregnancy loss
C. Hypothyroidism
D. Dichorionic-diamniotic twin gestation
E. All of the above

Q43: Define obesity.

A. BMI of 25 or more
B. BMI of 30 or more
C. BMI of 35 or more
D. BMI of 40 or more

Q44: Obesity affects fertility in all of the following ways EXCEPT:
A. Oligoovulation
B. Anovulation
C. Decreased response to ovulation induction
D. Anatomic barriers
E. All of the above are causes of infertility

Q45: According to ACOG, preterm labor is defined by which of the following in a 23-year-old G3P2002 at 33/0 weeks gestational age?
A. Symptomatic regular contractions and dilation of more than 1 cm
B. Regular contractions with a cervical dilation of 2/50/-3 stable over 3 h and two cervical exams
C. Regular contractions with a cervical dilation of 1/80/-2 stable over 3 h and two cervical exams
D. A and B
E. All of the above

Q46: A 35-year-old at 28 weeks gestational age is admitted with preterm labor. She is very concerned and asks how certain you are that she will delivery prematurely. What percent of women with the diagnosis of preterm labor give birth within 7 days of initial presentation?
A. 75%
B. 50%
C. 25%
D. 10%

Q47: Obesity during pregnancy is associated with having a higher risk of all of the following EXCEPT:
A. Gestational diabetes
B. Preeclampsia
C. Long labor with more oxytocin use
D. Operative morbidity
E. Spontaneous preterm birth

Q48: Which of the following is TRUE regarding the fetal risks associated with obese patients?

A. Higher risk for fetal cardiac defects in relation to increased risk of maternal diabetes
B. Increased risk of abnormal fetal growth, most commonly small for gestational age
C. The risk for stillbirth is eightfold greater in obese women
D. Infants born to obese women are at an increased risk for future childhood obesity
E. All of the above

Q49: A 17-year-old patient is 6 weeks postpartum from a cesarean section. She had a pregnancy complicated by class III obesity and asks what the best treatment is. You tell her:

A. Bariatric surgery is the most effective treatment for morbid obesity but is contraindicated in adolescents
B. Gastric banding is a malabsorptive procedure that may be an option for her
C. Roux-en-Y is a common procedure and can result in improved quality of life
D. Bariatric surgery is indicated for anyone with a BMI of 35 or more
E. All of the above

Q50: What are the diagnostic criteria for gestational diabetes using Carpenter and Coustan in mg/dL?

A. 100, 180, 150, 130
B. 95, 160, 155, 140
C. 100, 180, 150, 130
D. 95, 180, 155, 140

Q51: Between 1992 and 2013, the rate of cesarean sections ________ and rate of operative vaginal deliveries ________.

A. Increased; decreased
B. Increased; increased

C. Decreased; decreased
D. Decreased; increased

Q52: The choice to use forceps or vacuum extractor depends on the indication for operative delivery.
A. True
B. False

Q53: What cutoff is recommended per ACOG for the 1 h, 50 g glucose challenge?
A. 130
B. 135
C. 140
D. 130 for women who are high risk, 140 for women who are low risk
E. Individual practitioner should select a single consistent cut off

Q54: Pregnancies in women who have had bariatric surgery are at decreased risk for gestational diabetes and preeclampsia only if their postsurgery BMI is below 30.
A. True
B. False

Q55: This virus is transmitted through fecal-oral transmission, is an RNA virus, and does not lead to chronic infection.
A. Hepatitis A
B. Hepatitis B
C. Hepatitis C
D. Hepatitis D
E. Hepatitis B and D

Q56: What is the most common cause of thrombocytopenia during pregnancy?
A. Immune thrombocytopenia purpura (ITP)
B. Gestational thrombocytopenia
C. Pregnancy-induced hypertension (PIH)
D. Pseudothrombocytopenia

Q57: Which of the following would make a diagnosis of gestational thrombocytopenia less likely?
A. A platelet count of 60,000/μL
B. Thrombocytopenia incidentally detected during routine prenatal testing
C. No history of thrombocytopenia prior to pregnancy
D. Platelet count normalizes in the postpartum period
E. All of the above are consistent with gestational thrombocytopenia

Q58: Which psychiatric illness is associated with an increased risk of postnatal death?
A. Anxiety disorders
B. Major depression
C. Bipolar disorder
D. Schizophrenia
E. All of the above

Q59: Which of the following is TRUE in a pregnant woman with an elevated TSH but a normal free T4?
A. Treatment will not improve her pregnancy outcomes
B. Left untreated, she will likely develop overt hypothyroidism
C. Universal prenatal screening for this condition is recommended
D. B and C
E. All of the above

Q60: In which of the following scenarios would an operative vaginal delivery not be contraindicated?
A. A 22-year-old G3P2002 at term with a fetus suspected of having osteogenesis imperfecta
B. A 24-year-old G4P3003 with a term gestation has reached complete dilation and is at +1 station. Fetus is noted to be in occiput posterior position with Category III fetal heart tracing

C. A 27-year-old G2P1001 with term gestation has reached complete dilation though the head is not engaged in the pelvis. Category III fetal heart tracing noted
D. A 21-year-old G1P0 at term with known autosomal dominant bleeding disorder

Q61: Which of the following factors has been associated with an increased rate of failed operative vaginal delivery?
A. Increased birth weight
B. Primigravida
C. Increased duration of second stage of labor
D. Occiput posterior position
E. A and C

Q62: Which of the following pregnant women should have a thyroid laboratory evaluation?
A. A woman with a mildly enlarged thyroid
B. A woman with thyroid nodules
C. A woman with a family history of thyroid disorders
D. A woman with a BMI of 40
E. All of the above

Q63: A patient has bipolar disorder and asks which medication is safest for her to take during pregnancy. You counsel her toward:
A. Lithium
B. Valproic acid
C. Carbamazepine
D. Lamotrigine
E. All of the above have equal risks and benefits

Q64: Which of the following is FALSE regarding recurrent variable decelerations?
A. They are defined by occurring with more than 50% of contractions
B. Moderate variability or accelerations suggest the fetus is not academic

C. Management involves relieving the compression
D. Amnioinfusion decreases their recurrence and the rate of cesarean delivery
E. None of the above

Q65: Attempted ECV is associated with:
A. Lower risk of cesarean section
B. Low Apgar score
C. Low umbilical cord blood pH
D. B and C
E. All of the above

Q66: All of the following occur at rates of less than 1% of ECVs EXCEPT:
A. Fetal heart rate decelerations
B. Abruption
C. Rupture of membranes
D. Umbilical cord prolapse
E. All of the above occurred in less than 1% of cases

Q67: This virus is transmitted through sexual partners or needle sharing, and the intact virus is called the Dane particle.
A. Hepatitis A
B. Hepatitis B
C. Hepatitis C
D. Hepatitis D
E. Hepatitis B and D

Q68: Which of the following defines a modified biophysical profile?
A. Amniotic fluid assessment and nonstress test
B. Fetal breathing and fetal movement
C. Fetal tone and amniotic fluid assessment
D. Any of the above, but only valid in the third trimester

Q69: A 31-year-old G4P3003 presents to your office for umbilical artery Doppler velocimetry. She asks why this is being done. What do you tell her?

A. It is used to assess vascular resistance but correlates poorly with perinatal mortality
B. Abnormal flow is defined as absent or reversed end-diastolic flow
C. It can be used in the fetus with growth restriction or cardiac anomalies
D. B and C
E. All of the above are true

Q70: There is an increased risk of cesarean delivery in late-term and postterm pregnancies.

A. True
B. False

Q71: Membrane sweeping should not be performed in women who are Group B strep positive.

A. True
B. False

Q72: Which types of viral hepatitis can be prevented through vaccination?

A. Hepatitis A and B
B. Hepatitis B and C
C. Hepatitis A and C
D. Hepatitis C and D
E. Only hepatitis B

Q73: Antepartum fetal surveillance should begin:

A. When delivery would be considered for perinatal benefit
B. For most at-risk patients, 32/0 weeks gestation
C. For most at-risk patients, 34/0 weeks gestation
D. A and B
E. A and C

Q74: Your patient presents to clinic complaining of decreased fetal movement at 35 weeks gestation. Her pregnancy is otherwise uncomplicated. A biophysical profile is performed and the result is 8/10. The patient reports return of fetal movement. When should subsequent fetal testing be performed?

A. Weekly until delivery
B. In 1 week and then no further testing required if reassuring
C. No further testing is indicated
D. All of the above are reasonable options

Q75: Early amniocentesis is associated with all of the following, EXCEPT:

A. Increased risk of membrane rupture
B. Increased incidence of club foot
C. Increased risk of culture failure
D. All of the above are true

Q76: A 37-year-old woman presents to your office for her new OB visit. When discussing her specific risk of genetic disorders, it would be most accurate to explain to her:

A. If she has a prior history of having a child with an autosomal trisomy, her risk of recurrence is not increased above her risk based on age
B. Risk of aneuploidy increases with maternal age; however, this correlation is not seen with structural chromosomal abnormalities
C. Paternal age is inconsequential in the discussion of risk of genetic disorders
D. That discussing her screening options for genetic disorders should be deferred until the next visit

Q77: A former sex worker presents as a new patient. A viral hepatitis panel is obtained and results as positive for the viral hepatitis most associated with sexual transmission. What is her risk for long-term consequences?

A. Chronic infection is not a feature of this hepatitis
B. Her risk for chronic infection is 10–15%
C. It is associated with increased risk for hepatocellular carcinoma
D. A and C
E. B and C

Q78: Which of the following has been shown to decrease the risk of macrosomia?

A. Dietary regulation to prevent excess weight gain in nondiabetics
B. Daily exercise starting in the third trimester
C. Insulin therapy for diabetics
D. A and B
E. A and C

Q79: Which of the following is TRUE regarding the recommendations for cesarean delivery based on estimated fetal weight?

A. If the estimated fetal weight in a diabetic mother is above 4000 g, a cesarean delivery should be considered
B. If the estimated fetal weight in a diabetic mother is above 4500 g, a cesarean delivery is required
C. If the estimated fetal weight in a nondiabetic mother is above 4500 g, a cesarean delivery should be considered
D. If the estimated fetal weight in a nondiabetic mother is above 5000 g, a cesarean delivery should be considered
E. B and D

Q80: What are the most commonly used objective pulmonary function parameters used in pregnant patients with asthma?

A. Pulse oximetry and peak expiratory flow rate
B. Pulse oximetry and forced expiratory volume in the first second of inspiration
C. Methacholine challenge testing and peak expiratory flow rate
D. Forced expiratory volume in the first second of inspiration and peak expiratory flow rate

Q81: You counsel your patient that because of her high-risk thrombophilia, she will need to be on prophylactic anticoagulation. Which of the following are acceptable options for her?

A. Enoxaparin 40 mg SC daily
B. Unfractionated heparin 10000 units every 6 h in the third trimester
C. Unfractionated heparin 10000 units every 12 h in the second trimester
D. A and C
E. All of the above are acceptable

Q82: You receive a phone call as triage physician regarding a woman at 22 weeks gestation. She reports that she has tried scheduled doxylamine and pyridoxine; however, she has been unable to keep food down without vomiting for the last 5 days. She is able to tolerate liquids. She asks you if she needs to be admitted to the hospital. How do you respond?

A. Yes, because you have tried medicine and still cannot tolerate food
B. No, because you can still tolerate liquids
C. No, but I can prescribe additional antiemetics to assist you
D. Yes, because if we admit you, we may be able to prevent long-term hospitalization
E. B and C

Q83: A 35-year-old G5P3013 presents reporting that she is currently on therapeutic doses of unfractionated heparin. You are concerned that it may not be therapeutic. When do you measure an aPTT and what is your goal?

A. Check an aPTT 4 h after the injection, goal between 2 and 3
B. Check an aPTT 6 h after the injection, goal between 1.5 and 2.5
C. Check an aPTT just prior to the next injection, goal between 2 and 3
D. Check an aPTT 4 h after the injection, goal between 1.5 and 2.5
E. Check an aPTT 6 h after the injection, goal between 2 and 3

Q84: Hepatitis ____ can only cause disease if the patient is coinfected with hepatitis ___.

A. A; B
B. A; C
C. D; B
D. D; C
E. E; C

Q85: This viral hepatitis, when chronic, is associated with a mortality rate of 25% due to hepatic failure.

A. Hepatitis A
B. Hepatitis B
C. Hepatitis C
D. Hepatitis D
E. Hepatitis B and D

Q86: A pregnant patient has heard about the hepatitis A vaccine and asks if she should receive it. She is an IV drug user and has fatty liver disease. You counsel her:

A. Yes, it is recommended because of her drug use
B. Yes, it is recommended for all pregnant women
C. No, it is contraindicated during pregnancy. She may receive it at her postpartum visit
D. No, because it is contraindicated in patients who have chronic liver disease

Q87: A 26-year-old G2P0101 with a history of preterm birth at 28 weeks due to severe preeclampsia who is found to have a cervical length of 25 mm on her Level I ultrasound at 18 weeks.

A. Start 200 mg vaginal progesterone
B. Continue weekly IM progesterone injections
C. Place cerclage
D. Remeasure cervical length in 2 weeks

Q88: A 27-year-old G3P1101 with a history of preterm birth at 26 weeks who is found to have a cervical length of 24mm on her Level I ultrasound at 18 weeks.

A. Continue weekly IM progesterone injections
B. Place cerclage
C. Remeasure length in 2 weeks
D. A and B
E. A and C

Q89: A general surgery resident is panicked because she just had a needle stick during a surgical case on a patient with known hepatitis B. What should she receive to reduce risk of transmission?

A. Hepatitis B vaccine
B. Immune globulin
C. Hepatitis B vaccine and immune globulin as soon as possible
D. Hepatitis B vaccine and then immune globulin in 14 days
E. No prophylaxis is shows to decrease transmission rates

Q90: A 27-year-old G2P1001 has a fundal height concerning for macrosomia. She has an increased risk for all of the following complications EXCEPT:

A. Postpartum hemorrhage
B. Third- and fourth-degree lacerations
C. Cesarean delivery
D. Labor abnormalities
E. Risk is increased for all of the above

Q91: Which of the following is TRUE regarding brachial plexus injuries associated with macrosomia?

A. Cesarean section prevents brachial plexus injuries
B. 65% are resolved at 1 year of age
C. If there was no shoulder dystocia, the diagnosis of brachial plexus injury is likely false
D. Damage to C5 and C6 can produce Erb-Duchenne paralysis
E. None of the above

Q92: All of the following are symptoms of acute viral hepatitis EXCEPT:

A. Fatigue
B. Fever
C. Nausea
D. Darkened urine
E. Malaise

Q93: Dosing for unfractionated heparin in pregnancy should be twice daily.

A. True
B. False

Q94: What anticoagulation should be used in the case of a patient with heparin-induced thrombocytopenia in pregnancy?

A. Warfarin
B. Low-molecular-weight heparin
C. Fondaparinux
D. B or C
E. Any of the above are reasonable

Q95: This viral hepatitis progresses to a chronic infection in 50% of infected individuals.

A. Hepatitis A
B. Hepatitis B
C. Hepatitis C
D. Hepatitis D
E. Hepatitis B and D

Q96: Your 19-year-old primigravida presents for induction. You recommend a Foley catheter and she is nervous. What do you tell her the advantages are in comparison to other ripening agents?

A. Reduced risk of tachysystole without fetal heart rate changes
B. Painless placement
C. Associated with decreased risk of cesarean when compared to misoprostol
D. Low cost
E. A and D
F. All of the above

Q97: In which of the following scenarios is antibiotic prophylaxis appropriate?

A. To prolong labor in patients with preterm labor and intact membranes
B. For GBS prophylaxis in patients with preterm labor and intact membranes with unknown GBS status
C. For GBS prophylaxis in patients with preterm labor and intact membranes and known GBS-negative status 6 weeks ago
D. B and C
E. All of the above

Q98: Prophylactic antibiotic therapy for endocarditis may be considered for vaginal delivery in patients with the highest risk of adverse outcomes from endocarditis. These patients may include:

A. Patients with mitral valve prolapse
B. Patients with cyanotic cardiac disease
C. Patients with supraventricular tachycardia
D. Patients with atrial fibrillation
E. None of the above because prophylactic antibiotic therapy for endocarditis is no longer recommended in any patient undergoing a vaginal delivery

Q99: Which types of hepatitis are associated with travel?
- A. Hepatitis A and B
- B. Hepatitis B and D
- C. Hepatitis D and E
- D. Hepatitis A and E
- E. Hepatitis B and D

Q100: When is the risk of venous thromboembolism the greatest during pregnancy?
- A. First trimester
- B. Before 20 weeks gestation
- C. Third trimester
- D. After 30 weeks gestation
- E. The risk is the same throughout

Q101: Postpartum anticoagulation may be indicated for low-risk thrombophilias in certain situations even if not recommended antepartum.
- A. True, if they have additional risk factors including obesity or prolonged mobility
- B. True, if they have a history of a first-degree relative with a thrombotic episode before age 50 years
- C. False, if antepartum prophylaxis is not indicated than neither is postpartum prophylaxis
- D. False, anticoagulation is indicated for all low-risk thrombophilias both antepartum and postpartum
- E. A and B

Q102: What is the leading cause of chronic liver disease in the United States?
- A. Pancreatitis
- B. Hepatitis B
- C. Hepatitis C
- D. Alcoholism
- E. Gallstones

Q103: Toxoplasmosis is caused by:
A. A double-stranded DNA virus
B. A single-stranded RNA virus
C. An intracellular parasite
D. A gram-negative bacterium

Q104: Congenital transmission of toxoplasmosis is most likely to occur during the ______ trimester and most likely to cause severe disease if transmitted in the _____trimester.
A. First; first
B. Second; first
C. Third; third
D. Third; first

Q105: A pregnant patient is positive for HBsAg. What is most likely regarding her symptoms?
A. She may not have clinical symptoms yet
B. She may have acute symptoms currently
C. She may be a chronic carrier
D. A and B
E. All of the above

Q106: A 39-year-old G6P1311 presents to your clinic for a new OB visit at 8 weeks gestation. She reports that during her last pregnancy, she had a positive FTS and then had a cell-free fetal DNA test that showed a fetus with Down syndrome. She did not pursue diagnostic testing, and the baby was born with 46XX chromosomes. She conveys how much stress the false-positive cell-free fetal DNA testing caused her and requests counseling regarding what tests she should undergo for this pregnancy. As her provider, your next best step is to:
A. Counsel her regarding her options for screening for aneuploidy and order said tests
B. Refer her to a genetic counselor
C. Refer to a genetic counselor prior to ordering any testing
D. None of the above

Q107: Which of the following syndromes is most commonly missed by ultrasound screening alone?
A. Patau syndrome
B. Edwards syndrome
C. Down syndrome

Q108: Which of the following is TRUE regarding the hepatitis B core antibody?
A. Indicates a natural infection
B. Results in immunity to hepatitis B
C. Signals a chronic infection
D. Signifies evidence of prior vaccination
E. B and D

Q109: Which of the following factors make having a successful TOLAC LESS likely?
A. Indication for previous primary low transverse cesarean section was for non-reassuring fetal heart tones
B. African American ethnicity
C. Short pregnancy interval
D. B and C
E. All of the above

Q110: A patient presents to your office requesting information on TOLAC. She informs you of her previous obstetric history and gives pertinent factors regarding her current pregnancy. Using all this information, you quote her a TOLAC success rate of 55%. Given this, the best way to counsel her is:
A. Inform her that she would be a great candidate to attempt TOLAC
B. Recommend she have a repeat cesarean section given her low chance of success and greater chance of morbidity
C. Inform her that everybody has the same success rate regardless of their past history and she should make her own decision
D. None of the above

Q111: Which of the following are TRUE regarding lamotrigine?

A. It is effective at managing depressive episodes of bipolar depression
B. It should be avoided in the first trimester
C. Folate supplementation of 4 g/day should be offered preconceptually
D. Studies are lacking regarding its efficacy during pregnancy
E. None of the above

Q112: A person infected with parvovirus B19 is no longer infectious to others once a rash has developed.

A. True
B. False

Q113: A patient is considering paying for a nonmedical 3D ultrasound and asks your opinion. You counsel her that performing ultrasounds without a medical indication is:

A. Contrary to responsible medical practice
B. Known to cause fetal harm
C. Appropriate if only for keepsakes and patient is aware they are not for medical use
D. Outside the realm of ACOG recommendations and is a matter of personal preference

Q114: What is the latest gestational age a nuchal translucency should be performed at?

A. 12/0
B. 12/6
C. 13/0
D. 13/6
E. 14/0

Q115: A 39-year-old G3P2002 with 18 week gestation presents to your clinic reporting exposure to parvovirus

B19 with subsequent development of rash and arthritis. Serology studies confirm acute infection revealing:

A. Positive IgM antibodies and IgG antibodies
B. Positive IgM antibodies alone
C. Positive IgG antibodies alone
D. A and B

Q116: A patient has been unable to stop her benzodiazepine during pregnancy. Which potential neonatal syndromes should she be counseled about?

A. Floppy infant syndrome, particularly if she used benzodiazepines during the first trimester
B. Floppy infant syndrome, which is associated with feeding issues and hypothermia
C. Neonatal withdrawal syndrome, which is characterized by hyporeflexia and somnolence
D. Neonatal withdrawal syndrome, which may last up to 3 months postpartum
E. B and D

Q117: Why can results from FISH analysis be obtained within 2 days compared to the 7–14 days needed to complete karyotype analysis?

A. FISH analysis is cheaper and more accessible
B. FISH can be performed on uncultured cells
C. FISH analysis uses probes for specific chromosomes and chromosomal regions
D. None of the above

Q118: What two abnormalities can be detected by karyotype analysis but not chromosomal microarray analysis?

A. Unbalanced translocations and monosomy
B. Balanced translocations and monosomy
C. Unbalanced translations and triploidies
D. Balanced translocations and triploidies

Q119: How long after symptoms start do antibodies to hepatitis C usually appear?
A. 3–5 days
B. 2 weeks
C. 4 weeks
D. 6 weeks
E. 12 weeks

Q120: In general, which of the following is TRUE regarding nausea and vomiting of pregnancy?
A. It is overtreated, and patients should be reassured that 75% of pregnancy women experience nausea
B. Early treatment is recommended to prevent hospitalizations
C. Assessment tools to categorize degree of nausea in a patient can help distinguish who needs treatment
D. It is caused by excessive life stress

Q121: Hyperemesis gravidarum:
A. Is defined by a strict set of criteria involving specific lab abnormalities
B. Has an incidence of approximately 0.1% of pregnancies
C. Is a clinical diagnosis
D. Fifth most common cause of hospitalization during pregnancy

Q122: A pregnant patient has recently been diagnosed with hepatitis B. She asks about long-term consequences. You inform her:
A. Perinatal infection carries a decreased risk for chronic disease of approximately 5%
B. Perinatal infection carries an increased risk for chronic disease of approximately 90%
C. The risk for chronic disease in adults is 30%
D. HBsAg decreases the risk for vertical transmission
E. Vertical transmission risk is greatest if the mother is acutely infected in the first trimester

Q123: A 33-year-old G1P0 is 1 day postpartum and necessitates prophylactic anticoagulation. She is also breastfeeding and asks which medication is safest to use. You counsel her:

A. Only low-molecular-weight heparin is safe to use in women breastfeeding
B. Low-molecular-weight heparin and unfractionated heparin are safe to use in women breastfeeding
C. Low-molecular-weight heparin, unfractionated heparin, and warfarin are all safe to use in women breastfeeding
D. Unfortunately, none of the anticoagulant medications are safe in women who are breastfeeding so she will have to bottle-feed instead

Q124: Babies born to mothers who are HBsAg positive should receive:

A. Hepatitis B vaccine IM immediately
B. Immune globulin IM immediately
C. Hepatitis B vaccine and immune globulin immediately
D. Hepatitis B vaccine and then immune globulin in 14 days
E. No prophylaxis is shown to decrease transmission rates

Q125: Isolated structural birth defects are more common than chromosomal abnormalities.

A. True
B. False

Q126: Which of the following is TRUE regarding isolated structural birth defects?

A. Occur less within an affected family than in the general population
B. Diagnosis is rarely made by ultrasound or other imaging techniques
C. Usually determined by multiple genes in combination with environmental factors
D. Diagnosed using specific DNA methods

Q127: All of the following are associated with an increased risk for vertical transmission of hepatitis C EXCEPT:

A. HIV infection
B. Detectable viremia
C. Prolonged membrane rupture
D. Use of internal fetal monitoring
E. Vaginal delivery

Q128: Which of the following is TRUE regarding parental iron?

A. May be useful in patients with malabsorption syndromes
B. Associated with about a 1% rate of anaphylaxis
C. No significant difference between levels of hemoglobin after 40 days compared to those taking oral supplementation
D. All of the above are true

Q129: Which of the following are indications to screen for gestational diabetes at the first prenatal visit?

A. A BMI of 25 or above
B. A history of gestational diabetes
C. Chronic hypertension
D. A and B
E. All of the above

Q130: Your 25-year-old patient will undergo a primary cesarean section. She weighs 100 kg. What dose of cefazolin should she receive?

A. 1 g
B. 2 g
C. 3 g
D. 4 g

Q131: Iron supplementation does not decrease the prevalence of maternal anemia at the time of delivery.
- A. True
- B. False

Q132: Twins with isolated growth discordance are at no increased risk for morbidity or mortality.
- A. True
- B. False

Q133: IUGR twins have equivalent outcomes to singleton IUGR babies once gestational age is controlled for.
- A. True
- B. False

Q134: Dichorionic-diamniotic twin gestations should undergo growth ultrasounds every 4–6 weeks.
- A. True
- B. False

Q135: Dichorionic-diamniotic twin gestations should undergo antenatal testing starting at 32 weeks gestational age.
- A. True
- B. False

Q136: Which of the following patients should be screened for hepatitis C?
- A. A 19-year-old being treated for her first chlamydia infection
- B. A 45-year-old who has been happily married for 20 years but confesses to use of heroin once at age 19
- C. A 25-year-old who reports a postpartum hemorrhage with her first baby requiring massive transfusion protocol
- D. Any pregnant patient
- E. All of the above should be screened

Q137: A 32-year-old G2P1001 who is found to have a cervical length of 20 mm on her Level I ultrasound at 18 weeks.

A. Start 200 mg vaginal progesterone
B. Place cerclage
C. Remeasure length in 2 weeks
D. Continue routine obstetrical care
E. A and B

Q138: A 33-year-old G1P0 with a twin gestation who is found to have a cervical length of 25 mm on her Level II ultrasound at 18 weeks.

A. Start 200 mg vaginal progesterone
B. Place cerclage
C. Remeasure length in 2 weeks
D. Continue routine obstetrical care for twin gestation
E. A and B

Q139: During what time frame should a woman with a history of preterm birth be initiated on progesterone?

A. Between 12 and 24 weeks gestation
B. Between 18 and 24 weeks gestation
C. Between 16 and 28 weeks gestation
D. Between 16 and 24 weeks gestation
E. Between 12 and 28 weeks gestation

Q140: In which population is vaginal progesterone recommended as a management option to reduce the risk of preterm birth?

A. Asymptomatic women pregnant with a singleton without a history of preterm birth noted to have a shortened cervical length less than 25 mm before 24 weeks gestation
B. Asymptomatic women pregnant with a singleton without a history of preterm birth noted to have a shortened cervical length less than 20 mm before 24 weeks gestation

C. Asymptomatic women pregnant with twins without a history of preterm birth noted to have a shortened cervical length less than 25 mm before 24 weeks gestation
D. A and C
E. All of the above

Q141: What are the two most common causes of anemia in pregnancy and the puerperium period?
A. Hemoglobinopathies and iron deficiency
B. Iron deficiency and hemolysis
C. Acute blood loss and sickle cell anemia
D. Iron deficiency and acute blood loss

Q142: A 20-year-old G1P0 pregnant patient presents complaining of nausea and vomiting. She asks you to discuss the risks and benefits of ondansetron treatment. Which of the following is FALSE?
A. Ondansetron is more effective at decreasing nausea and vomiting than pyridoxine and doxylamine combined
B. High doses should be avoided to decrease the risk of torsades de pointes
C. It has been shown to cause a significant increase in birth defects
D. Continuous infusion pumps are associated with complications in approximately one third of patients
E. All of the above are true

Q143: Which of the following is a side effect of ondansetron?
A. Headache
B. Diarrhea
C. Hyperkalemia
D. Hypocalcemia
E. All of the above

Q144: To decrease risk of perinatal vertical transmission, cesarean delivery should be considered in patients with:

A. Hepatitis A
B. Hepatitis B
C. Hepatitis C
D. All of the above
E. None of the above

Q145: Severe and poorly controlled asthma is associated with all of the following EXCEPT:

A. Maternal morbidity and mortality
B. Prematurity
C. Cesarean delivery
D. Growth restriction
E. None of the above

Q146: In which of the following scenarios is delaying delivery until 38 0/7–39 6/7 weeks recommended?

A. A 24-year-old G1P0 diagnosed with IUGR and oligohydramnios
B. A 32-year-old G2P1001 diagnosed with IUGR and reverse end-diastolic flow on umbilical artery studies
C. A 18-year-old G1P0 diagnosed with IUGR and severe hypertension
D. A 28-year-old G3P2002 with a history of an SGA fetus diagnosed with IUGR and an inherited thrombophilia

Q147: The triple screen has been largely replaced by the quad screen because of its lower sensitivity for which of the following?

A. Open fetal defects
B. Down syndrome
C. Trisomy 13
D. Neural tube defects
E. None of the above

Q148: Ultrasonography is the best method for evaluating a growth-restricted fetus, and growth assessments should be performed every 2 weeks.

A. True
B. False

Q149: Which of the following medications can potentially worsen asthma symptoms during labor and delivery?

A. Indomethacin
B. Magnesium
C. Hemabate
D. A and C
E. All of the above

Q150: A 36-year-old G1P0 at 40 weeks gestation presents to the hospital loss of fluid starting 2 h ago and is confirmed to have rupture of membranes. Sterile vaginal exam is closed/thick/high. The patient reports cramping. Review of patient chart reveals a recent GBS-negative status. Fetus is cephalic and Category 1. The next BEST steps include:

A. Induction of labor
B. Induction of labor and administration of prophylactic antibiotics
C. Expectant management
D. Expectant management and administration of prophylactic antibiotics
E. Induction of labor and cesarean section for failed induction if still in latent phase 10–14 h later

Q151: Which of the following has NOT been shown to be useful in the monitoring of patients with preterm PROM?

A. Maternal temperature assessments
B. Ultrasound monitoring of fetal growth
C. Periodic fetal heart rate monitoring
D. Serial monitoring of maternal leukocyte count
E. None of the above

Q152: To decrease the risk of perinatal vertical transmission, breastfeeding should be avoided in patients with:
A. Hepatitis A
B. Hepatitis B
C. Hepatitis C
D. All of the above
E. None of the above

Q153: A laboring patient is suddenly noted to have fetal heart tones at 100 beats per minute for 3 min. All of the following EXCEPT which could be causative factors?
A. Maternal hypertension
B. Umbilical cord prolapse
C. Uterine rupture
D. Abruption
E. Tachysystole

Q154: In which of the following scenario(s) should a patient receive an additional intraoperative dose of prophylactic antibiotics?
A. A cesarean section that is lengthy
B. A cesarean section with excessive blood loss
C. A cesarean section with meconium noted at the time of delivery
D. A and B
E. All of the above

Q155: Routine screening of obstetric patients for MRSA colonization and subsequent treatment is recommended.
A. True
B. False

Q156: A prolonged deceleration is defined as:
A. A decrease in fetal heart rate of 10 beats per minute from baseline for 5 min
B. A decrease in fetal heart rate of 15 beats per minute from baseline for 2 min

C. A fetal heart rate below 110 beats per minute for 2 min
D. A fetal heart rate below 110 beats per minute for 5 min
E. A fetal heart rate below 110 beats per minute for 10 min

Q157: Which of the following are contraindicated during pregnancy?
A. Hepatitis A vaccine
B. Hepatitis A immune globulin
C. Hepatitis B vaccine
D. Hepatitis B immune globulin
E. None of the above

Q158: Operative vaginal delivery with vacuum should be abandoned after three vacuum detachments even if descent is noted with each pull.
A. True
B. False

For the following questions (159–164), designate the classification of asthma severity:

Q159: Patient reports daily symptoms and nighttime awakening more than once per week.
A. Intermittent (well controlled)
B. Mild persistent (not well controlled)
C. Moderate persistent (not well controlled)
D. Severe persistent (very poorly controlled)

Q160: Patient reports nighttime awakening twice per month and no interference with normal activity.
A. Intermittent (well controlled)
B. Mild persistent (not well controlled)
C. Moderate persistent (not well controlled)
D. Severe persistent (very poorly controlled)

Q161: Patient reports symptoms more than 2 days per week and has minor limitation with normal activity.
A. Intermittent (well controlled)
B. Mild persistent (not well controlled)
C. Moderate persistent (not well controlled)
D. Severe persistent (very poorly controlled)

Q162: Patient only requires albuterol as needed to control symptoms.
A. Intermittent (well controlled)
B. Mild persistent (not well controlled)
C. Moderate persistent (not well controlled)
D. Severe persistent (very poorly controlled)

Q163: Patient reports being prescribed high-dose inhaled corticosteroid and salmeterol in an effort to control symptoms.
A. Intermittent (well controlled)
B. Mild persistent (not well controlled)
C. Moderate persistent (not well controlled)
D. Severe persistent (very poorly controlled)

Q164: Patient reports daily symptoms and awakens at night with symptoms more than once per week but only reports some limitation on normal activity.
A. Intermittent (well controlled)
B. Mild persistent (not well controlled)
C. Moderate persistent (not well controlled)
D. Severe persistent (very poorly controlled)

Q165: What is the next BEST step when a growth-restricted fetus is diagnosed by ultrasound?
A. Repeat the study in a week due to the low sensitivity of ultrasound
B. Perform Doppler blood flow studies of the umbilical artery
C. Give steroids for fetal lung maturity and move toward delivery
D. Order weekly biophysical profiles for the fetus for the remainder of the pregnancy

Q166: What is the risk of recurrence of an SGA birth?
A. 10%
B. 20%
C. 30%
D. 40%

Q167: Which of the following carries the highest risk of transmission by occupational exposure?
A. Hepatitis A
B. Hepatitis B
C. Hepatitis C
D. Hepatitis D
E. HIV

Q168: To rehydrate a woman with hyperemesis gravidarum, what IV fluids should you give her?
A. First dextrose and then vitamins including thiamine
B. First thiamine and then vitamins and dextrose
C. First thiamine and dextrose and then vitamins and dextrose
D. First vitamins and then dextrose and thiamine

Q169: Obstetric lacerations are the most common cause of rectovaginal fistulas in the United States.
A. True
B. False

Q170: How should preterm labor with multifetal gestations be managed?
A. Hold tocolysis regardless of gestational age, give betamethasone if 23–34 weeks gestation, and hold magnesium sulfate for neuroprotection
B. Give tocolysis for steroid benefit, give betamethasone if 23–34 weeks gestation, and hold magnesium sulfate for neuroprotection
C. Give tocolysis for steroid benefit, give betamethasone if 23–34 weeks gestation, and give magnesium sulfate for neuroprotection up to 32 weeks gestation
D. Give magnesium for tocolysis and for neuroprotection up to 32 weeks gestation, and give betamethasone if between 23 and 34 weeks gestation

Q171: A pregnant patient has tried medical management and despite this is unable to maintain her weight. She begins to ask about other ways of getting nutrition. How do you counsel her?

A. Enteral nutrition is associated with sepsis and thromboembolic events
B. Enteral nutrition is not well tolerated during pregnancy
C. Enteral nutrition is indicated in her case
D. Parenteral nutrition is the preferred method
E. C and B

Q172: A Rh-negative woman should be screened for antibodies at all of the following times EXCEPT:

A. Prior to anti-D immune globulin at 28 weeks gestation
B. Postpartum
C. Abruption
D. Subsequent pregnancies
E. All of the above are recommended

Q173: A 33-year-old G3P2002 with intrauterine pregnancy at 21 weeks gestation presents to the emergency department with confirmed rupture of membranes. She is afebrile without evidence of infection. Fetal heart tones auscultated.

A. Immediate delivery should be offered
B. Outpatient surveillance should be offered
C. Latency antibiotic administration can be considered
D. A and C
E. All of the above are true

Q174: Patients with a previous history of preterm PROM with subsequent preterm birth are known to have an increased risk of recurrent preterm PROM and preterm delivery. Which of the following intervention(s) may be helpful to prevent recurrence?

A. Progesterone supplementation starting at 16–24 weeks gestation
B. Daily administration of ASA 81 mg with confirmation of fetal heart tones

C. Prophylactic cerclage placement
D. Progesterone supplementation starting with conception up to 10 weeks gestation
E. A and B
F. A, B, and C

Q175: Your 33-year-old G4P3003 with gestational diabetes controlled with insulin is concerned because her friend mentioned she may need a cesarean section if her baby gets too big. Which of the following is TRUE?
A. Fetal growth will be assessed by clinical exam or by ultrasound to identify macrosomia
B. Fifty-eight cesarean sections for an estimated fetal weight of 4500 g to prevent a single case of permanent brachial plexus palsy
C. Given the risks and benefits, women with gestational diabetes should be offered a cesarean section if the estimated fetal weight is 4500 g or more
D. A and B
E. A and C

Q176: Mediolateral episiotomy is associated with a ____ in third- and fourth-degree lacerations and an _____ likelihood of perineal pain.
A. Increase, increased
B. Decrease, increased
C. Increase, decreased
D. Decrease, decreased

Q177: The intern calls request assistance in the evaluation of a laceration following delivery. On exam, a hemostatic laceration on the labia that distorts the anatomy and a hemostatic first-degree laceration are noted. How should you proceed?
A. Repair the labial laceration to make it heal faster, and repair the first degree as sexual activity will be able to be resumed sooner
B. Do not repair either; there has been no evidence to support repair of lacerations that are hemostatic

C. Repair the labial laceration to restore anatomy, and repair the first degree as recommended by ACOG
D. Repair the labial laceration to restore anatomy, and defer repair on the first degree as it is hemostatic

Q178: Your 30-year-old patient presents for her postpartum checkup. Her pregnancy was complicated by gestational diabetes. All of the following are true EXCEPT:
A. She will need to be screened at this visit for diabetes or impaired fasting glucose
B. Fasting plasma glucose is less sensitive; hence, the 2 h glucose test is recommended
C. If she is found to have a normal screen, she should have her glycemic status assessed every 3 years
D. All of the above are true

Q179: A patient is Rh negative and known to be sensitized. She is counseled regarding titers. She read on the Internet about a "critical titer" and asks what it means. You tell her:
A. A critical titer is associated with a significant risk for severe erythroblastosis fetalis and hydrops
B. In most centers, it is between 8:1 and 32:1
C. Titers are reported as the lowest dilution with a positive agglutination reaction
D. A and C
E. B and C

Q180: Which of the following is TRUE regarding the commonly used terms "small for gestational age (SGA)" and "intrauterine growth restriction (IUGR)"?
A. SGA refers to a fetus in utero
B. IUGR is defined as a fetus with an estimated fetal weight of less than the fifth percentile for gestational age
C. The terms are interchangeable
D. SGA refers to a newborn whose birth weight is less than the 10% for gestational age

Q181: Which of the following are NOT associated with IUGR, preeclampsia, and fetal death in absence of structural abnormalities?

A. Elevated AFP
B. Elevated inhibin-A
C. Elevated unconjugated estriol
D. Elevated b-hCG

Q182: Which of the following maternal disorders have been associated with IUGR or SGA?

A. Hypertension
B. Hereditary thrombophilias
C. Antiphospholipid syndrome
D. A and C
E. All of the above

Q183: All of the following have been associated with IUGR and SGA EXCEPT:

A. Tobacco use during pregnancy
B. Extremely poor protein intake in the third trimester
C. Multiple gestation
D. Intrauterine infection
E. All of the above are true

Q184: A new obstetric patient presents for her initial visit. This is her first pregnancy, and review of her record reveals she is an insulin-dependent type II diabetic. She asks what changes she should expect in her insulin dosing during the pregnancy. You counsel her:

A. Her insulin dosage will increase until 28 weeks and then return to baseline
B. Her insulin dosage will increase throughout pregnancy, though most rapidly at about 30 weeks gestation
C. Her insulin dosage will increase throughout pregnancy, though most rapidly at about 20 weeks gestation
D. Her insulin dosage will gradually increase throughout pregnancy

Q185: There is evidence of increased neonatal morbidity associated with failed operative vaginal delivery followed by cesarean section in comparison to cesarean section or operative delivery alone.

A. True
B. False

Q186: Which of the following is an example of how regular insulin differs from insulin lispro?

A. Regular insulin carries a greater risk of hypoglycemia
B. Lispro should be taken 30 min prior to eating
C. Lispro has improved compliance and patient satisfaction
D. A and C
E. None of the above

Q187: Which of the following describes the correct repair of a cervical laceration?

A. A 3-0 polyglactin suture should be placed above the apex of the laceration. Running suture should then be continued incorporating half the thickness of the cervix
B. A 2-0 polyglactin suture should be placed above the apex of the laceration. Running locking suture should then be continued incorporating full thickness of the cervix
C. A 3-0 polyglactin suture should be placed at the apex of the laceration. Running suture should then be continued incorporating half the thickness of the cervix
D. A 2-0 polyglactin suture should be placed at the apex of the laceration. Running suture should then be continued incorporating half the thickness of the cervix
E. None of the above

Q188: Which of the following is TRUE regarding the ability of ultrasound to predict macrosomia?

A. The estimated fetal weight would need to exceed 4800 to have more than a 50% chance of being macrosomic
B. Hadlock's formula is most accurate in estimating fetal weight in the macrosomic fetus
C. The utility of ultrasound for obtaining fetal weight is operator and equipment dependent
D. Abdominal circumference is most predictive of macrosomia
E. None of the above

Q189: Twins are considered discordant when there is a 25% difference in fetal weight between larger and smaller fetus.

A. True
B. False

Q190: A 41-year-old G1P0 without diabetes has an estimated fetal weight of 5000 g on the day of her induction. She asks about a cesarean section. How do you counsel her?

A. A cesarean delivery is required given risk of brachial plexus injury of 30%
B. A cesarean section should be considered given brachial plexus injury rate of 10%
C. A cesarean delivery should not be offered given emphasis on preventing the primary cesarean section
D. None of the above are true
E. All of the above are reasonable

Q191: All of the following are important considerations in repairing the external anal sphincter EXCEPT:

A. Care should be taken to suture just the muscle, not the fascial sheath
B. End-to-end repair is most appropriate for 3a and 3b sphincter injuries

C. Allis clamps may be necessary to grasp the edges of the sphincter
D. 2-0 or 3-0 suture is recommended
E. For full-thickness external anal sphincter lacerations, either end-to-end or overlap repair is reasonable

Q192: Your 19-year-old primigravida presents for induction. You recommend a prostaglandin and she is nervous. What do you tell her the advantages are?
A. Likelihood of delivery within 24 h is increased compared with oxytocin alone
B. Decreased risk of cesarean section
C. Decreased risk of tachysystole with fetal heart rate changes
D. A and B
E. All of the above

Q193: Which of the following may decrease patient pain following OASIS repair?
A. Topical anesthetics
B. Local cooling treatments
C. Rectal suppositories
D. A and B
E. All of the above

Q194: A patient presents to clinic to establish prenatal care. She reports a history of a fourth-degree laceration with her previous delivery and requests a cesarean delivery with this pregnancy. What aspect of her history would justify this?
A. Reported anal incontinence
B. Reported need for repeat laceration repair
C. Reported psychological trauma from event
D. A and B
E. Any of the above could be indications for a cesarean delivery

Q195: At least one third of patients with a neural tube defect have a severe allergy to:
A. Penicillin
B. Latex

C. Sulfa
D. Peanuts

Q196: Patients with gestational diabetes should ideally have a caloric allotment of:
A. Carbohydrates 40%, protein 20%, fat 40%
B. Carbohydrates 60%, protein 20%, fat 20%
C. Carbohydrates 40%, protein 40%, fat 20%
D. Carbohydrates 60%, protein 30%, fat 10%
E. ACOG does not have a formal recommendation

Q197: Which of the following is FALSE in measuring amniotic fluid index (AFI)?
A. The width of the pocket must be 2 cm
B. ACOG favors using deepest vertical pocket to diagnose oligohydramnios
C. The transducer should be perpendicular to the floor
D. The maximum vertical pocket should be used in multiple pregnancies
E. None of the above

Q198: What percentage of fetuses with increased nuchal translucency will have a chromosomal abnormality?
A. 10%
B. 25%
C. 33%
D. 50%

Q199: Which of the following is TRUE regarding the initiation of pharmacologic treatment of gestational diabetes?
A. There is consensus regarding thresholds for starting medical therapy
B. Insulin and oral medications are equivalent in efficacy
C. Insulin and oral medications can be appropriate first-line therapy
D. Traditionally, insulin is standard therapy and is started if fasting or postprandials are persistently elevated
E. All of the above

Q200: What percent of neural tube defects occur in families with a positive family history?

A. 5%
B. 10%
C. 30%
D. 40%

Q201: Chronic immune thrombocytopenia is classified by a duration of symptoms:

A. Greater than 6 months
B. Greater than 8 months
C. Greater than 10 months
D. Greater than 12 months
E. Greater than three episodes requiring hospitalization

Q202: All of the following are examples of secondary causes of immune thrombocytopenia EXCEPT:

A. Systemic lupus erythematosus
B. Disseminated intravascular coagulation
C. Infection with human immunodeficiency virus
D. Drug-induced thrombocytopenia
E. Preeclampsia

Q203: Which of the following patients is at risk for developing an epidural or spinal hematoma following placement of regional anesthesia?

A. A patient who received their last dose of prophylactic low-molecular-weight heparin 8 h ago
B. A patient on unfractionated heparin with a normal activated partial thromboplastin time
C. A patient with a platelet count of 100,000/uL
D. A patient on low-dose aspirin

Q204: Which of the following is TRUE regarding dosage of insulin?
A. Typical starting dosage is 0.7–1.0 units/day given in divided doses
B. Insulin lispro has a peak action of 1–2 h and therefore may be helpful in postprandial glucose control
C. Insulin glargine has a peak action of 12 h
D. Insulin crosses the placenta
E. All of the above

Q205: Which of the following is TRUE regarding the usage of glyburide and metformin in gestational diabetes?
A. They are both FDA approved for this indication and can be considered for glycemic control in gestational diabetes
B. Metformin increases insulin secretion and insulin sensitivity of peripheral tissues
C. Glyburide should not be used in patients with a sulfa allergy
D. Glyburide inhibits hepatic gluconeogenesis and glucose absorption
E. All of the above are true

Q206: Depending on the type of anesthesia provided during labor and delivery, initiation of breastfeeding may need to be delayed.
A. True
B. False

Q207: Labor induction for suspected macrosomia is an effective strategy for decreasing the risk of shoulder dystocia.
A. True
B. False

Q208: She returns to your clinic pregnant and asks which interventions are most useful in avoiding excessive gestational weight gain. Which of the following appears to be most effective?

A. Dietary control
B. Exercise
C. None of the above

Q209: In a randomized controlled trial, interventions were able to reduce the risk of gestational weight gain by 20%. Which outcomes were also improved?

A. Decreased cesarean section rates
B. Decreased risk of preterm delivery
C. Decreased risk of macrosomia in obese women
D. Decreased risk of macrosomia in overweight women
E. All of the above

Q210: Outpatient cervical ripening with a PGE2 controlled release in the outpatient setting is currently not supported by ACOG as more research needs to be done.

A. True
B. False

Q211: What is the percent likelihood that after a patient is admitted for preterm labor she will ultimately deliver at term?

A. 75%
B. 50%
C. 25%
D. 10%

Q212: A 30-year-old G3P0202 at 30 weeks gestational age calls your office. She reports becoming increasingly nervous as she gave birth at 32 weeks in her previous pregnancy. She asks if she should go on bed rest and abstain from sexual activities. How should you counsel her?

A. Tell her to go on bed rest but that she may continue sexual activity
B. Tell her there is no need to go on bed rest but that she should abstain from sexual activity

C. Inform her that neither has been proven to be effective
D. Advise her that neither can hurt and with her history she should play it safe

Questions 213–214 pertain to the same patient:

Q213: A 31-year-old G3P2002 with intrauterine gestation at 16 weeks has recently confirmed acute toxoplasmosis infection. Spiramycin is immediately prescribed to the mother. You explain to your patient that the medication:
A. Reduces transplacental parasitic transfer
B. Does not readily cross the placenta
C. Cannot prevent fetal infection
D. A and B
E. All of the above

Q214: Which of the following are appropriate recommendations for pregnant patients to prevent toxoplasmosis infection?
A. Avoid consuming undercooked meat or dairy products
B. Avoid working in the soil without gloves
C. Avoid handling cat litter
D. A and C
E. All of the above

Q215: You are just starting an induction on your G3P002 patient. Her cervix is 4/80/-1, and you tell her your plans to start oxytocin at 2 mU/min and increase by 2 every half hour. She asks about a high-dose protocol and mentions her nurse friend told her about it. How do you counsel her?
A. High-dose regimens are associated with shorter labor and less frequent cases of chorioamnionitis
B. High-dose regimens are associated with increased rates of cesarean section for dystocia
C. High-dose protocol is not currently recommended
D. A and C
E. All of the above

Q216: You attempt an ECV on your patient, however, are unsuccessful. Which of the following are acceptable options?

A. Schedule a cesarean section at 39 weeks gestation with plans to confirm breech prior to the surgery
B. Schedule a retrial of ECV prior to delivery planning
C. Monitor through 41 weeks for spontaneous version with plans to deliver by cesarean section then if still breech
D. A and C
E. All of the above

Q217: In general, it is recommended that a platelet transfusion be employed in patients undergoing cesarean delivery to increase the count above ___________ prior to surgery.

A. 10,000/μL
B. 30,000/μL
C. 50,000/μL
D. 70,000/μL

Q218: What treatment modality is an option for the management of patients with ITP if first-line treatment fails?

A. Platelet transfusion
B. Intravenous steroids
C. Intravenous immunoglobulins
D. Splenectomy

Q219: Which of the following patients would NOT be a candidate for an ECV?

A. A 29-year-old G2P1001 at 37/3 weeks gestation with a previous classical cesarean section
B. A 37-year-old G1P0 with a BMI of 40 at 38 weeks gestation
C. A 23-year-old G2P1001 at 40/3 weeks gestation presenting with contractions and I kept found to be 3 cm dilated
D. A and C
E. None of the above would be candidates

Q220: Prophylactic cesarean section should be considered for estimated fetal weights greater than 5000 g in women without diabetes.

A. True
B. False

Q221: What is the risk of vertical transmission at the time of delivery with primary and recurrent HSV, respectively?

A. 30–50%; 3%
B. 50–70%; 6%
C. 20–40%; 3%
D. 30–50%; 6%

Q222: A single course of corticosteroids can be considered in women as early as _____ weeks gestation in the setting of preterm PROM.

A. 20 weeks gestation
B. 21 weeks gestation
C. 22 weeks gestation
D. 23 weeks gestation
E. 24 weeks gestation

Q223: For women at higher risk of having a fetus affected with a neural tube defect, what is the daily recommended folic acid intake?

A. 400 mg
B. 4 mg
C. 40 mg
D. 4 g

Q224: Your patient asks about the possibility of using methylprednisolone to decrease her nausea and vomiting of pregnancy. You tell her that it is effective and:

A. It should only be used in the third trimester to decrease the risk of anomalies
B. If no improvement is seen after 3 days of use, the dose should be increased
C. It is associated with fetal cardiac defects

D. It should only be used in refractory patients as a last resort treatment
E. All of the above

Q225: Delayed pushing has been shown to:
A. Decrease third- and fourth-degree lacerations
B. Decrease operative deliveries
C. Decrease the risk of lacerations requiring repair
D. Decrease rates of episiotomy
E. None of the above

Q226–228: In uncomplicated pregnancies, choose the latest recommended gestational age to deliver at:

Q226: Dichorionic-diamniotic twin gestations
A. 34 weeks
B. 35 weeks
C. 36 weeks
D. 37 weeks
E. 38 weeks
F. 39 weeks

Q227: Monochorionic-diamniotic twin gestations
A. 34 weeks
B. 35 weeks
C. 36 weeks
D. 37 weeks
E. 38 weeks
F. 39 weeks

Q228: Monochorionic-monochorionic twin gestations
A. 34 weeks
B. 35 weeks
C. 36 weeks

D. 37 weeks
E. 38 weeks
F. 39 weeks

Q229: Episiotomy is indicated in which of the following situations?
A. Routine use is advocated
B. Shoulder dystocia
C. Vacuum-assisted vaginal delivery
D. Restricted use is recommended
E. B and C

Q230: Which of the following medications are contraindicated for patients taking ondansetron?
A. Diuretics
B. Metronidazole
C. HIV protease inhibitors
D. Oxycodone
E. All of the above

Q231: How can dyspnea of pregnancy be differentiated from a new diagnosis of asthma during pregnancy?
A. Dyspnea of pregnancy is not associated with a cough
B. Dyspnea of pregnancy often has evidence of airway obstruction
C. Dyspnea of pregnancy does not exhibit wheezing on auscultation
D. A and C
E. All of the above

Q232: The risk of a fetus developing congenital varicella syndrome is high.
A. True
B. False

Q233: A 25-year-old G1P0 is noted to develop a maculopapular rash and vesicles 24 h after vaginally delivering a term infant. You counsel her:

A. There is no need for concern since her infant has already been delivered
B. Her infant is at risk of developing neonatal varicella-zoster virus infection which has a high neonatal death rate
C. Her infant may have been exposed to varicella zoster but the robust neonatal immune system will likely prevent infection from developing
D. As long as the patient is placed in isolation from her infant until her vesicles resolve, the infant should be safe from developing infection

Q234: How should a patient be counseled regarding the use of allergen immunotherapy during pregnancy?

A. Allergen immunotherapy should be immediately discontinued upon confirmation of pregnancy due to risk of anaphylaxis
B. If a patient is tolerating allergen immunotherapy prior to pregnancy, increasing the dose generally provides improve control
C. Due to the benefit of allergen immunotherapy, it is reasonable to start therapy while pregnant
D. The risk of anaphylaxis associated with allergen immunotherapy is a reason not to initiate therapy during pregnancy

Q235: A successful VBAC can have several advantages for patients in comparison to a scheduled repeat cesarean section, including:

A. Lower rates of hemorrhage
B. Shorter recovery period
C. Lower rates of infection

D. B and C
E. All of the above

Q236: A patient presents to your clinic requesting information regarding the success rates of TOLAC. Without knowing anything about the patient, it would be reasonable to tell her that success rate ranges between:
A. 40 and 50%
B. 50 and 70%
C. 60 and 80%
D. 70 and 90%

Q237: Your pregnant patient has epilepsy and is taking carbamazepine. What is she at an increased risk for?
A. Fetal neural tube defects
B. Increased seizure activity due to folic acid supplementation
C. Both of the above
D. None of the above

Q238: Which of the following is FALSE regarding a limited obstetric ultrasound examination?
A. Performed when a specific question requires investigation
B. Can be used to confirm fetal presentation
C. Can only be performed in the second or third trimester
D. Does not replace a standard examination
E. None of the above

Q239: First-trimester ultrasound is performed before 12/0 weeks gestation, can be performed transabdominally or transvaginally, and should include an evaluation of the uterus and cervix.
A. True
B. False

Q240: Regarding regional anesthesia during ECV attempts, which is true?
A. Data supports its utility in increasing success
B. Data are inconclusive
C. Data does not support its use

Q241: The recommendation that a single dose of antibiotics should be given for repair of an OASIS is based on what evidence?
A. Cohort investigation
B. Randomized controlled trial
C. Retrospective case series
D. Expert opinion

Q242: Following repair of an OASIS, a patient should be counseled regarding the ______ risk of wound infection.
A. 3%
B. 5%
C. 10%
D. 15%
E. 20%

Q243: Choose the correct sequence for performing an ECV:
A. Informed consent; elevate breech fetal part; attempt forward roll; NST
B. NST; informed consent; attempt forward roll; elevate breech fetal part; NST
C. NST; informed consent; elevate breech fetal part; attempt forward roll
D. NST; informed consent; elevate breech fetal part; attempt forward roll; NST

Q244: A 32-year-old G2P0101 at 27 weeks gestation is admitted for suspected preterm labor as a transfer. She has received butorphanol, betamethasone, and magnesium at the outside hospital. On initial monitor, the fetus has a baseline of 140 with minimal variability, no accelerations, and no decelerations. You suspect the minimal variability is likely due to maternal medications or a fetal sleep cycle. How do you proceed?

A. Expectant management for up to 60 min
B. Proceed with scalp stimulation
C. Proceed with maternal repositioning and administration of oxygen and IV fluids
D. B and C
E. Any of the above are appropriate

Questions 245–250 all refer to the same patient:

Q245: A 25-year-old G2P1001 comes to your office for her first prenatal visit. Her BMI is 41. What class of obesity is she?

A. Class I
B. Class II
C. Class III
D. Class IV

Q246: Based on her obesity, she has an increased risk of all of the following EXCEPT:

A. Spontaneous abortion
B. Fetal gastroschisis
C. Fetal neural tube defects
D. Fetal limb reduction
E. Her risk for all of the above is increased

Q247: Her first delivery was a cesarean section, and she asks you about the possibility of a trial of labor after cesarean section. How do you counsel her on her risks compared to a nonobese woman?

A. Her risk of maternal morbidity is increased
B. She has an equal chance of having a successful vaginal delivery
C. Her risk of neonatal injury is increased
D. A and C
E. All of the above

Q248: Which of the following is TRUE regarding her risk of stillbirth?

A. Antepartum surveillance has been shown to improve outcomes
B The risk for stillbirth increases with each class of obesity
C. Her risk of stillbirth decreases at term; thus, she should be induced due to her obesity
D. Obese women are 30% more likely to experience stillbirth than nonobese women
E. All of the above are true

Q249: Which of the following are potential consequences for her baby?

A. Fetal macrosomia
B. Impaired fetal growth
C. Childhood obesity
D. A and C
E. All of the above

Q250: Postpartum she is at increased risk for which of the following?

A. Postpartum depression
B. Mastitis
C. Retained products of conception
D. A and B

Q251: A 27-year-old G3P2002 presents to your office distraught because the thyroid ultrasound you ordered showed a nodule which is suspicious for malignancy. Which of the following are true?

A. Fine needle aspiration is the next step in diagnosis
B. Thyroid cancer is generally an extremely aggressive cancer
C. Radioiodine scanning should be utilized to aid in diagnosis
D. Surgery should always be postponed until postpartum if needed

Q252: Your patient presents to her postpartum visit and you suspect postpartum thyroiditis. After confirming the diagnosis with labs, how will you treat her?

A. Methimazole then T4 replacement
B. Beta blockers then T4 replacement
C. Propylthiouracil then T4 replacement
D. T4 replacement then propylthiouracil
E. T4 replacement then methimazole

Q253: Which of the following is associated with the lowest risk of aneuploidy?

A. Thickened nuchal fold
B. Echogenic bowel
C. Renal pelvis dilation
D. Echogenic intracardiac focus
E. They are all equally associated with aneuploidy

Q254: For which of the following isolated findings are follow-up ultrasounds recommended?

A. Echogenic bowel
B. Renal pelvis dilation
C. Echogenic intracardiac focus
D. A and B
E. A and C

Q255: A 25-year-old patient will undergo a primary cesarean section. She weighs 100 kg. In planning for her surgery, you remember:

A. The best incision for primary cesarean sections in obese women is a vertical midline
B. Drains should be left in place if there is 4 cm or more of subcutaneous tissue
C. The subcutaneous tissue should be closed if it is greater than 2 cm
D. A and B
E. A and C

Q256: Your patient with postpartum thyroiditis would like to know how long her condition will last. You tell her:

A. The hyperthyroid phase generally lasts 6–12 months
B. The hypothyroid phase generally lasts 6–12 months
C. One half of patients develop overt hypothyroidism
D. All of the above are true

Q257: Tachysystole is defined as:

A. Five or more contractions over 10 min averaged over 20 min
B. More than five contractions over 10 min averaged over 20 min
C. Five or more contractions over 10 min averaged over 30 min
D. More than five contractions over 10 min averaged over 30 min

Q258: Your patient was just told that her fetus has a neural tube defect. She inquires about fetal surgery. Which of the following is FALSE?

A. It significantly raises the risk for preterm labor
B. It is currently considered investigational
C. Studies show an increased rate of hindbrain herniation
D. Patients require delivery by cesarean section if they proceed with the surgery
E. All of the above are true

Q259: Which of the following is TRUE regarding first-trimester screening in obese women?

A. The detection rate for trisomy 18 is decreased by analyte screening
B. It is equally as effective in women who are obese as those who are not
C. The detection of neural tube defects is decreased with analyte screening
D. Nuchal fold measurements are not affected by obesity
E. All of the above are true

Q260: Which of the following is true in the setting of preterm PROM?

A. Prophylactic tocolysis is associated with a longer latency period
B. Prophylactic tocolysis increases risk of chorioamnionitis
C. Prophylactic tocolysis is not recommended in preterm PROM
D. A and B
E. All of the above

Q261: Administration of magnesium for neuroprotection should be considered in preterm PROM patients:

A. At less than 28 weeks gestational age
B. At less than 30 weeks gestational age
C. At less than 32 weeks gestational age
D. At less than 34 weeks gestational age

Q262: Your patient complains of daytime sleepiness, and you suspect she may have obstructive sleep apnea. If she does, which of the following does she have an increased risk of?

A. Preeclampsia
B. In-hospital mortality
C. Cardiomyopathy
D. A and B
E. All of the above

Q263: A 28-year-old G2P1001 presents for her first obstetrical visit in the first trimester. In review of her history, you note that her last delivery was complicated by a shoulder dystocia. The patient reports that her newborn suffered no long-term complications from the delivery. She is now asking you what mode of delivery you recommend for her current pregnancy. You counsel her:

A. Due to the increased risk of recurrence, she should undergo primary cesarean section for delivery
B. As the true risk of recurrence is unknown, depending on the factors present at her previous delivery and how this pregnancy progresses, it may be reasonable to have vaginal delivery or cesarean section
C. As the true risk of recurrence is unknown, she should undergo a vaginal delivery
D. Since there is no increased risk of recurrence, she should undergo a vaginal delivery

Q264: Ideal timing for ECV is based on all of the following EXCEPT:

A. The fetus is unlikely to spontaneously turn to vertex after this gestation
B. After a successful version, the fetus is unlikely to spontaneously turn to breech at this gestation
C. If complications necessitate delivery, there is low fetal morbidity at given gestation
D. All of the above are true

Q265: A 26-year-old G3P2002 at 36/0 weeks gestation presents to your office for routine prenatal care. On ultrasound, her fetus is breech. She has had one previous term cesarean section and one successful VBAC and strongly desires a vaginal delivery. How should you counsel her?

A. ECV is known to be higher risk in patients with previous cesarean section
B. ECV is thought to be safe only if attempted prior to the start of labor

C. Small studies show no increased rate in adverse events in ECV in patients with previous cesarean section
D. ECV success rates are lower in patients with prior cesarean section

Q266: What is the intended goal of obtaining an anesthesia consultation antepartum?
A. To help streamline the flow of patients on labor and delivery
B. To help reduce the risk of anesthesia complications in certain patients
C. To educate patients regarding their anesthesia options during labor and delivery
D. All of the above

Q267: Which of the following antibiotics do not cross the placenta adequately?
A. Aminoglycosides and azithromycin
B. Clindamycin and ampicillin
C. Erythromycin and cephalosporin
D. Azithromycin and erythromycin

Q268: Fetal parvovirus infection is diagnosed. What specific ultrasound measurement will be important in monitoring for signs of developing sequelae?
A. Femur length
B. Biparietal diameter
C. Umbilical artery systolic to diastolic ratio
D. Middle cerebral artery Doppler assessment

Q269: Administration of varicella-zoster immune globulin (VZIG) should be considered in the following situation(s):
A. To an infant when maternal infection develops 36 h following delivery
B. To a nonimmune pregnant mother who has been exposed to someone with active varicella-zoster infection within the past 5 days

C. To a pregnant mother who has personal history of varicella-zoster infection as a child who has been exposed to someone with active varicella zoster within the past 2 days
D. A and B
E. All of the above

Q270: It is reasonable to increase single-dose preoperative antibiotic prophylaxis in patients with a BMI of:
A. BMI > 25
B. BMI > 30
C. BMI > 35
D. BMI > 40

Q271: A 32-year-old G3P2002 presents to the office as a transfer of care for pregnancy. She is Rh negative and is found to be alloimmunized. She is newly married and does not know the blood type of her husband. What is the next best step?
A. Schedule serial titers
B. Order assessment of the peak systolic velocity in the fetal middle cerebral artery
C. Obtain paternal genotype
D. A and C
E. A and B

Q272: What is the preferred method to analyze cells from cases of fetal death or still birth?
A. FISH
B. Karyotype analysis
C. Chromosomal microarray analysis
D. No single method is preferred

Q273: Which of the following statements is FALSE regarding chromosomal microarray analysis?
A. Should not be the primary diagnostic test offered for a fetal structural anomaly detected by ultrasound
B. Low-level mosaicism may not be identified

C. Best suited to detect copy number variants in the fetus
D. Results can be obtained within 3–7 days

Q274: A 40-year-old G2P1001 presents at 28 weeks gestation with complaints of acute abdominal pain. Upon review of her surgical history, it is noted that she has had bariatric surgery and a previous cesarean section. Which of the following is she at increased risk for?
A. Uterine rupture
B. Gastrointestinal hemorrhage
C. Intestinal obstruction
D. A and C
E. All of the above

Q275: A 37-year-old with polycystic ovarian syndrome is referred to you. She reports taking metformin but denies a history of diabetes. How do you counsel her?
A. Metformin should be stopped now as it was only helpful in achieving pregnancy
B. Metformin should be continued until the end of the first trimester
C. Metformin should be continued throughout the entire pregnancy given her diagnosis of polycystic ovarian syndrome
D. Metformin should be continued and patient can defer screening for gestational diabetes

Q276: A 24-year-old women presents for her Level I ultrasound at which time her fetus is noted to have a major structural abnormality that is not strongly suggestive of a particular aneuploidy. What is the BEST next step?
A. CVS with karyotype analysis with or without FISH should be offered
B. Amniocentesis with karyotype analysis with or without FISH should be offered

C. CVS with chromosomal microarray should be offered
D. Amniocentesis with chromosomal microarray should be offered

Q277: Which of the following is FALSE regarding treatment options for gestational diabetes?
A. Glyburide, metformin, and insulin are all acceptable first-line treatments
B. Glyburide may be superior to metformin in that less women require the addition of insulin
C. Glyburide is known to cross the placenta, as opposed to insulin, which does not
D. Insulin can be added to both metformin and glyburide if needed
E. All of the above are true

Q278: A 17-year-old patient recently underwent bariatric surgery. At her annual exam, you counsel her:
A. Expert opinion recommends waiting 6 months after surgery before attempting pregnancy
B. Oral contraceptives are safe and effective in the absence of uncontrolled hypertension
C. Were she to become pregnant, growth ultrasounds should be considered
D. Adolescents after bariatric surgery are still at lower risk for pregnancy than the general adolescent population
E. All of the above

Q279: At what gestational ages should steroid administration be considered?
A. 23/0–36/6 weeks gestational age
B. 24/0–33/6 weeks gestational age
C. 23/0–33/6 weeks gestational age
D. 24/0–36/6 weeks gestational age

Q280: A patient presents to triage at 29 weeks gestational age and is found to be in preterm labor. Betamethasone is administered and a tocolytic is started. Eleven hours later, she has progressed to 8/100/-1. A medical student asks if we can administer the second dose of steroids 12 h after the first. What is your response?

A. There is no proven benefit; hence, second dose will not be given early despite probable imminent delivery
B. Yes, it is called accelerated dosing. Please notify nursing and I'll place the order

Q281: What is the risk of thrombosis in pregnancy or postpartum in women who have APS?

A. Less than 1%
B. 10%
C. 25%
D. 50%
E. None of the above

Q282: Delivery via cesarean section is safer for the fetus in patients with maternal ITP.

A. True
B. False

Q283: What defines a "high-risk" pregnancy for intracranial hemorrhage?

A. Fetal platelet count less than 30,000/μL at 30 weeks of gestation
B. History of a sibling with a perinatal intracranial hemorrhage
C. Fetal platelet count less than 20,000/μL at 20 weeks of gestation
D. B and C
E. All of the above

Q284: Which method of amniotic fluid measurement is associated with a reduction in unnecessary interventions without an increase in adverse perinatal outcomes?

A. Measurement of a 2 cm by 2 cm pocket
B. Measurement of a single vertical pocked of 2 cm, not containing umbilical cord
C. An amniotic fluid index of 5 cm or less
D. All of the above are equivalent, and decision made may be based on provider's preference

Q285: Your 30-year-old G3P0030 has just been diagnosed with APS. She states that she was previously diagnosed with ITP. How do you counsel her?

A. Autoimmune thrombocytopenia occurs in up to 50% of patients with APS
B. A simple blood test will distinguish if she had ITP as well as APS
C. Treatment does not differ
D. A and B
E. A and C

For questions 286–293, designate which fetal heart rate tracing category is being described:

Q286: Recurrent late decelerations with moderate baseline variability

A. Category I
B. Category II
C. Category III

Q287: Recurrent variable decelerations with absent fetal heart rate variability

A. Category I
B. Category II
C. Category III

Q288: Bradycardia with minimal baseline variability
A. Category I
B. Category II
C. Category III

Q289: Moderate baseline variability with accelerations and early decelerations
A. Category I
B. Category II
C. Category III

Q290: Baseline tachycardia
A. Category I
B. Category II
C. Category III

Q291: Sinusoidal pattern
A. Category I
B. Category II
C. Category III

Q292: Moderate baseline variability without decelerations or accelerations
A. Category I
B. Category II
C. Category III

Q293: Tracing that requires prompt evaluation due to association with abnormal fetal acid-base status
A. Category I
B. Category II
C. Category III
D. Category II and III

Q294: Which of the following is FALSE regarding thrombocytopenia and platelet counts?

A. The normal range of platelet count in nonpregnant individuals is approximately 150–400/μL
B. Excessive bleeding associated with trauma or surgery is uncommon unless the patient's platelet count is less than 50,000/μL
C. Thrombocytopenia is often caused by increased platelet destruction during pregnancy
D. The mean platelet count in pregnant women is higher than in nonpregnant individuals

Q295: Clinically significant spontaneous bleeding is usually limited to patients with platelet counts less than ______.

A. 50,000/μL
B. 30,000/μL
C. 20,000/μL
D. 10,000/μL
E. Is often not predicted by platelet counts due to variable function

Q296: In pregnancies achieved after bariatric surgery, micronutrients should be tested at the beginning of pregnancy. If normal, no further laboratory testing is indicated.

A. True
B. False

Q297: Which of the following are effective treatments for cervical insufficiency?

A. Bed rest
B. Pelvic rest
C. Activity restriction

D. None of the above
E. All of the above

Q298: Choose the most correct description of the three different types of cerclage:
A. Transabdominal is reserved for patients who have failed other types of cerclages; Shirodkar involves placing a single suture around the cervix; McDonald involves placing a double suture around the cervix
B. Transabdominal may be a first choice option in Mullerian anomalies; Shirodkar involves dissection of the vesicocervical mucosa; McDonald involves placing a single suture around the cervix
C. Transabdominal is reserved for patients who have failed other types of cerclages; Shirodkar involves dissection of the vesicocervical mucosa; McDonald involves placing a double suture around the cervix
D. None of the above are correct

Q299: How should pregnant patients who have had bariatric surgery be counseled in regard to nutrition and vitamin intake?
A. They should take two prenatal vitamins per day
B. They should double their protein intake
C. Breastfed infants should be closely monitored by their pediatrician as they may have nutritional deficiencies
D. All repletion should be parenteral due to decreased absorption
E. None of the above

Q300: A 34-year-old G1P0 at 36 weeks gestational age presents to your office for a routine OB visit. During this visit, you discuss the potential circumstances and associated risks that accompany an operative vaginal delivery. While comparing the two different instruments available to perform an operative delivery, you inform her that if an operative vaginal delivery is indicated:

A. She would be more likely to achieve a vaginal birth with use of a vacuum extractor
B. She would be more likely to sustain a third- or fourth-degree laceration with forceps
C. Her infant would be more likely to develop a cephalohematoma with use of a forceps extractor
D. She would be more likely to have anal sphincter dysfunction 5 years after delivery with use of forceps
E. All of the above

Q301: The best technique for use of vacuum extraction includes:

A. Placing the cup 2 cm posterior to anterior fontanelle
B. Centering the cup over the lambdoid suture
C. Placing the cup 2 cm anterior to the posterior fontanelle
D. Centering the cup over the coronal suture

Q302: Dumping syndrome:

A. Is caused by ingestion of protein
B. May cause patients to not tolerate the 50 g glucose screen
C. Causes hypoinsulinemia and hyperglycemia
D. A and B
E. B and C

Q303: Which of the following is TRUE regarding preterm birth?

A. Spontaneous preterm birth does not include birth that follows cervical insufficiency
B. After the first year of life, infants born prematurely have similar outcomes as those born at term
C. Preterm labor precedes approximately 20% of preterm birth
D. The risk of poor birth outcomes generally increases with advancing gestational age
E. None of the above

Q304: Which is true regarding monitoring fetal heart tones during an attempted ECV?

A. It is only indicated if the attempt lasts more than 5 min
B. Ultrasound monitoring of fetal heart tones intermittently is recommended
C. Continually monitoring fetal heart tones using a Doppler is recommended
D. There is no recommendation to guide fetal monitoring during the procedure

Q305: Which of the following Rh-negative patients should receive anti-D immune globulin immediately after the ECV attempt?

A. A woman who undergoes a failed ECV at 39 weeks gestation and will undergo a primary cesarean section tomorrow
B. A woman who undergoes a successful ECV at 37 weeks gestation and will return at 39 weeks gestation for induction
C. A woman who undergoes a failed ECV at 38 weeks gestation and will return at 39 weeks gestation for her cesarean section
D. B and C
E. All of the above

Questions 306–307 pertain to the same patient:

Q306: A 39-year-old G3P2002 with 18 weeks gestation presents to your clinic reporting exposure to parvovirus B19. She is confirmed to have an acute infection. You inform the patient that the risk of her male fetus having severe effects if vertical transmission occurs is more likely due to:

A. The severity of her symptoms
B. Her gestational age
C. Sex of her fetus
D. All of the above

Q307: This same patient has now progressed to 27 weeks gestation, and there is no ultrasound evidence of parvovirus B19 infection in her fetus. You tell her:

A. Until the fetus is born, she cannot be assured that her fetus will not suffer severe effects
B. Since more than 8 weeks have passed since her infection, it is unlikely that severe manifestations such as hydrops will occur
C. Repeat serology is necessary to confirm maternal infection
D. Serology will need to be drawn on fetus once it is born to determine newborn sequelae

Q308: Which of the following interventions could decrease a patients' risk for preterm birth?

A. Smoking cessation
B. Improved dental care during pregnancy
C. Having an interpregnancy interval of 36 months
D. A and B
E. All of the above

Q309: Which of the following medications should be avoided in patients who have had malabsorptive procedures?

A. NSAIDs
B. Multivitamins
C. Extended release formulations
D. A and B
E. A and C

Q310: Which of the following has been shown to reduce the risk of late-term and postterm pregnancies?
A. Confirmation of menstrual dating with ultrasonography
B. Membrane sweeping
C. Walking and frequent intercourse
D. A and B
E. All of the above

Q311: Which of the following factors are necessary to attempt a vaginal delivery in dichorionic-diamniotic twin gestations?
A. No prior cesarean sections
B. Gestational age 32 weeks or greater
C. Presenting twin is vertex
D. A and C
E. B and C
F. All of the above

Q312: If all criteria are met, planned vaginal delivery compared to planned cesarean section in dichorionic-diamniotic twin gestations is associated with:
A. Increased risk of fetal death
B. Increased risk of serious neonatal morbidity
C. Increased risk of cerebral palsy
D. B and C
E. None of the above

Q313: A 27-year-old G2P1001 with intrauterine gestation at 40 weeks presents for her OB visit. She is scheduled for induction in 12 days. She asks if there are any special precautions that need to be taken starting at her next visit in 1 week. You counsel her:
A. Yes, antenatal testing should be instituted, though the frequency is provider dependent due to insufficient data
B. Yes, ultrasound measurement of amniotic fluid should be considered with nonstress test or biophysical profile

C. Yes, antenatal testing should be started due to the increased risk of stillbirth in postterm pregnancies
D. B and C
E. All of the above

Q314: Bariatric surgery lowers the rate of cesarean sections.
A. True
B. False

Q315: A 35-year-old woman with a BMI of 52 presents to your office for preconceptual counseling. What do you recommend for weight loss?
A. Anoretics
B. Weight loss surgery
C. Behavioral interventions
D. B and C
E. All of the above

Q316: Gestational thrombocytopenia and immune thrombocytopenia purpura (ITP) can be differentiated by antiplatelet antibody testing.
A. True
B. False

Q317: Given the risk for preterm delivery, all women with multifetal gestations should be screened using the following method:
A. Serial cervical lengths
B. Cervical length at growth US
C. Fetal fibronectin at visits between 24 and 34 weeks gestational age
D. All of the above
E. B and C
F. None of the above

Q318: Which of the following interventions have been shown to prolong pregnancy in women with multifetal gestations without a history of cervical insufficiency?
A. Bed rest
B. Prophylactic cerclage

C. Prophylactic tocolysis
D. Vaginal progesterone in setting of a shortened cervix
E. Prophylactic pessary
F. None of the above

Q319: In a patient diagnosed with gestational thrombocytopenia, how often should a provider check the platelet count antepartum?
A. Weekly starting at 34 weeks gestational age
B. Every other week starting at 34 weeks gestational age
C. Weekly starting at 37 weeks gestational age
D. Once at term

Q320: Your patient has a BMI of 52. You counsel her that a weight loss of ___ % will improve her metabolic health.
A. 3%
B. 5%
C. 10%
D. The percentage is unknown

Q321: A 20-year-old G2P1001 is found to be Rh negative and is alloimmunized. She is unsure who the father is. What is the next best step in management?
A. Schedule serial titers
B. Order assessment of the peak systolic velocity in the fetal middle cerebral artery
C. Perform amniocentesis if gestational age is appropriate
D. Perform chorionic villus biopsy if gestational age is appropriate
E. A and B

Q322: A 20-year-old G1P0 is at 34 weeks gestation and asks what adjustments will need to be made in preparation for delivery. You counsel her:

A. At 40 weeks, she will be changed from low-molecular-weight heparin to unfractionated heparin
B. That neuraxial anesthesia generally needs to be done 12 h after the last prophylactic dose or 24 h after the last therapeutic dose
C. In cases of planned delivery, therapeutic anticoagulation may be stopped, and labor may be induced within 48 h
D. If there is concern for delivery, recommendation is for low-molecular-weight heparin as it has a shorter half-life and can be reversed
E. A and C

Q323: Which of the following is most consistently associated with increased rate of success for ECV?

A. Nulliparous patient
B. Low fetal station
C. Normal amniotic fluid index
D. Parous patient

For the following statements (Q324–Q330), choose which one BEST applies:

Q324: Should be performed between 10–13 weeks gestational age.

A. CVS
B. Amniocentesis
C. Neither

Q325: Obtains sample of placental villi without entering the amniotic sac.

A. CVS
B. Amniocentesis
C. Neither

Q326: When performed at the appropriate gestational age, it has a higher risk of limb reduction defects.
A. CVS
B. Amniocentesis
C. Neither

Q327: Associated with a 2% procedure-related pregnancy loss rate.
A. CVS
B. Amniocentesis
C. Neither

Q328: Viable cells obtained by this process require shorter processing time of 5–7 days compared to 7–14 days.
A. CVS
B. Amniocentesis
C. Neither

Q329: Most frequently performed between 15–20 weeks gestational age.
A. CVS
B. Amniocentesis
C. Neither

Q330: The perinatal outcomes following spontaneous preterm rupture of membranes are equivalent to the outcomes for membrane rupture after amniocentesis at a similar gestational age.
A. True
B. False

Q331: The use of terbutaline was shown in a randomized controlled trial to ____ of ECV. ACOG states that the evidence _______ the use of tocolytics in ECV.
A. Increase the success; is inconclusive regarding
B. Increase the success; is in support of
C. Have no effect on the success; is inconclusive regarding
D. Have no effect on the success; does not support

Q332: Which of the following reflects the upper limit of normal for TSH in the first trimester?

A. 2.0 mlU/L
B. 2.5 mIU/L
C. 3.0 mIU/L
D. There is no consensus

Q333: Which type of incontinence was reported to be more prevalent at 1 year postpartum than before delivery in patients who had an operative vaginal delivery without anal sphincter laceration?

A. Urinary incontinence
B. Anal incontinence of flatus and liquids
C. Anal incontinence of solids
D. None of the above

Q334: Studies have shown that the rates of newborn intracranial hemorrhage are similar between infants delivered by forceps, vacuum, and cesarean section during labor.

A. True
B. False

Q335: A 30-year-old patient complains of sweating, weight loss, heat intolerance, and insomnia. Her TSH is found to be suppressed and her free T4 is normal. Which of the following is TRUE?

A. A free T3 should be obtained
B. She currently meets criteria for subclinical hyperthyroidism
C. She should be tested for antithyroid peroxidase and antithyroglobulin antibodies
D. A and B
E. All of the above

Q336: What is the soonest anticoagulation which can be restarted following delivery?

A. 4 h after a vaginal delivery, 6 h after a cesarean delivery
B. 6 h after a vaginal delivery, 12 h after a cesarean delivery
C. 12 h after a vaginal delivery, 24 h after a cesarean delivery
D. 24 h after a vaginal delivery or a cesarean delivery
E. 12 h after if using enoxaparin, 24 h after if heparin

Q337: NSAIDs used postpartum have been shown to decrease maternal opioid consumption by what percent?

A. 30%
B. 40%
C. 50%
D. 60%

Q338: Which of the following increase the risk for venous thromboembolism?

A. Preeclampsia
B. Fetal growth restriction
C. Infection
D. All of the above

Q339: You elect to start prophylactic low-molecular-weight heparin on your patient. Her BMI is 52. What dose should you use?

A. 40 mg once a day
B. 40 mg twice a day
C. 60 mg once a day
D. 60 mg twice a day
E. 0.5 mg/kg twice a day

Q340: All of the following are known neonatal complications due to poorly controlled pregestational diabetes EXCEPT:
A. Hypoglycemia
B. Hypobilirubinemia
C. Respiratory distress syndrome
D. Electrolyte disturbances
E. All of the above are known complications

Q341: How is discordance calculated?
A. (Larger twin–smaller twin) × 100/smaller twin
B. (Larger twin–smaller twin) × 100/larger twin

Q342: You are taking care of a partner's patient who is a type I diabetic with nephropathy. She is concerned because her blood pressure has been increasing over the past several weeks and asks what it could mean. You counsel that her risk of developing preeclampsia is:
A. 10%
B. 20%
C. 30%
D. 40%
E. 50%

Q343: What is the most efficient method of induction at less than 28 weeks if second-trimester dilation and evacuation are unavailable?
A. Pitocin regardless of Bishop score and previous cesarean section history
B. Misoprostol regardless of Bishop score and previous cesarean section history
C. Misoprostol regardless of Bishop score and in patients without a previous history of cesarean section
D. Transcervical Foley catheter regardless of Bishop score and previous cesarean section history

Q344: Which of the following adverse effects is associated with inadequately treated maternal hyperthyroidism?
A. Severe preeclampsia
B. Fetal hypothyroidism
C. Fetal hyperthyroidism
D. A and C
E. All of the above

Q345: In which of the following scenarios would umbilical cord blood sampling be reasonable if disease could not be excluded based on clinical or ultrasound findings?
A. Any mother with Graves' disease should be offered umbilical cord sampling
B. Mothers with uncontrolled Graves' disease
C. Fetal growth restriction and hydrops
D. Fetal macrosomia and tachycardia
E. Patients with any of the above should be offered umbilical cord sampling to assess fetal thyroid status.

Q346: Timing of delivery is critical following diagnosis of stillbirth due to the association of coagulopathies with prolonged fetal retention being common.
A. True
B. False

Q347: Which of the following is the cutoff for when 10 by 10 accelerations appear to sufficiently predict fetal well-being?
A. 28 weeks or less
B. 30 weeks or less
C. 32 weeks or less
D. 34 weeks or less
E. Exact week is not known

Q348: Which of the following is FALSE regarding the components of a biophysical profile?

A. Amniotic fluid volume as defined by measurement of four pockets
B. Fetal breathing movements defined as one or more of 30 s
C. Fetal movement including three or more body or limb movements
D. Fetal tone defined as one or more episodes of extension than flexion
E. A nonstress test can be omitted if other components are normal

Q349: The rate of early stillbirth has ______ and the rate of late stillbirth has ______ since 1990.

A. Increased; decreased
B. Increased; increased
C. Decreased; decreased
D. Remained stable; decreased

Q350: How can ultrasound be used to assess for fetal anemia?

A. Diastolic velocity of the fetal middle cerebral artery
B. Systolic velocity of the fetal middle cerebral artery
C. Diastolic velocity of the umbilical artery
D. Systolic velocity of the umbilical artery
E. B and C

Q351: All of the following are recommended if IUGR is diagnosed EXCEPT:

A. Amniotic fluid assessment
B. Doppler blood flow of the umbilical artery
C. Assessment for structural abnormalities
D. Assessment for genetic abnormalities
E. All of the above are recommended

Q352: How frequently should monochorionic twins be monitored by ultrasound?

A. Every week starting at 20 weeks gestational age
B. Every 2 weeks starting at 16 weeks gestational age
C. Every 4 weeks starting at 20 weeks gestational age
D. Every week starting at 16 weeks gestational age

Q353: In Rh-negative women who have not received immune globulin prophylaxis, the most common time to become alloimmunized is:

A. At the time of delivery
B. With third-trimester bleeding
C. After therapeutic first-trimester abortion
D. With amniocentesis

Q354: A 23-year-old presents to your office as a transfer of care at 12 weeks gestation stating that another practitioner diagnosed her with hyperemesis gravidarum. You review her labs and note a suppressed TSH. She requests that you start treatment as it may help with her nausea and vomiting. Which of the following are appropriate?

A. Thyroid exam with initiation of treatment only if a goiter is present
B. Initiation of treatment for symptomatic hyperthyroidism
C. No initiation of treatment given she has an established diagnosis which accounts for her suppressed TSH
D. None of the above are correct

Q355: Which of the following should you discuss with your patient regarding possible causes for nausea and vomiting during pregnancy?

A. Estrogen ad human chorionic gonadotropin levels
B. Psychological predisposition
C. Smoking
D. A and C
E. All of the above

Q356: Which of the following is FALSE regarding pain associated with labor and delivery?

A. Pain experienced with uterine contractions is mediated by T-10 through the L-1 portions of the spinal cord
B. Cervical dilation and descent of the fetal head generate somatic pain
C. The pudendal nerve is responsible for transmitting the pain felt in the pelvic floor and perineum
D. A medical indication is not necessary to provide maternal pain relief
E. None of the above

Q357: Fetal fibronectin is a specific test for ruptured membranes.

A. True
B. False

Q358: In regard to labor induction in term patients with PROM, which of the following is TRUE?

A. Induction with prostaglandins has been shown to be more effective than induction with Pitocin
B. Induction with Pitocin has been shown to be more effective than induction with prostaglandins
C. Induction with prostaglandins is associated with a higher risk of chorioamnionitis
D. Induction with Pitocin versus prostaglandins has been shown to have equal risks for chorioamnionitis
E. A and C

Use the following scenario for Q359–Q360:

A 36-year-old G4P3003 presents for her new OB visit. In reviewing her records, you note a history of a term vaginal delivery followed by a primary low transverse cesarean section for non-reassuring fetal heart tones. The patient's last delivery was complicated by an attempted TOLAC with uterine rupture necessitating an emergent cesarean delivery.

Q359: She is contemplating TOLAC with her current gestation; you counsel her:

A. Given her history of having had a successful vaginal delivery previously, she is a reasonable candidate to attempt TOLAC
B. If her uterine rupture was located at the level of the previous uterine incision, then her risk of repeat rupture during labor is approximately 3%
C. If her uterine rupture extended to the upper segment of the uterus, then her risk of repeat rupture during labor may be as high as 32%
D. B and C

Q360: Based on her history, you recommend delivery before ______ weeks gestation.

A. 41
B. 40
C. 39
D. 34

Q361: Which of the following is FALSE regarding the herpes simplex virus?

A. Is transmitted through direct contact
B. Most people who are infected with HSV are unaware that they have the virus
C. Antibodies to HSV can be detected within 2–3 weeks after infection
D. Genital lesions caused by HSV-1 are becoming more common
E. All of the above are true

Q362: The risk of procedure-related bleeding is limited with administration of regional anesthesia after how many hours after the last dose of low-molecular-weight heparin?

A. 4 h after prophylactic dosing; 8 h after therapeutic dosing
B. 6 h after prophylactic dosing; 12 h after therapeutic dosing

C. 12 h after prophylactic dosing; 24 h after therapeutic dosing
D. 18 h after prophylactic dosing; 36 h after therapeutic dosing

A patient is trying to decide between the first-trimester screen and the quad screen. Choose the best test for the patient in the following scenarios:

Q363: A 27-year-old G1P0 with pregnancy at 11 weeks gestational age
A. FTS
B. Quad screen

Q364: A 38-year-old at her new OB appointment whose doctor does not have a professional ultrasonographer on staff
A. FTS
B. Quad screen

Q365: A 37-year-old who is especially concerned about her risk of neural tube defects
A. FTS
B. Quad screen

Q366: A 32-year-old who would consider termination if her fetus is diagnosed with an aneuploidy
A. FTS
B. Quad screen

Q367: How soon after a cesarean section can unfractionated heparin or low-molecular-weight heparin be restarted?
A. 4–6 h
B. 6–12 h
C. 12–16 h
D. 20–24 h

Q368: Which of the following is an example of a nonprimary first episode?

A. HSV-2 is isolated from a genital lesion and HSV-2 antibodies are present in the blood
B. HSV-2 is isolated from a genital lesion and no HSV-1 or HSV-2 antibodies are present in the blood
C. No genital lesions are present and HSV-1 antibodies are present in the blood
D. HSV-1 is isolated from a genital lesion and HSV-2 antibodies are present in the blood

Q369: Patients with antiphospholipid syndrome (APS) are at risk for all of the following EXCEPT?

A. Arterial thrombosis
B. Stroke
C. Autoimmune thrombocytopenia
D. Fetal loss
E. All of the above

Q370: What lab criteria are required in diagnosing APS?

A. All three antiphospholipid antibodies must be positive once
B. Two out of three antiphospholipid antibodies must be positive on more than one occasion 6 weeks apart
C. One antiphospholipid antibody must be positive on more than one occasion 12 weeks apart
D. A and C
E. Any of the above

Q371: Which of the following accurately describes the timing of new HSV-2 infections in pregnant patients?

A. Most occur in the first trimester
B. Most occur in the second trimester
C. Most occur in the third trimester
D. Approximately one third occur in each trimester

Q372: A 33-year-old G1P0 is noted to have a hemoglobin of 9.8 g/dL in the second trimester. Her mean corpuscular volume (MCV) is 88fL. Which of the following is NOT a possible cause of her anemia?

A. Early iron deficiency
B. Chronic disease
C. Autoimmune hemolysis
D. Lead poisoning

Q373: Patients with APS have an increased risk for which of the following disorders involving pregnancy and hypertension?

A. Severe preterm preeclampsia
B. Pregnancy-induced hypertension
C. Severe pregnancy-induced hypertension
D. A and C
E. All of the above

Q374: Which of the following pregnancy loss scenarios are concerning for APS?

A. Losses greater than 10 weeks
B. Sporadic embryonic loss
C. Recurrent embryonic loss
D. A and C
E. All of the above

Q375: Why are hemoglobin and hematocrit levels typically decreased in a pregnant woman?

A. Due to blood volume expansion
B. Due to a decrease in red blood cell production
C. Due to increased iron requirement
D. A and C
E. All of the above

Q376: A 37-year-old G3P2002 comes to your office for a return OB visit. You had previously counseled her on screening for aneuploidy, and she elected for cell-free fetal DNA. The result is "no reportable result." How do you counsel her?

A. Given no result, repeat free-cell DNA or diagnostic testing is recommended
B. From baseline, her risk for aneuploidy is decreased
C. From baseline, her risk for aneuploidy is increased
D. A and B
E. A and C

Q377: Which of the following is TRUE regarding fetal kick counts?

A. Decreases in fetal movement are seldom correlated with clinical outcomes
B. The optimal number of movements and duration for counting is evidence based
C. One method includes counting fetal movement for 1 h every day
D. It is considered a form of antepartum fetal surveillance

Q378: Approximately what percent of live-born infants in the United States have birth weights of more than 4500 g?

A. 1%
B. 2%
C. 5%
D. 8%
E. 10%

Q379: What is the sensitivity of fundal height measurement for detecting macrosomia?

A. 50% or less
B. 60%
C. 75%
D. 90%

Q380: The majority of HSV-infected infants are born to mothers who reported no history of HSV infection.
A. True
B. False

Q381: Examples of the morbidity and mortality associated with fetal growth restriction include all of the following EXCEPT?
A. Increased risk of stillbirth
B. Cognitive delay in childhood
C. Hypoglycemia
D. Seizures
E. All of the above are true

Q382: Fundal height measurements are most useful at what gestational age?
A. 20–40 weeks
B. 20–36 weeks
C. 24–38 weeks
D. 28–42 weeks

Q383: Which of the following is TRUE regarding neonatal herpes infection?
A. Usually acquired during the intrapartum period
B. Over half of all cases are caused by HSV-1
C. Approximately 70% of survivors will have long-term neurologic sequelae
D. Risk of development is equivalent with recurrent and nonprimary first episodes of infections
E. None of the above

Q384: What is the single most important risk factor for infection in the postpartum period?
A. Obesity
B. Prolonged rupture of membranes
C. Group B strep-positive status
D. Cesarean delivery

Q385: Why would cefazolin, a first-generation cephalosporin, be a better choice for single-dose antibiotic prophylaxis for cesarean section than a second-generation cephalosporin or ampicillin?

A. Cefazolin has greater efficacy compared to the other drugs
B. Cefazolin is cheaper than a second-generation cephalosporin
C. Cefazolin has a much longer half-life than ampicillin
D. B and C
E. All of the above

Q386: In order to report a stillbirth as being caused by a cord accident, there must be evidence of:

A. Obstruction on umbilical cord examination
B. Circulatory compromise on umbilical cord examination
C. A nuchal cord upon delivery of fetus
D. A or B
E. All of the above

Q387: An obese patient presents to the ER and requires a viability scan for further evaluation. Which ultrasound settings would likely be most helpful?

A. High frequency as it provides better resolution and penetration
B. Low frequency as it provides worse resolution but better penetration
C. Low frequency as it provides better resolution but worse penetration
D. High frequency as it provides better resolution and penetration

Q388: Which of the following is NOT included in the standard obstetric ultrasound examination?

A. Fetal biometry
B. Anatomic survey
C. Cervix and adnexa

D. Placental position
E. All of the above are included

Q389: What measurement can be useful to help estimate gestational age, especially before 23 weeks?
A. Humerus length
B. Foot length
C. Chest circumference
D. Femur length

Q390: An 18-year-old G1P0 presents to your office and is found to have a new diagnosis of overt hypothyroidism. She asks you what your treatment plan is and you tell her:
A. She'll start at a dose of approximately 100 mcg of T4 replacement per day
B. Her TSH will be checked every 2 weeks until it is within normal limits
C. After initiation of treatment, if her TSH remains high, her dose will be increased by 25–50 mcg
D. A and B
E. A and C

Q391: Third- and fourth-degree lacerations are quality care measures.
A. True
B. False

Q392: Perineal massage has been shown to:
A. Decrease perineal trauma that required suture repair when done at 34 weeks gestation and further
B. Decrease third- and fourth-degree lacerations when done during the second stage of labor
C. Increase the rate of women with intact perineum after delivery
D. A and B
E. All of the above

Q393: All of the following regarding classic thyroid storm are true EXCEPT:

A. Thyroid storm is a hypermetabolic state
B. Symptoms include fever, central nervous dysfunction, and cardiac dysrhythmia
C. It has an insidious onset leading to multi-organ decompensation
D. It is a life-threatening condition
E. Treatment should not be delayed until laboratory confirmation

Q394: Which of the following is FALSE in regard to the techniques used to diagnose herpes?

A. May include viral detection and antibody detection techniques
B. Polymerase chain reaction (PCR) techniques have increased sensitivity over cultures
C. The presence of HSV-1 antibodies alone may be indicative of either genital or orolabial infection
D. A negative genital culture excludes the presence of an infection

Q395: Fetal growth restriction has been associated with both chromosomal abnormalities and structural malformations.

A. True
B. False

Q396: The most common pathology associated with fetal growth restriction is the finding of a single umbilical artery.

A. True
B. False

Q397: It is possible to differentiate between a primary herpes infection and a nonprimary first episode during pregnancy based on clinical findings alone.

A. True
B. False

Q398: Which of the following is FALSE regarding a patient wanting to attempt a TOLAC?

A. External cephalic version is not contraindicated; however, the chances of success are lower
B. Regional anesthesia is not recommended due to it decreasing the chances of a successful TOLAC
C. Regional anesthesia is not recommended due to the concern it may mask the symptoms of uterine rupture
D. None of the above
E. All of the above

Q399: A 22-year-old G1P0 with intrauterine pregnancy at 24 weeks gestation has confirmed fetal cytomegalovirus infection. The next best steps include:

A. Administration of ganciclovir
B. Passive immunization with CMV-specific hyperimmune globulin
C. Serial ultrasound surveillance
D. A and C
E. B and C

Q400: All of the following have been shown in studies to decrease nausea and vomiting in pregnancy EXCEPT:

A. Small frequent meals
B. Multivitamins at the time of conception
C. Ginger pills
D. All of the above have been proven to decrease nausea and vomiting

Q401: Which of the following is TRUE regarding the use of pyridoxine combined with doxylamine for the treatment of nausea and vomiting of pregnancy?

A. It is shown to decrease nausea and vomiting of pregnancy compared to placebo
B. It should be used as a second-line therapy
C. Fetal effects are unlikely; however, there is not enough data yet to know
D. It should be taken as soon as nausea begins for greatest decrease in symptoms

Q402: For which of the following infectious diseases should women undergo routine serologic screening prior to or during pregnancy?
A. Cytomegalovirus
B. Parvovirus B19
C. Toxoplasmosis
D. All of the above
E. None of the above

Q403: Following successful VBAC, it is important to vaginally palpate the integrity of previous lower uterine incision.
A. True
B. False

Q404: Which of the following is FALSE regarding electronic fetal monitoring (EFM)?
A. Has poor interobserver and intraobserver reliability
B. Has uncertain efficacy
C. Fetal heart rate tracing patterns provide information on current acid-base status of fetus
D. Has low false-positive rates

Q405: When measuring the biparietal diameter, which of the following is TRUE?
A. It should be measured at the level of the cerebellar hemispheres
B. Measurement should be taken from the inner edge of the proximal skull to the inner edge of the distal skull
C. It may be affected by fetal head shape in which case circumference may be more reliable
D. A and B
E. All of the above

Q406: Which of the following is TRUE regarding measurement of the femoral diaphysis?
A. It can be used for dating after 12 weeks gestation
B. It should include the femoral epiphysis
C. All of the above
D. None of the above

Q407: When measuring the abdominal circumference, all of the following should be in the transverse ultrasound view EXCEPT:

A. The umbilical vein
B. The portal sinus
C. The fetal stomach
D. The renal vessels

Match the following tests with the current knowledge of their use in multiple gestations:

Q408: CVS

A. Not as sensitive because average of values can mask abnormal values
B. Can be technically challenging but is equally as sensitive in singletons and multiples
C. Insufficient evidence to recommend its use
D. Can be performed for definitive diagnosis, higher risk of sampling error
E. Can be performed for definitive diagnosis, lower risk of sampling error

Q409: Nuchal translucency

A. Not as sensitive because average of values can mask abnormal values
B. Can be technically challenging but is equally as sensitive in singletons and multiples
C. Insufficient evidence to recommend its use
D. Can be performed for definitive diagnosis, higher risk of sampling error
E. Can be performed for definitive diagnosis, lower risk of sampling error

Q410: Amniocentesis

A. Not as sensitive because average of values can mask abnormal values
B. Can be technically challenging but is equally as sensitive in singletons and multiples

C. Insufficient evidence to recommend its use
D. Can be performed for definitive diagnosis, higher risk of sampling error
E. Can be performed for definitive diagnosis, lower risk of sampling error

Q411: Cell-free fetal DNA
A. Not as sensitive because average of values can mask abnormal values
B. Can be technically challenging but is equally as sensitive in singletons and multiples
C. Insufficient evidence to recommend its use
D. Can be performed for definitive diagnosis, higher risk of sampling error
E. Can be performed for definitive diagnosis, lower risk of sampling error

Q412: Serum screening
A. Not as sensitive because average of values can mask abnormal values
B. Can be technically challenging but is equally as sensitive in singletons and multiples
C. Insufficient evidence to recommend its use
D. Can be performed for definitive diagnosis, higher risk of sampling error
E. Can be performed for definitive diagnosis, lower risk of sampling error

Q413: When describing uterine contractions, it is important to do which of the following:
A. To note whether the contractions are associated with fetal decelerations
B. To describe whether or not hyperstimulation is occurring
C. To quantify the number of contractions in a 10 min window, averaged over a 60 min period
D. A and C
E. All of the above

Q414: A 34-year-old G3P1103 presents for her new OB visit. She has a past surgical history significant for a LEEP procedure. Her pregnancy history includes a term singleton vaginal delivery followed by a 28 week vaginal delivery of twins due to preterm labor. The patient is concerned about her risk of having a preterm birth with her current pregnancy. You counsel her:

A. Her risk is only increased due to her history of LEEP and not her previous preterm delivery because it was a twin gestation
B. The evidence is not clear whether or not a LEEP procedure puts her at risk of having a preterm birth
C. She is at an increased risk for preterm birth due to her pregnancy history
D. She is not at an increased risk for preterm birth, especially since her first pregnancy delivered at term
E. B and C

Q415: Which of the following is NOT associated with an increased risk for aneuploidy?

A. Choroid plexus cyst
B. Shortened femur length
C. Pyelectasis
D. Echogenic bowel
E. Ventriculomegaly

Q416: How is an occult OASIS defined?

A. Laceration of the anal sphincter that is only palpated on a rectal exam but is unable to be visualized
B. A laceration that is visualized without needing to perform a rectal exam
C. A laceration that involves the perineal skin and the rectal mucosa but spares much of the perineal body
D. A laceration that has no clinical findings but is identified on endoanal ultrasonography
E. None of the above

Q417: Endoanal ultrasonography has a high:
A. False-positive rate
B. False-negative rate
C. Positive predictive value
D. Negative predictive value

Q418: Regarding cell-free fetal DNA testing, which of the following statements is FALSE?
A. It can detect Down syndrome at a rate of 93%
B. It is more effective at detecting trisomy 18 than trisomy 13
C. It has not been proven to detect microdeletions
D. All of the above are true

Q419: What is the most reliable and reproducible way to assess cervical length?
A. Digital examination
B. Transvaginal ultrasound
C. Transabdominal ultrasound
D. Magnetic resonance imaging (MRI)

Q420: Which of the following are TRUE regarding the baseline of electronic fetal monitoring?
A. Baseline must be a minimum of 4 min over any 10 min segment
B. Normal fetal heart rate baseline includes 120–160 beats per minute
C. Tachycardia is defined as baseline rate greater than 160 beats per minute
D. B and C
E. All of the above

For the following types of infant injuries, please indicate which type of delivery is more associated with their occurrence in comparison to delivery by cesarean section:

Q421: Facial nerve palsy
A. Vacuum extractor
B. Forceps
C. A and B

Q422: Brachial nerve palsy
- A. Vacuum extractor
- B. Forceps
- C. A and B

Q423: Minimal baseline variability refers to when:
- A. Amplitude range is undetectable
- B. Amplitude range is detectable but 5 beats per minute or fewer
- C. Amplitude range is 6–25 beats per minute
- D. Amplitude range is greater than 25 beats per minute

Q424: Which of the following describes the correct way to measure a cervical length?
- A. Patient should have a full bladder
- B. The shortest of three measurements should be used
- C. Calipers should be placed at the internal and external os
- D. B and C
- E. All of the above are correct

Q425: A 27-year-old G1P0 who is found to have a cervical length of 25 mm on her Level I ultrasound at 18 weeks. What is the best option for management?
- A. Start 200 mg vaginal progesterone
- B. Start weekly IM progesterone injections
- C. Place cerclage
- D. Remeasure cervical length in 2 weeks

Q426: What is the risk of vertical transmission to the neonate with a primary genital HSV outbreak at the time of delivery?
- A. Less than 3%
- B. 10–20%
- C. 20–40%
- D. 30–60%
- E. As high as 80%

Q427: A 32-year-old G2P0101 with history of preterm birth at 32 weeks who is found to have a cervical length of 30mm on her growth ultrasound at 24 weeks.

A. Continue weekly IM progesterone injections
B. Place cerclage
C. Remeasure cervical length in 2 weeks
D. A and B

Q428: Which definition of oligohydramnios may reduce unnecessary interventions without compromising perinatal outcomes?

A. Amniotic fluid index of 5 cm or less
B. Maximum vertical pocket of 2 cm or less
C. Maximum vertical pocket of 3 cm or less
D. Amniotic fluid index of 7 cm or less

Q429: Which of the following is FALSE in regard to secondary infection with CMV?

A. The incidence of secondary infection is higher than primary infection in pregnant women
B. Rate of vertical transmission after a secondary infection is much lower than after a primary infection
C. Unlikely to cause multiple sequelae in the fetus
D. Congenital hearing loss is the most common severe sequelae
E. All of the above are true

Q430: A 33-year-old G1P0 is known to have contracted CMV, and vertical transmission to her fetus is strongly suspected. You counsel her regarding the potential clinical manifestations of congenital CMV telling her that her newborn may have:

A. Jaundice, petechiae, and thrombocytopenia
B. Chorioretinitis
C. Periventricular calcifications and ventriculomegaly
D. Microcephaly

Q431: Which of the following is FALSE in regard to oligohydramnios in postterm pregnancies?
A. Associated with an increased risk of fetal demise
B. Is an indication for delivery
C. Increased risk of fetal heart rate abnormalities
D. All of the above are true

Q432: A 25-year-old G2P0102 with a history of preterm birth of twin gestation at 34 weeks who is found to have a cervical length of 40 mm on her Level I ultrasound at 18 weeks.
A. Continue weekly IM progesterone injections
B. Remeasure cervical length in 2 weeks
C. Continue routine obstetrical care
D. Place cerclage
E. A and D

Q433: A woman who is pregnant for the first time presents with her husband. He reports that she has developed a flat affect, has stopped functioning well at work, and even seems paranoid at times. What is the most likely diagnosis?
A. Anxiety disorder
B. Major depression
C. Bipolar disorder
D. Schizophrenia
E. Pregnancy-associated mood changes

Q434: A patient presents to triage in active labor. Review of fetal heart tones reveals a baseline of 110, moderate variability, accelerations, early decelerations, and no late or variable decelerations. What category does this tracing represent?
A. Category I
B. Category II
C. Category III
D. Unable to determine

Q435: A term patient is currently laboring. Upon review of the fetal heart tracing, it is noted that the baseline is

100 with moderate variability and recurrent late decelerations. What category does this tracing represent?

A. Category I
B. Category II
C. Category III
D. Unable to determine

Q436: What is the most common fetal heart rate anomaly during labor?

A. Intermittent variable decelerations
B. Recurrent variable decelerations
C. Intermittent late decelerations
D. Recurrent late decelerations
E. Minimal variability

Q437: A 28-year-old G1P0 presents for her first obstetrical visit at 8 weeks gestation. In review of her medications, it is noted that she is currently taking paroxetine for depression. What is your recommendation regarding use of this medication?

A. Continue use given the risk of relapse
B. Discontinue use as it is associated with fetal cardiac malformations
C. Taper the medication to avoid withdrawal
D. A and C
E. B and C

Q438: A 33-year-old G2P1001 with intrauterine pregnancy at 38 weeks gestational age presents to labor and delivery in active labor. Review of her antenatal records reveals a diagnosis of gestational thrombocytopenia which was made at 35 weeks. The patient's platelet count is 80,000/μL prior to delivery. The risk of bleeding complications in this fetus compared to a fetus delivered by a patient without gestational thrombocytopenia is:

A. 50% greater
B. 20% greater
C. The same
D. 20% less

Q439: Which of the following is TRUE regarding preeclampsia and thrombocytopenia?
A. Thrombocytopenia may be the first clinical sign of preeclampsia
B. In the setting of new-onset hypertension, it can be a diagnostic indicator of preeclampsia if platelet count is less than 120,000/μL
C. Clinical hemorrhage is common
D. A and B
E. All of the above

Q440: What are possible reasons for increased vertical transmission of genital HSV at the time of delivery associated with primary compared to recurrent outbreaks?
A. There is increased transplacental passage of protective HSV-2-specific antibodies with recurrent outbreaks
B. Cervical shedding may be increased with primary outbreaks
C. Primary outbreaks are associated with shorter duration yet higher concentrations of viral shedding
D. A and B
E. All of the above

Q441: Which of the following patients should NOT be offered a TOLAC?
A. Patient with a history of an extensive abdominal myomectomy
B. Patient with a current twin gestation pregnancy
C. Patient with a history of a previous low vertical incision
D. A and D
E. All of the above

Q442: A patient with a previous cesarean section of unknown scar type may still be offered a TOLAC.
A. True
B. False

Q443: Your 32-year-old G2P1001 presents at term, SROM, and is found to be 2 cm dilated. All of the following EXCEPT which are reasonable:

A. Misoprostol
B. Oxytocin
C. Intravaginal PGE2
D. Expectant management
E. All of the above are reasonable

Q444: Digital examinations are discouraged in preterm PROM patients unless absolutely necessary due to:

A. Increased risk of infection
B. Add little information to sterile speculum exam
C. Increased risk of bleeding
D. A and B
E. All of the above

Q445: Which of the following can cause a false-negative test result for membrane rupture?

A. Prolonged rupture
B. Blood or semen
C. Bacterial vaginosis
D. Continued leakage of fluid

Q446: In women with a previous uterine incision with an intrauterine fetal demise, 800 mcg every 6 h up to 28 weeks gestation does not appear to be associated with an increase in complications.

A. True
B. False

Q447: Doppler has lower energy delivery and is therefore preferable to ultrasound in the first trimester.

A. True
B. False

Q448: The office has obtained a transvaginal ultrasound to use for patient care. How is microbial prevention accomplished when the same probe is used?

A. Single use disposable covers
B. High-level disinfection
C. Either A or B
D. Both A and B must be performed

Q449: Cesarean delivery is indicated in any woman with a history of genital HSV, regardless of current outbreak status.

A. True
B. False

Q450: Pregnancy is characterized by increased thrombotic potential. Which of the following factors contribute to this known state?

A. Decreased fibrinolysis
B. Increased insulin resistance and hyperlipidemia
C. Compression of the aorta by the pregnant uterus
D. A and B
E. All of the above

Q451: Venous thromboembolism is a leading cause of maternal mortality in the United States.

A. True
B. False

Q452: At what gestational age should women with active recurrent genital herpes be offered suppressive viral therapy?

A. 36 weeks
B. 34 weeks
C. 32 weeks
D. 28 weeks

Q453: A 32-year-old women has a QUAD screen which results with an increased risk of trisomy 13. When you call her to discuss the results, what testing in particular should be offered?

A. CVS with karyotype analysis with or without FISH
B. Amniocentesis with karyotype analysis with or without FISH
C. CVS with chromosomal microarray
D. Amniocentesis with chromosomal microarray

Q454: Which of the following statements is FALSE in regard to counseling patients about prenatal diagnostic testing for genetic disorders who have blood-borne infections?

A. Women who are positive for hepatitis B e antigen have a lower risk of vertical transmission with amniocentesis
B. Risk of vertical transmission of hepatitis B with amniocentesis is related to viral load
C. Risk of vertical transmission of HIV with amniocentesis is related to viral load
D. Risk of vertical transmission is higher in patients with multiple infections, i.e., HIV and hepatitis C

Q455: The three antiviral agents most commonly used to treat HSV infection in pregnancy are FDA pregnancy Category A medications.

A. True
B. False

Q456: Which of the following are components of a first-trimester screen?

A. PAPP-A
B. Inhibin A
C. b-hCG
D. A and C
E. B and C

Q457: In which of the following is it possible for a patient be told she has low risk for aneuploidy without completion of a quad screen?

A. Integrated
B. Contingent
C. Sequential
D. A and B
E. A and C

Q458: Routine HSV screening of pregnant women is not recommended.

A. True
B. False

Q459: Which of the following is TRUE regarding a transabdominal cerclage?

A. Can be placed in any trimester; must be removed at the time of delivery
B. Can be placed in any trimester; can be left in place between pregnancies
C. Requires delivery by cesarean section
D. A and C
E. B and C

Q460: A 25-year-old G2P0101 presents with a cervical length of 23 mm at 23 weeks gestation. What type of cerclage would you offer her?

A. History indicated
B. Physical exam indicated
C. Ultrasound indicated
D. Do not offer cerclage
E. Do not offer cerclage but would offer her vaginal progesterone therapy

Q461: A 34-year-old G1P0 at 39 weeks gestational age presents to labor and delivery in active labor. On exam, the patient is noted to have a painful ulcer on her outer thigh. When the patient is questioned about this, she says that she has had such lesions "come and go" on her thigh previously. She denies ever having genital lesions. What is the next best step in her management?

A. Due to likely HSV infection, proceed with cesarean section for delivery
B. Due to unlikely HSV infection, proceed with vaginal delivery if otherwise indicated
C. Due to concern for HSV infection, perform thorough vaginal and cervical examination to rule out presence of additional lesions. If exam is negative, proceed with vaginal delivery if otherwise indicated
D. Start IV acyclovir immediately and proceed with cesarean section for delivery

Q462: Ideally, the BEST time to screen a patient for an inherited thrombophilia is:
A. At least 4 weeks from the acute thrombotic event
B. While the patient is not pregnant
C. While the patient is on anticoagulation
D. A and B
E. All of the above

Q463: Estimated fetal weight by ultrasound can yield errors as high as:
A. 10%
B. 20%
C. 30%
D. 40%

Q464: Three-dimensional ultrasonography provides a clear clinical advantage in prenatal diagnosis.
A. True
B. False

Q465: Unfractionated heparin is the preferred agent for prophylaxis in pregnancy.
A. True
B. False

Q466: Which of the following is TRUE regarding active herpes simplex virus infection and preterm premature rupture of membranes in a pregnant patient?

A. Expectant management is reasonable depending upon gestational age and associated risk of prematurity
B. Treatment with an antiviral medication is contraindicated
C. Administering corticosteroids for fetal lung maturity is contraindicated due to increased risk of worsening infection
D. Immediate cesarean section should be performed as long as fetus is greater than 24 weeks gestational age
E. None of the above

Q467: Which of the following patients should have early screening for gestational diabetes?

A. A woman with a BMI of 28
B. A woman with gestational diabetes during her past pregnancy who passed her postpartum glucose screen
C. A woman with gestational diabetes during her past pregnancy who did not have a postpartum glucose screen
D. A and C
E. B and C

Q468: Which of the following would give the highest risk for an obstetric anal sphincter injury?

A. Midline episiotomy combined with forceps
B. Vacuum-assisted delivery
C. Increased fetal birth weight
D. Persistent occiput posterior position
E. Duration of the second stage of labor

Q469: Which of the following is associated with increased risk for an obstetric anal sphincter injury?

A. Maternal age
B. Maternal BMI
C. Duration of the second stage of labor
D. Epidural anesthesia
E. Occiput transverse

Q470: Which of the following describes the correct method of diagnosis of gestational diabetes?

A. Screening should be performed at 24–30 weeks gestation
B. A 1 h, 50 g oral glucose test followed by a 3 h, 100 g glucose test
C. A one-step approach with a 2 h, 75 g oral glucose test
D. A and B
E. All of the above are acceptable

Q471: Breastfeeding is contraindicated in the following scenario:

A. Active primary HSV genital lesions
B. Mother is currently taking valacyclovir
C. Recurrent HSV genital lesions
D. Active HSV breast lesions
E. All of the above

For the following scenarios choose:

Q472: A type 1 diabetic patient at 31 weeks gestation in diabetic ketoacidosis with a biophysical profile of 4/10.

A. Immediate delivery
B. Repeat biophysical profile in 24 h or extended monitoring

Q473: A healthy woman at 36 weeks gestation with a biophysical profile of 6/10.
A. Immediate delivery
B. Repeat biophysical profile in 24 h or extended monitoring

Q474: A healthy woman at 33 weeks gestation with a biophysical profile of 4/10.
A. Immediate delivery
B. Repeat biophysical profile in 24 h or extended monitoring

Q475: A healthy woman at 31 weeks gestation with a biophysical profile of 4/10.
A. Immediate delivery
B. Repeat biophysical profile in 24 h or extended monitoring

Q476: A healthy woman with a fetus with intrauterine growth restriction at 38 weeks gestation who is found to have presence of diastolic flow with an elevated S/D ratio.
A. Immediate delivery
B. Repeat biophysical profile in 24 h or extended monitoring

Q477: A woman at 38 weeks with a new finding of oligohydramnios.
A. Immediate delivery
B. Repeat biophysical profile in 24 h or extended monitoring

Q478: What percent of pregnant women with recurrent genital HSV have at least one recurrence during pregnancy?
A. 25%
B. 40%

C. 50%
D. 75%
E. 90%

Q479: A 34-year-old patient presents for her 6 week postpartum visit. She underwent an operative vaginal delivery due to non-reassuring fetal status and examination of the newborn afterward revealed no obvious defects. Today in your clinic, she asks you about the likelihood of her baby having long-term effects stemming from her mode of delivery. You tell her:

A. Her child may have slightly impaired scholastic performance
B. Her child may have delayed speech
C. The long-term outcomes of operative vaginal delivery are not well understood
D. Her mode of delivery will not have long-term effects on her child

Q480: Which of the following statements regarding operative vaginal delivery and fetal macrosomia are TRUE?

A. Macrosomic infants delivered by operative vaginal delivery had an overall higher injury rate compared to those in a lower birth weight group
B. The risk of persistent injury in infants does not differ between operative vaginal delivery and spontaneous vaginal delivery in birth weights greater than 4000 g
C. Use of operative vaginal delivery in a macrosomic infant is not contradicted
D. A and C
E. All of the above

Q481: Your patient presents for a postpartum visit. She had recurrent genital HSV, used suppression therapy, and delivered vaginally after having an exam showing no lesions. She presents upset because her baby was readmitted at 2 weeks age due to neonatal HSV. She wonders if she may have infected her baby. How do you counsel her?

A. Intrapartum infection is extremely unlikely given the above scenario
B. The infection may have been acquired from a family member through oropharyngeal disease
C. The infection may have been acquired from a family member through cutaneous disease
D. A and B
E. All of the above

Q482: Which of the following strategies have been proven to be effective in preventing fetal growth restriction?

A. Daily aspirin
B. Dietary supplementation
C. Bed rest
D. Nutritional counseling
E. None of the above

Q483: Operative vaginal delivery should not be attempted if provider feels chances of success are low.

A. True
B. False

Q484: It is reasonable to attempt both forceps and vacuum extraction on the same patient to avoid cesarean delivery.

A. True
B. False

Q485: Use of umbilical artery Doppler velocimetry is associated with improved outcomes in fetuses with fetal growth restriction.

A. True
B. False

Q486: A patient presents for a routine prenatal visit at 34 weeks gestational age. She is wondering about the differences between parental and regional anesthesia during labor and delivery. You counsel her:

A. Regional anesthesia has been shown to be more effective at controlling pain during labor and delivery than parental agents but may have greater risks to the fetus
B. Shorter-acting parental agents may decrease some of the neonatal risks associated with longer-acting agents
C. Parental anesthesia has been shown to be as effective as regional anesthesia in providing pain relief during labor and delivery but may have greater risks to the fetus
D. A and B
E. None of the above

Q487: Which of the following is most accurate when estimating gestational age?

A. Crown-rump length
B. Mean gestational sac diameter
C. Both are equivalent

Q488: Which of the following is diagnostic of a nonviable pregnancy?

A. A mean gestational sac of 20 mm or greater
B. Lack of cardiac motion with a 10 mm embryo
C. Lack of cardiac motion with a 5 mm embryo
D. A and C
E. All of the above

Q489: All of the following are factors that are associated with the development of neural tube defects EXCEPT:

A. Diet
B. Maternal diabetes
C. High maternal core temperature
D. Ethnicity
E. All of the above are associated with the development of neural tube defects

Q490: A 23-year-old G1P0 at 39 weeks gestational age is currently in labor with a cervical exam of 5 cm. She is painfully contracting and interested in regional anesthesia, but she is concerned about how this may affect her fetus and labor course. You counsel her:

A. She is at an increased risk of cesarean delivery due to fetal heart rate abnormalities associated with regional anesthesia use
B. She may experience fewer fetal heart rate abnormalities if she has a combined spinal-epidural versus epidural
C. She may develop hypotension secondary to regional anesthesia which can lead to fetal heart rate abnormalities
D. A and C
E. All of the above

Q491: Parents of a child affected by a neural tube defect are more likely to be homozygous for the ________ mutation in comparison to the unaffected population.

A. Protein C
B. Factor V Leiden
C. MTHFR
D. PKU

Q492: Which of the following statement is FALSE regarding Down syndrome?

A. The severity of the syndrome can be predicted prenatally
B. It is the most common autosomal aneuploidy
C. It occurs at a rate of 1/800 live births
D. It is usually due to nondisjunction
E. Detection rates are roughly equivalent between first-trimester screen and quad screen

Q493: Which of the following women should be offered screening for aneuploidy at the first prenatal visit?

A. A 36-year-old G1P0 at 6 weeks gestational age by LMP
B. A 36-year-old G3P2002 at 16 weeks gestational age with history of a baby with Down syndrome

C. A 25-year-old G1P0 at 19 weeks gestational age who has a normal Level 1 ultrasound
D. A and B
E. All of the above

Q494: The amount of fetomaternal hemorrhage at which women can become alloimmunized is approximately:
A. 0.1 mL
B. 1 mL
C. 5 mL
D. 10 mL

Q495: A 23-year-old G1P0 with intrauterine pregnancy at 22 weeks has just been informed by the maternal fetal medicine specialist that her fetus has spina bifida. She calls the office wanting to know if her baby will have disabilities. In addition to referring her for additional MFM counseling, you tell her:
A. The extent of disability will depend on the level of the lesion
B. 90% of infants born with a sacral lesion will be wheelchair bound
C. Her infant will likely have some impairment of bowel and bladder function
D. Her infant will likely be severely mentally handicapped
E. A and C

Q496: What is the recommended rescue therapy for asthma during pregnancy?
A. Short-acting beta-2 agonists
B. Short-acting beta-2 antagonists
C. Inhaled mild corticosteroids
D. Oral corticosteroids

Q497: Which of the following is a severe maternal effect related to nausea and vomiting of pregnancy?
A. Esophageal rupture
B. Splenic avulsion
C. Psychosocial morbidity

D. A and B
E. All of the above

Q498: A 36-year-old G1P0 presents for a routine obstetric. She is followed for hyperemesis gravidarum and is worried about what effect this will have on her baby. How do you counsel her?

A. It often portends well for pregnancy outcome, may be associated with low birth weight, gives a lower risk of miscarriage, and is unlikely associated with malformations
B. Its impact on the fetus is unknown overall. It may be associated with low birth weight, but it is unlikely associated with malformations
C. The risk for miscarriage is decreased, the risk for low birth weight infants is significantly increased, and long-term health of children appears to be unaffected
D. It often portends well for pregnancy outcomes. Although it is associated with low birth weight, it is also associated with a lower risk of miscarriage and is unlikely associated with malformations. Long-term health of children is unaffected

Q499: A 28-year-old G2P1001 with intrauterine gestation at 28 weeks calls the triage phone stating that she has had an acute exacerbation of her asthma symptoms. She has used her rescue treatment as her physician advised in the office, and now her peak expiratory flow rate (PEFR) has reached 60% of her personal best, and her symptoms have overall improved. You counsel her:

A. To continue to monitor her symptoms from home and reinitiate rescue therapy as needed
B. To lay on her left side and monitor for appropriate fetal movement

C. Her asthma exacerbation has resolved appropriately and to follow-up in clinic as previously scheduled
D. To come into the hospital for medical attention as soon as possible

Q500: Intellectual ability of patients with by spina bifida is influenced by:
A. Presence of increased intracranial pressure
B. Intraoperative complications of an Arnold-Chiari malformation repair
C. Ventricular size regardless of intracranial pressure
D. A and B
E. All of the above

Q501: A 22-year-old G2P1001 Caucasian patient is found to have a hemoglobin of 9.8 g/dL in the second trimester. She has no known medical issues. Which of the following is a reasonable next step in her management?
A. Obtain iron studies
B. Treat empirically with iron supplementation and monitor for improvement
C. Screen for hemoglobinopathies
D. A or B
E. All of the above are reasonable options

Q502: A patient presents to urgent care with cardiomyopathy and is diagnosed with thyrotoxic heat failure. She is transferred to the ICU, and her husband asks why this happened and what will happen to his wife. You counsel him that:
A. Her condition is due to an elevated TSH which caused heart failure and pulmonary hypertension
B. Her condition is unfortunately not reversible
C. She has a rare form of thyroid storm
D. Decompensation generally has an additional underlying cause such as sepsis or anemia
E. All of the above are true

Q503: When treating thyroid storm, all of the following medications should be administered EXCEPT:
A. Propylthiouracil
B. Methimazole
C. Lugol solution
D. Dexamethasone
E. Propranolol

Q504: What is the most likely diagnosis in an anemic pregnant patient based on the following lab indices: iron level, decreased; total iron-binding capacity, decreased; and ferritin level, increased?
A. Iron deficiency anemia
B. Thalassemia
C. Anemia of chronic disease
D. None of the above

Q505: Episiotomies are no longer routinely performed with operative vaginal deliveries because:
A. Of the association between midline episiotomies and increased risk of injury to the anal sphincter
B. Of poor healing and increased likelihood of dyspareunia with use of mediolateral episiotomies
C. Of the increased risk of perineal infection with either type of episiotomy
D. A and B
E. All of the above

Q506: Which type of incontinence was reported to be more prevalent at 6 weeks postpartum than before delivery in patients who had an operative vaginal delivery without anal sphincter laceration?
A. Urinary incontinence
B. Anal incontinence of flatus and liquids
C. Anal incontinence of solids
D. None of the above

Q507: A 32-year-old patient presents for a return obstetric visit. She is worried because her cervix is closed at 36 weeks gestation. She is a type II diabetic, controlled on insulin, with glucose logs demonstrating excellent control. Assuming no other complications, what is the latest gestational age ACOG recommends delivery?

A. 37/0 weeks gestational age
B. 38/0 weeks gestational age
C. 39/0 weeks gestational age
D. 40/0 weeks gestational age
E. 41/0 weeks gestational age

Q508: What is the goal for blood glucose levels during labor?

A. Less than 140 mg/dL
B. Less than 130 mg/dL
C. Less than 120 mg/dL
D. Less than 110 mg/dL
E. Less than 100 mg/dL

Q509: All of the following anticoagulants are compatible with breastfeeding EXCEPT:

A. Low-molecular-weight heparin
B. Unfractionated heparin
C. Warfarin
D. None of the above are safe with breastfeeding
E. All of the above are safe with breastfeeding

Q510: Women who are heterozygous for factor V Leiden are candidates for all of the following contraceptive methods EXCEPT:

A. Progestin-only pills
B. Intrauterine devices
C. Barrier methods
D. Progestin-only implant
E. All of the above are acceptable

Q511: The rate of primary cesarean delivery is increased in pregestational diabetics.
A. True
B. False

Q512: The development of chronic back pain is a known adverse outcome to epidural placement during labor and delivery.
A. True
B. False

Q513–517: For the following thrombophilias, indicate whether it is high risk or low risk:

Q513: Factor V Leiden heterozygote
A. Low risk
B. High risk

Q514: Protein C deficiency
A. Low risk
B. High risk

Q515: Double heterozygote for prothrombin G20210A and factor V Leiden
A. Low risk
B. High risk

Q516: Factor V Leiden homozygote
A. Low risk
B. High risk

Q517: Protein S deficiency
A. Low risk
B. High risk

Q518: Epidural-related fever is benign.
A. True
B. False

Q519: Postpartum administration of a single dose of anti-D immune globulin can reduce the alloimmunization rate by 90% if given within:
A. 12 h of delivery
B. 24 h of delivery
C. 48 h of delivery
D. 72 h of delivery

Q520: Your intern asks you how to interpret the results of a contraction stress test. You answer:
A. A negative test means that there are no variable or late contractions
B. A positive test indicates the presence of late decelerations after every contraction
C. An equivocal test means that the decelerations occur if contractions are longer than 90 s or more frequent than every 2 min
D. A and C
E. All of the above

Q521: Acute maternal infection with CMV can be diagnosed by:
A. Seroconversion from negative to positive anti-CMV IgG
B. Greater than twofold increase in anti-CMV IgG titers
C. Presence of anti-CMV IgM antibodies
D. A and B
E. All of the above

Q522: Amniocentesis with positive culture for CMV is predictive of severe congenital infection.
A. True
B. False

Q523: How is a nonstress test conducted?
A. The patient is placed in the semi-Fowler position
B. The test should be conducted for 20 min but may last as long as 40 min

C. Vibroacoustic stimulation safely reduces the frequency of nonreactive tests
D. Accelerations are defined as 15 beats per minute above the baseline for 15 s for term pregnancies
E. All of the above are true

Q524: The current standard prophylactic dose of anti-D immune globulin given in the United States is:
A. 50 μg
B. 100 μg
C. 200 μg
D. 300 μg

Q525: One prophylactic dose of anti-D immune globulin can prevent Rh D alloimmunization after exposure of up to ____ mL of Rh D-positive blood or ____mL of fetal cells.
A. 30 mL of Rh D- positive blood and 15 mL of fetal cells
B. 40 mL of Rh D-positive blood and 25 mL of fetal cells
C. 50 mL of Rh D-positive blood and 35 mL of fetal cells
D. 60 mL of Rh D-positive blood and 45 mL of fetal cells

Q526: Risk for various outcomes should be assessed by calculating the patient's BMI at each trimester.
A. True
B. False

Q527: How many pounds should an overweight patient gain during her pregnancy?
A. 10–20 pounds
B. 15–25 pounds
C. 20–30 pounds
D. 30–40 pounds

Q528: Shoulder dystocia results in persistent brachial plexus injury in 15% of deliveries.
A. True
B. False

Q529: Which of the following statement(s) are TRUE regarding preterm PROM and antibiotic administration?
A. Can prolong pregnancy and reduce maternal and neonatal infections
B. Regimen includes 7 day course of IV erythromycin and ampicillin combined with oral erythromycin and amoxicillin—clavulanic acid
C. Should be administered in pregnancies less than 34 weeks gestation
D. A and C
E. All of the above

Q530: The macrosomic fetus of a diabetic mother would likely have ____ compared to the macrosomic fetus of a nondiabetic mother?
A. Lesser upper-extremity skinfold measurement
B. Larger head to abdominal circumference
C. Greater total body fat
D. A and C
E. All of the above

Q531: Which of the following is superior for prediction of macrosomia?
A. Ultrasound in the third trimester
B. Clinical palpation maneuvers
C. Multiparous mothers' estimate
D. A and C
E. None of the above has been proven superior

Q532: Due to lack of adequate evidence regarding the management of patients with preterm PROM and cerclage, no recommendation can be made as to whether or not cerclage should be removed following preterm PROM.

A. True
B. False

Q533: Bipolar disorder:

A. Affects men and women equally
B. Typically first manifests itself in women in their early 30s
C. Carries an increased risk for postpartum psychosis of 20%
D. A and B
E. All of the above

Q534: How frequently does a live birth involve some type of chromosomal abnormality that results in an abnormal fetal or neonatal phenotype?

A. 1 in 50 live births
B. 1 in 100 live births
C. 1 in 150 live births
D. 1 in 200 live births

Q535: Which of the following statements regarding chromosomes is FALSE?

A. Chromosome irregularities are more common early in pregnancy
B. The most common abnormality of chromosome number is aneuploidy
C. Balanced translocations are often associated with a normal phenotype
D. Epigenetics means an abnormal number of chromosomes are not present in all cell lines

Q536: When do most exacerbations of panic disorders occur?
A. First trimester
B. Second trimester
C. Third trimester
D. Postpartum

Q537: A Rh-negative pregnant patient presents for her routine OB visit at 28 weeks. The father of the baby has documentation revealing that he is also Rh negative. As her physician, you should advise her to:
A. Receive the standard prophylactic dose of anti-D immune globulin
B. Forgo the prophylactic dose of anti-D immune globulin because it is unnecessary
C. Receive a smaller dose of anti-D immune globulin
D. Receive the prophylactic dose of anti-D immune globulin only if she has had a history of antepartum bleeding

Q538: Fetal-neonatal alloimmune thrombocytopenia affects women and fetuses.
A. True
B. False

Q539: A 33-year-old G2P1001 at 31 weeks gestational age presents for routine obstetrical visit. Her pregnancy has been complicated by maternal immune thrombocytopenia purpura (ITP). Her most recent platelet count was 90,000/μL. She asks you how her diagnosis will affect her fetus. You counsel her:
A. Maternal antibodies do not cross the placenta, protecting her fetus from the risk of thrombocytopenia
B. There is no relationship between maternal platelet count at the time of delivery and infant platelet count at birth

C. Up to one half of infants born to mothers with ITP will develop platelet counts less than 150,000/μL
D. The risk of severe hemorrhagic complications in newborns is high in neonates born to mothers with ITP
E. None of the above

Q540: Which of the following is NOT an example of an absolute contraindication to regional anesthesia?
A. Patient with positive blood cultures for *E. coli* that resulted within the past 3 h
B. Patient with a history of an Arnold-Chiari malformation with a functioning ventricular shunt in place
C. Patient had her last dose of low-molecular-weight heparin 10 h ago
D. Patient with a fibrinogen level of 110 mg/liter

Q541: Your patient presents to triage complaining of a headache at 38 weeks gestation. She is diagnosed with preeclampsia and is admitted for induction. Which of the following should be avoided?
A. Regional anesthesia
B. General anesthesia
C. Butorphanol
D. Nalbuphine
E. Fentanyl

Q542: A patient has an ultrasound with an estimated fetal weight of 4200 g. She should be informed that newborn weights of ____ and more are associated with increased stillbirth and neonatal mortality.
A. 3500 g
B. 4000 g
C. 4500 g
D. 5000 g
E. There are no data to support a cut off

Q543: A 28-year-old G2P1001 presents for her first prenatal visit at 12 weeks gestational age. A type and screen are performed, and the patient is found to be Rh negative with a positive anti-D antibody screen. As her physician, in addition to increased antenatal surveillance, you should:

A. Administer a prophylactic dose anti-D immune globulin immediately
B. Obtain a Kleihauer-Betke test immediately, and administer a sufficient amount of anti-D immune globulin accordingly
C. Administer the standard prophylactic dose of anti-D immune globulin at 28 weeks
D. Not administer anti-D immune globulin during this pregnancy

Q544–Q547: Match the tocolytic class or agent to its associated characteristics:

Q544: Calcium channel blocker

A. Maternal side effect: gastritis and platelet dysfunction. Fetal adverse effect: oligohydramnios
B. Maternal side effect: flushing and elevation of transaminases. Contraindications: preload-dependent maternal cardiac lesions
C. Maternal side effect: diaphoresis, respiratory depression, and suppresses heart rate. Fetal adverse effect: neonatal depression
D. Maternal side effect: palpitations, shortness of breath, and pulmonary edema. Fetal adverse effect: tachycardia. Contraindication: poorly controlled diabetes

Q545: Nonsteroidal anti-inflammatory drugs

A. Maternal side effect: gastritis and platelet dysfunction. Fetal adverse effect: oligohydramnios
B. Maternal side effect: flushing and elevation of transaminases. Contraindications: preload-dependent maternal cardiac lesions

C. Maternal side effect: diaphoresis, respiratory depression, and suppresses heart rate. Fetal adverse effect: neonatal depression
D. Maternal side effect: palpitations, shortness of breath, and pulmonary edema. Fetal adverse effect: tachycardia. Contraindication: poorly controlled diabetes

Q546: Beta-adrenergic receptor agonists
A. Maternal side effect: gastritis and platelet dysfunction. Fetal adverse effect: oligohydramnios
B. Maternal side effect: flushing and elevation of transaminases. Contraindications: preload-dependent maternal cardiac lesions
C. Maternal side effect: diaphoresis, respiratory depression, and suppresses heart rate. Fetal adverse effect: neonatal depression
D. Maternal side effect: palpitations, shortness of breath, and pulmonary edema. Fetal adverse effect: tachycardia. Contraindication: poorly controlled diabetes

Q547: Magnesium sulfate
A. Maternal side effect: gastritis and platelet dysfunction. Fetal adverse effect: oligohydramnios
B. Maternal side effect: flushing and elevation of transaminases. Contraindications: preload-dependent maternal cardiac lesions
C. Maternal side effect: diaphoresis, respiratory depression, and suppresses heart rate. Fetal adverse effect: neonatal depression
D. Maternal side effect: palpitations, shortness of breath, and pulmonary edema. Fetal adverse effect: tachycardia. Contraindication: poorly controlled diabetes

Q548: Uterine response to Pitocin starts ________ after infusion of oxytocin, and a steady state is reached at ________.

A. 1–2 min, 10 min
B. 2–3 min, 20 min
C. 2–3 min, 30 min
D. 3–5 min, 30 min
E. 3–5 min, 40 min

Q549: Membrane stripping is commonly practiced, but is not supported by evidence.

A. True
B. False

Q550: A 33-year-old G1P0 is scheduled for a primary low transverse cesarean section at 38 weeks gestation due to breech presentation of Twin A. In reviewing her history, it is noted that she has a severe penicillin allergy. What alternative antibiotic(s) should she receive for prophylaxis?

A. Cefazolin and clindamycin
B. An aminoglycoside and clindamycin
C. An aminoglycoside
D. Vancomycin and clindamycin

Q551: Ideally, when should antibiotic prophylaxis for cesarean section be administered?

A. More than an hour before skin incision
B. Before clamping of the umbilical cord
C. Prior to skin closure
D. Within an hour prior to skin incision

Q552: Diabetic nephropathy, when in the setting of pregnancy, can lead to end-stage renal disease particularly if:

A. Serum creatinine is above 1.0 mg/dL or 24 h protein is 300 mg per 24 h
B. Serum creatinine is above 1.5 mg/dL or 24 h protein is 3000 mg per 24 h
C. Serum creatinine is above 2.0 mg/dL or 24 h protein is 300 g per 24 h
D. Serum creatinine is above 2.5 mg/dL or 24 h protein is 3000 g per 24 h
E. Urine protein is not predictive of progression to end-stage renal disease

Q553: When is antenatal surveillance recommended?

A. In women with pregestational diabetes
B. In all women with gestational diabetes
C. In women with gestational diabetes with poor glycemic control
D. At the discretion of the provider in women with well-controlled gestational diabetes
E. A and C

Q554: When does ACOG recommend delivery of pregestational diabetics who are well controlled?

A. 37th week
B. 38th week
C. 39th week
D. 40th week
E. There are insufficient data to make a recommendation

Q555: Diabetic ketoacidosis occurs more commonly in pregnancy and can even occur in patients who have normal blood glucose readings.

A. True
B. False

Q556: You are monitoring fetal heart tones on labor and delivery when you notice a deceleration. It coincides with the uterine contraction and is abrupt, and the total deceleration is noted to be 45 s. What type of deceleration is this?

A. Early deceleration
B. Late deceleration
C. Variable deceleration
D. Prolonged deceleration
E. Unable to classify based on the information given

Q557: A medical student on labor and delivery asks how baseline fetal heart rate is defined and what value is considered to be normal. You explain:

A. The baseline is given in increments of 10 beats per minute and must be present for a minimum of 3 min in a 10 min segment. Normal is defined as 120–160
B. The baseline is given in increments of 5 beats per minute and must be present for a minimum of 2 min in a 10 min segment. Normal is defined as 120–160
C. The baseline is given in increments of 10 beats per minute and must be present for a minimum of 3 min in a 10 min segment. Normal is defined as 110–160
D. The baseline is given in increments of 5 beats per minute and must be present for a minimum of 2 min in a 10 min segment. Normal is defined as 110–160

Q558: A 33-year-old Rh-negative G3P2002 with intrauterine pregnancy at 11 weeks gestational age presents for chorionic villus sampling (CVS). The patient should be given ______ prior to the procedure.

A. 50 μg anti-D immune globulin
B. 150 μg anti-D immune globulin
C. 300 μg anti-D immune globulin
D. No anti-D immune globulin

Q559: The same patient in Question #558 goes on to have a miscarriage at 15 weeks gestational age. The patient should now be given _____.

A. 50 μg anti-D immune globulin
B. 150 μg anti-D immune globulin
C. 300 μg anti-D immune globulin
D. No anti-D immune globulin

Q560: In a patient who continues to bleed after being administered prophylactic anti-D immune globulin, what test can be used to monitor persistent presence of the immune globulin?

A. Kleihauer-Betke test
B. Repeat type and screen
C. Direct Coombs test
D. Indirect Coombs test

Q561: Two pregnant patients, a 23-year-old and a 47-year-old, present to their NOB visit requesting cell-free DNA because they both desire to know the sex of their fetus as early as possible. Both have unremarkable past OB histories. Both have cell-free fetal DNA results that are positive for T18. Which of the following is true?

A. The 23-year-old is more likely to have a T18 fetus
B. The 47-year-old is more likely to have a T18 fetus
C. They are equally both likely to have a T18 fetus

Q562: A critically ill OB patient is being transferred to another hospital due to the availability of ICU services. Which of the following are true?

A. Patient needs to have secure IV access prior to transfer
B. Minimal maternal monitoring during transfer includes pulse oximetry, electrocardiography, and frequent assessment of vital signs
C. Minimal fetal assessment during transfer includes continuous external fetal monitoring
D. A and B
E. All of the above

Q563: The most common causes for ICU admission for obstetric patients are hemorrhage and sepsis.

A. True
B. False

Q564: Key differences in laboratory values during pregnancy include all of the following EXCEPT:

A. Decreased blood pressure
B. Increased serum creatinine levels
C. Increased heart rate
D. Increased D-dimer levels
E. All of the above are true

Q565: A 32-year-old patient has a positive first-trimester screen. Which of the following are acceptable options for follow-up assessment?

A. Cell-free fetal DNA
B. CVS
C. Amniocentesis
D. Any of the above

Q566: A patient presents to the obstetrical triage on postpartum day 3 reporting a headache that is worsened when in the sitting or standing position. Upon review of her chart, you note that she was delivered by cesarean section and had a spinal placed for analgesia. You suspect she has a postdural puncture headache. You counsel her:

A. A blood patch has minimal effectiveness in treating postdural headaches
B. A postdural puncture headache only occurs in patients who have had spinal anesthesia
C. It is reasonable to try conservative measures first including supine positioning, hydration, and analgesics
D. Having a postdural puncture headache increases her risk of having persistent back pain in the upcoming years

Q567: Treatment for gestational diabetes is associated with a decrease in which of the following EXCEPT:

A. Hypertensive disorders
B. Shoulder dystocia
C. Cesarean section
D. Neonatal hypoglycemia
E. All of the above were decreased

Q568: Your patient was recently diagnosed with gestational diabetes. She asks you what you recommend in terms of management of gestational diabetes for the rest of her pregnancy. You counsel her:

A. To eat three meals a day and limit snacks
B. To check her glucose three times a day, 1 or 2 h postprandial
C. To initiate a moderate exercise program
D. A and C
E. All of the above

Q569: What is the most common side effect of regional analgesia?

A. Transient neurological symptoms
B. Pruritus
C. Postdural puncture headache
D. Hypotension

Q570: Which of the following is FALSE regarding twin-twin transfusion syndrome?

A. Ultrasounds should be performed to monitor for twin-twin transfusion syndrome starting at 20 weeks gestational age
B. Twin-twin transfusion syndrome occurs in 10–15% of monochorionic-diamniotic twin gestations
C. Twin-twin transfusion syndrome is generally diagnosed in the second trimester
D. Twin-twin transfusion syndrome results from AV anastomoses in the placenta

Q571: Which of the following is the correct sequence for the progression of twin-twin transfusion?

A. Absent bladder in the donor; abnormal Doppler ultrasonography; oligohydramnios/polyhydramnios; hydrops; death
B. Oligohydramnios/polyhydramnios; absent bladder in the donor; abnormal Doppler ultrasonography; hydrops; death
C. Oligohydramnios/polyhydramnios; abnormal Doppler ultrasonography; absent bladder in the donor; death
D Absent bladder in the donor; oligohydramnios/polyhydramnios; abnormal Doppler ultrasonography; hydrops; death
E. Oligohydramnios/polyhydramnios; absent bladder in the donor; abnormal Doppler ultrasonography; death

Q572: Asthma symptoms consistently worsen with pregnancy.

A. True
B. False

Q573: Your 23-year-old patient was previously very nervous as her nuchal translucency measurement was 4 mm. She then underwent an amniocentesis revealing a normal XY fetus. In regard to her current risk for abnormalities, you counsel her that:

A. Her fetus has a decreased risk for genetic syndromes
B. Her risk for adverse outcome is comparable to having a nuchal translucency of 6mm
C. A fetal ECHO should be performed
D. None of the above

Q574: Your patient comes to her return OB appointment and is very concerned following the finding of a cystic hygroma on her first-trimester ultrasound. How do you counsel her?

A. Her risk for aneuploidy is approximately 50%
B. Her risk for structural malformation in the absence of aneuploidy is 50%
C. Her chance for a healthy live-born term infant is approximately 50%
D. A and B
E. A and C

Q575: Which of the following does NOT point toward a new diagnosis of asthma in pregnancy?

A. Symptoms fluctuate in intensity and are often worse at night
B. Symptoms do not respond to typical asthma therapy
C. Symptoms are triggered by allergens
D. Wheezing can be heard on auscultation
E. FEV1 improves after bronchodilator

Q576: A MFM physician calls regarding a patient who had middle cerebral artery Doppler testing today. The testing revealed that the measurement was two times the median for gestational age. How should the patient be counseled?

A. This test is somewhat sensitive for fetal anemia and the baby may be anemic
B. This is a very specific test for fetal anemia and shows the baby is anemic
C. This is a very sensitive test for fetal anemia and currently the baby is not anemic
D. This test is interpreted as part of a calculation; no meaningful results can be given at this time

Q577: A patient is diagnosed with alloimmunization that is non-Rh-D. Which of the following is TRUE regarding this?

A. Most are due to prior incompatible blood transfusions
B. There has been a relative decrease in this due to anti-D immune globulin
C. They occur in approximately 10% of obstetric patients
D. None of the above

Q578: Which of the following is true regarding the effects of teratogen exposure on IUGR?

A. The effect is dependent on the timing, duration, exposure, and dosage of the drug
B. Drugs commonly associated with IUGR include cyclophosphamide, valproic acid, warfarin, and lisinopril
C. Individual genetic predisposition for drug metabolism can mediate the effect of a teratogen
D. A and B
E. A and C

Q579: All of the following infections are associated with IUGR EXCEPT:

A. HSV
B. CMV
C. Rubella
D. Malaria
E. Varicella

Q580: Which of the following tests are predictive of fetal anemia in Kell alloimmunization?

A. Amniotic fluid bilirubin measurements
B. Middle cerebral Doppler measurements
C. Antibody titers
D. A and B
E. B and C

Q581: Decreased variability seen with use of magnesium sulfate is related to early gestational age not the serum magnesium level.

A. True
B. False

Q582: Woman with pregnancies complicated by gestational diabetes is at increased risk for hypertensive disorders of pregnancy, cesarean section, macrosomia, and:

A. Neonatal hyperglycemia
B. Hyperbilirubinemia
C. Fetal hypoinsulinemia
D. All of the above
E. None of the above

Q583: Gestational diabetes is defined by:

A. Carbohydrate intolerance with onset or recognition during pregnancy
B. Carbohydrate intolerance at 20 or more weeks gestation
C. Glucose intolerance with onset or recognition during pregnancy
D. Glucose intolerance at 20 or more weeks gestation
E. None of the above

Q584: Use of which medication during labor can cause a transient sinusoidal fetal heart rate pattern?

A. Butorphanol
B. Morphine
C. Bupivacaine
D. Magnesium

Q585: Fetal heart rate findings which are strongly reassuring of a normal acid-base status include:

A. Moderate variability with decelerations
B. Moderate variability with no decelerations
C. Presence of accelerations
D. All of the above
E. B and C

Q586: Which of the following is TRUE regarding lupus anticoagulant?

A. It is an anticoagulant
B. Testing involves screening and then a second confirmatory test
C. Results are reported as low, medium, or high levels
D. It can be tested, while the patient is treated with anticoagulation
E. All of the above

Q587: Which of the following is TRUE regarding anticardiolipin antibodies and anit-B2 glycoprotein I?

A. Only IgG should be tested
B. Testing involves screening and then a second confirmatory test
C. A positive result is greater than the 99th percentile for normal population
D. IgA can be tested in patients that test negative when clinical suspicion is high
E. All of the above

Q588: A 42-year-old G3P2002 at term is currently laboring on the maternal care unit. Her most recent cervical exam is 8/90/-1. Review of her fetal heart rate tracing reveals minimal variability without accelerations. Which of the following techniques can be performed to illicit an acceleration to give reassurance that academia is unlikely?

A. Allis clamp stimulation
B. Vibroacoustic stimulation
C. Digital scalp stimulation
D. All of the above

Q589: Maternal supplemental oxygen has been shown to be effective in improving fetal heart rate tracings.

A. True
B. False

Q590: Transcervical amnioinfusion has been shown to be effective at reducing which of the following fetal heart rate abnormalities?

A. Recurrent late decelerations
B. Recurrent variable decelerations
C. Recurrent early decelerations
D. A and B
E. All of the above

Q591: Which of the following has an increased risk for aneuploidy above that of the mother's age-adjusted risk?

A. A dizygotic twin
B. A monozygotic twin
C. Both
D. Neither

Q592: Nuchal translucency is:

A. If discordant in monochorionic gestations, may be a marker for twin-twin transfusion syndrome
B. A reliable way to evaluate twins and higher-order multifetal gestations independently
C. Useful if cutoffs are adjusted for twins and higher-order gestations
D. A and B
E. All of the above

Q593: In which scenario is tocolytic therapy thought to be most appropriate?

A. With any fetal heart rate abnormality
B. When tachysystole is present with associated fetal heart rate changes
C. When Pitocin is currently being administered and a Category II tracing is noted
D. There is not an appropriate scenario for tocolytic therapy

Q594: Excluding ART use, the likelihood of a multifetal gestation increases with maternal age.

A. True
B. False

Q595: Which of the following ART techniques may have the most significant effect on the increase of multifetal pregnancies?
A. In vitro fertilization
B. Ovulation induction with clomiphene
C. Controlled ovarian hyperstimulation with gonadotropins
D. A and C
E. All of the above

Q596: Initial evaluation of a Category II or Category III fetal heart tracing should include all of the following EXCEPT:
A. Monitoring of maternal blood pressure
B. Placement of intrauterine pressure catheter
C. Evaluation for umbilical cord prolapse
D. Cessation of labor-inducing agent
E. All of the above are appropriate initial evaluations

Q597: Which of the following fetal complications is more likely to be seen with preterm PROM pregnancies than preterm deliveries due to other causes?
A. Intraventricular hemorrhage
B. White matter damage
C. Necrotizing enterocolitis
D. Respiratory distress

Q598: Which of the following is FALSE regarding fetal pulmonary hypoplasia?
A. Associated with a high risk of mortality
B. Less common after 23–24 weeks gestation
C. Early gestational age at membrane rupture and low residual amniotic fluid volume are primary determinants
D. All of the above are true

Q599: What is the latest gestational age that pregnancies complicated by alloimmunization should be delivered?
A. 34 weeks gestational age
B. 35 weeks gestational age

C. 36 weeks gestational age
D. 37 weeks gestational age
E. 38 weeks gestational age

Q600: What percent of women who have venous thromboembolism have a thrombophilia?
A. 5–10%
B. 10–20%
C. 20–50%
D. 50–70%

Q601: At what gestation does the fetal thyroid begin to synthesize its own thyroid hormone?
A. 8 weeks gestation
B. 12 weeks gestation
C. 20 weeks gestation
D. 24 weeks gestation
E. At birth

Q602: In which of the following cases is the fetus at the highest risk for fetal thyrotoxicosis?
A. A woman with Graves' disease being treated with methimazole
B. A woman with Graves' disease who was previously treated with a thyroidectomy
C. A woman with a suppressed TSH but normal free T4 who is on no medications
D. All of the above have equal risk for adverse outcomes

Q603: Dosing of heparin compounds in pregnancy is impacted by the following:
A. Crosses the placenta but appears to be safe during pregnancy
B. Renal excretion is increased
C. Protein-bound fraction is decreased
D. B and C
E. All of the above

Q604: A patient is given a dose of prophylactic anti-D immune globulin at 37 weeks gestational age due to abdominal trauma sustained during a motor vehicle accident. Patient is discharged home after extended monitoring without evidence of abruption. The patient goes on to have an uncomplicated vaginal delivery at 39/4 weeks gestational age. Does the patient need postpartum anti-D immune globulin?

A. Yes because this represents a separate event at which time fetomaternal hemorrhage can occur
B. Yes because anti-D immune globulin half-life is only 14 days; thus, a redosing is needed
C. No because the anti-D immune globulin half-life is 24 days; thus, a redosing is not needed
D. No because it was an uncomplicated vaginal delivery without hemorrhage

Q605: Fetal tissue sampling after birth has a greater tissue culture rate than amniocentesis before delivery.

A. True
B. False

Q606: Which of the following is TRUE regarding infection as it relates to stillbirth?

A. May be caused by malaria in developing countries
B. More likely to occur before the third trimester in developed countries
C. May be associated with the pathogens parvovirus and syphilis
D. A and B
E. All of the above

Q607: Which inherited thrombophilia accounts for the greatest percentage, as high as 40%, of thromboembolism in pregnancy?

A. Antithrombin deficiency
B. Factor V Leiden heterozygote
C. Protein C deficiency
D. Prothrombin gene homozygote

Q608: Which of the following confers the greatest risk for thromboembolism?
A. A 32-year-old pregnant patient who is a heterozygote for factor V Leiden and has a personal history of thromboembolism
B. A 32-year-old pregnant patient with protein C deficiency
C. A 32-year-old pregnant patient who is a homozygote for factor V Leiden and has a sister with a history of thromboembolism
D. A and C have the same risk

Q609: A G2P1001 Rh-negative patient presents for her initial prenatal visit and reports that she never received Rh prophylaxis with her previous pregnancy. What are the chances that she is currently alloimmunized?
A. 0–5%
B. 15–20%
C. 30–40%
D. 50–70%

Q610: Tocolytics should be considered in which of the following situations?
A. A 37-year-old G5P0040 presents at 32 weeks gestational age with moderate contractions; cervical exam is 2/50/-2. She is not ruptured
B. A 37-year-old G5P0040 presents to triage at 26 weeks gestation. She is found to be ruptured. The first dose of betamethasone is administered. The patient has mild contractions, her abdomen is soft and nontender to palpation, and she has no leukocytosis. She requests tocolysis until steroid benefit has been reached
C. An 18-year-old G1P0 at 18 weeks gestation who has just had an appendectomy
D. All of the above
E. None of the above

Q611: A 30-year-old G2P0101 at 32 weeks gestation in your office. She is your patient and also your coworker. She reports contractions throughout the day that interfere with her ability to focus on her job and requests nifedipine for symptomatic relief to use as needed.

A. You tell her that the use of chronic tocolytics does not prevent preterm delivery
B. You empathize with her symptoms and give her a prescription for nifedipine prn
C. Tell her that there is no indication to give her nifedipine and do not write a prescription
D. A and B
E. A and C

Q612: Fetal spina bifida increases the risk for oligohydramnios.

A. True
B. False

Q613: A 33-year-old G2P1001 presents for her routine obstetrical visit at 32 weeks gestation. Diagnostic tests have previously revealed her fetus to be affected with spina bifida. She asks you about plans for delivery. You counsel her:

A. She will need a cesarean section at term
B. She will likely be able to have a vaginal delivery at term
C. She will need a cesarean section at 37 weeks
D. She will be offered induction of labor at 37 weeks

Q614: How should a pregnancy at "high risk" for fetal intracranial hemorrhage be managed?

A. Combination of maternal intravenous immunoglobulin and intravenous prednisone should be given
B. Direct fetal administration of intravenous immunoglobulin
C. Cesarean section should be performed if fetal platelet count is less than 50,000/μL at the time of delivery

D. A and C
E. All of the above

Q615: If platelet count is stable, it is reasonable to provide epidural or spinal anesthesia if maternal platelet count is equal to or above ________.
A. 60,000/μL
B. 70,000/μL
C. 80,000/μL
D. 90,000/μL
E. 100,000/μL

Q616: Thrombocytopenia in pregnancy is defined as:
A. 100,000/μL
B. 120,000/μL
C. 130,000/μL
D. 140,000/μL
E. 150,000/μL

Q617: What is the difference between primary and secondary postpartum hemorrhage?
A. Primary postpartum hemorrhage occurs within the first 12 h of delivery, and secondary hemorrhage occurs between 12 h and 6–12 weeks postpartum
B. Primary postpartum hemorrhage occurs within the first 24 h of delivery, and secondary hemorrhage occurs between 24 h and 6–12 weeks postpartum
C. Primary postpartum hemorrhage occurs within the first 48 h of delivery, and secondary hemorrhage occurs between 48 h and 6–12 weeks postpartum
D. Primary postpartum hemorrhage occurs within the first 72 h of delivery, and secondary hemorrhage occurs between 72 h and 6–12 weeks postpartum

Q618: A patient is currently taking risperidone for schizophrenia. Which of the following is TRUE regarding this medication?

A. It is a typical antipsychotic
B. It is not associated with teratogenic effects
C. It is associated with an increase in low birth weight of exposed infants
D. It has a long reproductive safety profile
E. B and D

Q619: A 36-year-old G4P3003 is found to be 2 cm dilated at 20 weeks gestation. She denies complaints. What type of cerclage would you offer her?

A. History indicated
B. Physical exam indicated
C. Ultrasound indicated
D. Do not offer cerclage
E. Do not offer cerclage but would offer her vaginal progesterone therapy

Q620: A 28-year-old G2P0101 at 13 weeks gestation presents for routine obstetric care. What type of cerclage would you offer her?

A. History indicated
B. Physical exam indicated
C. Ultrasound indicated
D. Do not offer cerclage
E. Do not offer cerclage but would offer her vaginal progesterone therapy

Q621: Which of the following is TRUE regarding the fetal and neonatal effects of typical antipsychotics?

A. Their use is associated with minimal risk
B. Oral clefts are associated with their use
C. Hypertonia may persist up to 1 year of age
D. Their use is associated with floppy infant syndrome

Q622: Higher levels of SSRI medications are found in breast milk than the fetus was exposed to by transplacental exposure during pregnancy.

A. True
B. False

Q623: Which of the following medication is associated with fetal cholestatic hepatitis and hyperbilirubinemia?

A. Lithium
B. Valproate
C. Carbamazepine
D. Doxepin

Q624: An ultrasound is performed on a patient who is 10/5 weeks gestational age by LMP, and the crown-rump length measures larger. At what difference would you change her estimated date of delivery?

A. More than 5 days
B. More than 6 days
C. More than 7 days
D. More than 10 days

Q625: Which single measurement is most predictive of gestational age during the second and third trimester, respectively?

A. Femur length, head circumference
B. Head circumference, femur length
C. Biparietal diameter, femur length
D. Femur length, biparietal diameter
E. None is superior

Q626: What is the most common cause of primary postpartum hemorrhage?

A. Retained placenta
B. Defects in coagulation

C. Vaginal laceration
D. Uterine atony

Q627: Which of the following is NOT an example of an atypical antidepressant?
A. Bupropion
B. Duloxetine
C. Mirtazapine
D. Nefazodone
E. All of the above are atypical antidepressants

Q628: Which of the following lab value is NOT consistent with a diagnosis of hyperemesis gravidarum?
A. Amylase ten times normal
B. Ketonuria
C. Increased liver function tests in the 100s
D. Elevated serum bilirubin of 3
E. Hypochloremic metabolic alkalosis

Q629: Which of the following is a characteristic of a mediolateral episiotomy?
A. It starts within 10 mm of midline
B. It is angled at least 30°
C. It is aimed toward the ischial tuberosity
D. It is more common in the United States
E. It is associated with increased rates of pelvic organ prolapse

Q630: Episiotomy is associated with:
A. Increased risk of anal incontinence if there is extension into the anal sphincter complex
B. Increased risk of anal incontinence regardless of extension
C. No increased risk of anal incontinence
D. Decreased risk of anal incontinence
E. Increased risk or stress urinary incontinence

Q631: All of the following are options to consider in the differential for nausea and vomiting of pregnancy EXCEPT:
A. Acute pancreatitis
B. Chronic hepatitis
C. Helicobacter pylori
D. Gastric ulcer

Q632: A patient presents for a well-woman exam who has a history of bipolar disorder. She is currently well controlled on lithium. Prior to starting the medication, she had severe episodes, though they were infrequent. What would you recommend she do prior to attempting to conceive?
A. Stop lithium immediately given teratogenicity
B. Taper off of lithium given teratogenicity
C. Taper off of lithium, and then restart it after organogenesis
D. Taper off of lithium, and then restart it in the third trimester
E. Continue throughout pregnancy due to high risk of relapse

Q633: Perioperative antibiotic prophylaxis is not recommended at the time of prophylactic or emergent cerclage placement.
A. True
B. False

Q634: Vertical transmission of CMV:
A. Has the same probability of occurring in all trimesters
B. Is more likely to occur in the third trimester
C. Is more likely to cause severe disease if it occurs in the first trimester
D. A and C
E. B and C

Q635: Which of the following is FALSE regarding parvovirus B19?
A. Is a single-stranded DNA virus
B. Causes "fifth disease" in children

C. Serious manifestation is more likely to occur in patients with a hemoglobinopathy
D. Most common symptoms in adult include reticular rash on trunk and peripheral arthropathy
E. All of the above are true

Q636: What dose of prophylactic antibiotic is recommended at the time of manual placenta extraction following a vaginal delivery?
A. 2 g cefazolin
B. 1 g cefazolin
C. 2 g ampicillin
D. No data supports prophylactic antibiotic usage in this scenario

Q637: Examples of causes of secondary postpartum hemorrhage include all of the following EXCEPT:
A. Infection
B. Subinvolution of placental site
C. Inherited coagulation defects
D. Retained products of conception
E. All of the above are causes of secondary postpartum hemorrhage

Q638: Management of a subsequent pregnancy in a patient with a history of prior stillbirth may include all of the following EXCEPT:
A. Antepartum fetal surveillance starting at 34 weeks gestational age or 1–2 weeks earlier than prior stillbirth
B. Support and reassurance
C. Kick counts starting at 28 weeks gestational age
D. Screening for fetal growth restriction by ultrasound after 28 weeks gestation
E. None of the above

Q639: How is cervical insufficiency diagnosed?
A. Painless cervical dilation at any time during pregnancy
B. Shortened cervical length in the second trimester

C. History of a second-trimester delivery after painless dilation
D. Balloon elastin test
E. B and C

Q640: Which of the following are risk factors for cervical insufficiency?
A. Cold knife cone
B. In utero exposure to DES
C. Mullerian anomalies
D. A and B
E. All of the above

Q641: A 34-year-old G2P1000 presents for her routine prenatal visit at 30 weeks gestation. She has an obstetrical history significant for a stillbirth in her previous pregnancy at 37 weeks gestational age with unknown cause. She has no current medical issues. Patient is asking at what gestational age she will be delivered this pregnancy. You counsel her:
A. She will be scheduled for an elective induction at 39 weeks gestation
B. She will be scheduled for an elective induction at 37 weeks gestation
C. She will be scheduled for an elective induction at 35 weeks gestation
D. A or B
E. Any of the above are reasonable given her history

Q642: Inherited thrombophilias are associated with which of the following?
A. Fetal loss
B. Preeclampsia
C. Placenta abruption
D. All of the above
E. None of the above

Q643: In which of the following patient(s) would it be appropriate to screen for an inherited thrombophilia at their first obstetrical visit?

A. A 32-year-old G2P1001 with a first cousin with a known antithrombin deficiency
B. A 29-year-old G1P0 with a history of a DVT following a pelvic fracture sustained in a motor vehicle accident
C. A 42-year-old G6P5005 with bulging varicose veins on exam
D. A 23-year-old G2P1001 whose brother is known to be a homozygote for factor V Leiden
E. All of the above
F. B and D

Q644: A 24-year-old G2P1001 is status post spontaneous vaginal delivery 5 min ago. The placenta has delivered without issue. The patient begins to have heavy vaginal bleeding. What FIRST steps should be taken to evaluate the patient?

A. Lacerations should be ruled out with thorough visual assessment of vaginal area
B. The vagina should be packed immediately
C. The bladder should be emptied and a bimanual pelvic exam should be performed
D. Ultrasound should be performed to assess for retained placenta

Q645: Which of the following is FALSE regarding a genital tract hematoma?

A. Interventional radiology should be considered for management
B. Often times a single source of bleeding will be identified when the hematoma is incised
C. It may be appropriate to place a drain in situ after a hematoma is drained
D. Can lead to large blood loss
E. Can occur in the absence of a vaginal laceration

Q646: Which of the following is NOT part of the perineal body?

A. Deep muscle of the perineal membrane
B. Transverse perineal muscle
C. Bulbocavernosus muscle
D. External anal sphincter
E. The perineal body includes all of the above

Q647: The internal anal sphincter is under autonomic control and provides 80% of the resting pressure of the anal canal.

A. True
B. False

Q648: Which of the following makes the diagnosis of a retained placenta less likely?

A. Echogenic mass within the uterus visualized on ultrasound
B. History of previous uterine surgery
C. Manual extraction of the placenta
D. All of the above increase the likelihood of retained placenta

Q649: Which of the following principles are recommended when prescribing psychotropic medications to pregnant patients?

A. Prescribe multiple medications at their lowest doses to avoid possible teratogenic consequences of higher doses
B. Prescribe medications with higher protein binding properties to decrease placental passage
C. Continue to change medications as needed if the lowest dose is ineffective
D. Prioritize medications with more metabolites to increase efficacy at lower doses

Q650: Which class of drugs is associated with floppy infant syndrome and neonatal withdrawal syndrome?

A. Benzodiazepines
B. SSRIs
C. Lithium
D. Antiepileptic drugs
E. Antipsychotic medications

Q651: An amniotic fluid embolism can be associated with clotting abnormalities leading to hemorrhage.

A. True
B. False

Q652: Which of the following is TRUE regarding a clot observation test?

A. Can provide a rough estimate of fibrinogen level within 10 min
B. The blood will not clot within 10 min if fibrinogen level is less than 200 mg/dL
C. Blood with normal levels of fibrinogen will clot within 10 min and remain intact
D. A and C
E. All of the above

Q653: Asthma medications should be continued during labor and delivery, and fluids should be given sparingly to decrease the risk of bronchospasm.

A. True
B. False

Q654: Pregnant patients receiving systemic corticosteroids require additional IV dosing of steroids during labor and after delivery to prevent adrenal crisis.

A. True
B. False

Q655: Which of the following asthma medications are contraindicated with breastfeeding?
A. Prednisone
B. Cromolyn
C. Theophylline
D. Inhaled corticosteroids
E. None of the above

For the following questions, choose the uterotonic drug which best matches the description given.

Q656: Should be avoided in asthmatics.
A. Pitocin
B. Methergine
C. Hemabate
D. Misoprostol

Q657: Can cause diarrhea.
A. Pitocin
B. Methergine
C. Hemabate
D. Misoprostol

Q658: Can cause hypotension.
A. Pitocin
B. Methergine
C. Hemabate
D. Misoprostol

Q659: Dosing is 0.2 mg IM q 2–4 h.
A. Pitocin
B. Methergine
C. Hemabate
D. Misoprostol

Q660: A maximum of eight doses may be given.
A. Pitocin
B. Methergine

C. Hemabate
D. Misoprostol

Q661: Should be avoided in hypertensive patients.
A. Pitocin
B. Methergine
C. Hemabate
D. Misoprostol

Q662: Which of the following tests provide no information regarding risk stratification until the second trimester?
A. Integrated
B. Contingent
C. Sequential
D. A and B
E. A and C

Q663: A 19-year-old G1P0 has completed a normal first-trimester screen. She now presents to her 16 week appointment with concerns regarding neural tube defects because she has a friend who had a baby with spina bifida. What test would you offer her?
A. AFP
B. Quad screen
C. Sequential screen
D. Detailed anatomy scan
E. None of the above

Q664: Sickle cell disease:
A. Is an autosomal dominant disorder
B. Occurs most commonly in people of Caucasian descent
C. Involves a single nucleotide substitution on the alpha-globin gene
D. A and C
E. None of the above

Q665: A 33-year-old G1P0 presents to the office for her first obstetrical visit. In reviewing her history, you note a history of Crohn's disease. You counsel her that she is most at risk for which kind of anemia?

A. Macrocytic anemia caused by folate deficiency
B. Macrocytic anemia caused by vitamin B12 deficiency
C. Microcytic anemia caused by iron deficiency
D. Normocytic anemia caused by bone marrow suppression

Q666: Which of the following is TRUE regarding preterm PROM?

A. Delivery will occur within 1 week in 50% of patients regardless of management
B. Latency after membrane rupture is directly correlated with gestational age at the time of membrane rupture
C. Incidence of infection is higher at earlier gestational age
D. B and C
E. A and C

Q667: What is the most common complication of prematurity for the fetus?

A. Sepsis
B. Necrotizing enterocolitis
C. Intraventricular hemorrhage
D. Respiratory distress

Q668: Not all women should be screened for anemia during pregnancy.

A. True
B. False

Q669: Hemoglobin A is composed of:

A. Two alpha and two beta chains
B. Two beta and two delta chains
C. Two alpha and two gamma chains

D. Four beta chains
E. Four alpha chains

Q670: Varicella zoster is a highly contagious virus that has a period of infectivity lasting:
A. 24 h before a rash appears until the first vesicles form
B. 24 h before a rash appears until the vesicles crust over
C. 48 h before a rash appears until the first vesicles form
D. 48 h before a rash appears until the vesicles crust over

Q671: A 29-year-old G2P1001 with intrauterine pregnancy at 31 weeks gestation develops symptoms of acute varicella-zoster infection including rash and vesicle formation. You counsel her that she is at risk of developing _______ which is a significant risk factor for maternal mortality.
A. pneumonia
B. coagulopathy
C. SIRS
D. myocarditis

Q672: Acute chest syndrome includes all of the following EXCEPT:
A. Pulmonary infiltrates
B. Fever
C. Hypoxemia
D. Infection
E. All of the above are present in acute chest syndrome

Q673: Which of the following is TRUE regarding vaginal births after cesarean section for the macrosomic fetus?
A. Macrosomia is a contraindication
B. Success rates are less than 50%
C. All of the above
D. None of the above

Q674: Large for gestational age is defined as:
A. Birth weight at or above 4000 g
B. Birth weight at or above 5000 g
C. Birth weight at or above the 90th percentile
D. Birth weight at or above the 95th percentile
E. None of the above

Q675: Which of the following will NOT have clinical implications?
A. Hb SC disease
B. Hb SS
C. Hb S/beta-thalassemia
D. Deletion of one alpha-globin gene
E. All of the above have clinical consequences

Q676: In a patient attempting a TOLAC, which of the following is TRUE?
A. Misoprostol should not be used for cervical ripening or labor induction in the third trimester
B. Misoprostol should not be used as a cervical ripening or labor induction agent in the second trimester
C. Misoprostol is never safe for a patient with a previous cesarean section
D. Misoprostol may be safe for term inductions when used at lower doses in a tertiary care facility
E. None of the above are true

Q677: What is the most common sign associated with uterine rupture?
A. Fetal heart rate abnormality
B. Increased uterine contractions
C. Vaginal bleeding
D. Loss of fetal station
E. New-onset intense uterine pain

Q678: What is the genotype of alpha-thalassemia carriers?
A. α-/αα
B. αα/--

C. α-/α-
D. B and C
E. All of the above

Q679: Hb Bart is:
A. Associated with abnormalities on the beta globin
B. Associated with hydrops fetalis
C. More common in patients of African origin
D. B and C
E. All of the above are true

Q680: Which of the following is a feature of beta-thalassemia major?
A. Precocious sexual development
B. Rapid growth
C. Extramedullary erythropoiesis
D. Decreased levels of Hb F
E. Death by age 30

Q681: Which of the following is TRUE regarding beta-thalassemia minor?
A. Severity depends on amount of beta chain production
B. Commonly associated with HB S
C. Common in individuals of Mediterranean descent
D. All of the above
E. None of the above

Q682: A 19-year-old African American G1P0 presents for her first obstetrical visit. She denies any known history of hemoglobinopathies in her family. What initial testing should be obtained?
A. CBC
B. Hemoglobin electrophoresis
C. Solubility tests
D. A and B
E. A and C

Q683: A patient presents for her first prenatal visit. She reports a history of depression and is currently taking an antidepressant. She asks about her overall risk of depression during pregnancy if she were to continue versus discontinue the medication. You counsel her that ______ % of women who discontinued their medications reported a relapse in depression compared to ________% of women who continued their medications.

A. 39%, 15%
B. 49%, 10%
C. 59%, 20%
D. 69%, 25%

Q684: Untreated depression during pregnancy is associated with:

A. Premature birth
B. Low birthweight
C. Fetal growth restriction
D. B and C
E. All of the above

Q685: How is alpha-thalassemia diagnosed?

A. Hemoglobin electrophoresis
B. Solubility testing
C. Molecular genetic testing
D. MCV
E. A or C

Q686: All of the following patients meet clinical criteria for antiphospholipid syndrome testing EXCEPT?

A. A 29-year-old with a DVT who is 36 weeks pregnant
B. A 60-year-old with retinal arterial thrombosis
C. An 18-year-old with three missed abortion at 6 weeks
D. A 30-year-old with a history of severe preeclampsia requiring delivery at 35 weeks gestation
E. All of the above meet criteria for testing

Q687: A 30-year-old G4P0030 presents for a new obstetrical visit at 10 weeks gestation and asks if you recommend anticoagulation. She has never had a thrombotic event. You counsel here that:

A. Clinical surveillance is recommended
B. Prophylactic anticoagulation until 6 weeks postpartum
C. Aspirin is recommended
D. A and C
E. All of the above are reasonable

Q688: How can thalassemias be diagnosed prenatally?

A. Preimplantation genetic diagnosis
B. Chorionic villus sampling
C. Amniocentesis
D. B and C
E. All of the above

Q689: Which of the following is TRUE regarding the risk for thromboembolic events associated with pregnancy?

A. All trimesters carry increased risk
B. Third trimester has a higher risk than any trimester or postpartum
C. The risk of thromboembolic event begins to increase in the second trimester
D. Approximately 75% of thromboembolic events associated with pregnancy occur during pregnancy, with 35% occurring postpartum
E. B and C

Q690: All of the following EXCEPT which increase the potential for thromboembolic events during pregnancy?

A. Increased venous stasis
B. Compression of the pelvic arteries
C. Compression of the inferior vena cava
D. Decreased mobility
E. All of the above contribute to an increased risk

Q691: Your 21-year-old G1P0 presents in active labor. At 7 cm dilation, she is noted to have tachysystole. Her fetus is Category 1. How is this defined?

A. 5 contractions or more per 10 min, averaged over 20 min
B. 5 contractions or more per 10 min, averaged over 30 min
C. more than 5 contractions per 10 min, averaged over 20 min
D. more than 5 contractions per 10 min, averaged over 30 min
E. Tachysystole is only diagnosed in induced or augmented labor

Q692: Your patient requests to be induced as she lives 4 h away from the hospital. How do you counsel her?

A. This is not an indication supported by ACOG
B. This is reasonable if an ultrasound done prior to 20 weeks confirms a gestational age of 37 weeks or greater
C. This is reasonable if it has been 36 weeks since a positive urine pregnancy test
D. This is reasonable if fetal heart tones have been documented for 20 weeks by Doppler
E. None of the above are true

Q693: Patients with sickle cell anemia are at increased risk for:

A. Gestational diabetes
B. Preterm labor
C. Macrosomia
D. Multifetal gestations
E. All of the above

Q694: What percentage of term fetuses are breech?

A. 1–2%
B. 3–4%
C. 5–6%
D. 7–8%

Q695: Patients are ideal candidates for external cephalic version (ECV) starting at:
A. 35/0 weeks
B. 36/0 weeks
C. 37/0 weeks
D. 38/0 weeks
E. 39/0 weeks

Q696: Which of the following therapies is recommended in pregnant patients with sickle cell disease?
A. 1 mg folate a day
B. 4 mg folate a day
C. Prophylactic cesarean section
D. Avoidance of regional anesthesia
E. Hydroxyurea

Q697: Which of the following is FALSE regarding macrocytic anemia?
A. Reticulocytosis may be decreased
B. Associated with a mean corpuscular volume greater than 100 fL
C. May be associated with folic acid deficiency
D. May be associated with liver disease
E. None of the above

Q698: Which of the following is TRUE regarding prothrombin G20210A mutations?
A. Is a point mutation that results in decreased circulating prothrombin levels
B. Has a synergistic hypercoagulable effect when also present with factor V Leiden mutations
C. Having a personal history of thromboembolism increases the risk for thromboembolism in carriers during pregnancy
D. B and C
E. All of the above are true

Q699: Screening for which thrombophilia is less reliable during pregnancy?

A. Protein C deficiency
B. Protein S deficiency
C. Factor V Leiden mutation
D. Prothrombin G20210A mutation
E. Antithrombin deficiency

Q700: What is the most common cause of microcytic anemia?

A. Acute blood loss
B. Iron deficiency
C. Sickle cell anemia
D. Thalassemia

Q701: In a patient attempting TOLAC, cervical ripening with a transcervical Foley catheter has been associated with uterine rupture rates similar to spontaneous labor.

A. True
B. False

Q702: In a patient attempting TOLAC, cervical ripening with misoprostol for an intrauterine fetal demise in the third trimester is recommended.

A. True
B. False

Q703: Your 32-year-old patient had planned for a TOLAC. She presents in spontaneous labor at term and her fetus is estimated to be 4500 g. She has an otherwise uncomplicated pregnancy. How do you counsel her?

A. If her fetus is macrosomic, her likelihood of a successful VBAC is lower, and her risk for uterine rupture is higher
B. If her fetus is macrosomic, her likelihood of a successful VBAC is unchanged, and her risk for uterine rupture is higher

C. If her fetus is macrosomic, her likelihood of a successful VBAC is unchanged as is her risk for uterine rupture
D. If her fetus is macrosomic, her likelihood of a successful VBAC is lower, but her risk for uterine rupture is unchanged

Q704: Which of the following accurately describes the care of a pregnant patient with a sickle cell pain crisis?
A. Diagnosis of medical problems causing predisposition
B. Control of pain while avoiding opiates
C. Oxygen to keep O2 saturation 90% or more
D. A and B
E. B and C

Q705: What is the most common complication encountered in multifetal gestations?
A. Neonatal death
B. Stillbirth
C. Preeclampsia
D. Spontaneous preterm birth

Q706: Multifetal gestations are associated with all of the following, EXCEPT:
A. Increased prevalence of cerebral palsy
B. Higher costs
C. Increase in short-term morbidity neonatal morbidity
D. Increase in long-term infant morbidity
E. All of the above are true

Q707: What is the goal of transfusion in pregnant patients with sickle cell disease?
A. Lower the Hb S to 30% and raise the total hemoglobin to 8 g/dL
B. Lower the Hb S to 40% and raise the total hemoglobin to 10 g/dL

C. Lower the Hb S to 30% and raise the total hemoglobin to 10 g/dL
D. Lower the Hb S to 40% and raise the total hemoglobin to 8 g/dL

Q708: Which of the following is TRUE regarding the treatment of overt hyperthyroidism in pregnancy?
A. Labs should be checked every trimester and doses adjusted accordingly
B. Doses should be adjusted to keep TSH at the upper limit of normal or just above
C. Patients should be given precautions regarding symptoms of agranulocytosis
D. Propylthiouracil should be used in the first and second trimester, and then the patient should be transitioned to methimazole
E. A and C

Q709: Which of the following statements are TRUE regarding thioamides in the treatment of overt hyperthyroidism of pregnancy?
A. Propylthiouracil is associated with aplasia cutis
B. Propylthiouracil inhibits the conversion of T3 to T4
C. Methimazole is associated with choanal atresia
D. Methimazole is associated with maternal hepatotoxicity
E. All of the above are true

Q710: Which of the following is FALSE regarding a gradual fetal heart rate decrease?
A. Includes early decelerations
B. Defined as from the onset of the fetal heart rate nadir of 30 s or more
C. Includes late decelerations
D. All of the above are false
E. All of the above are true

Q711: Which of the following is TRUE regarding inherited thrombophilias and contraception?

A. The risk of venous thromboembolism is not appreciably increased in factor V Leiden heterozygotes using estrogen-containing oral contraceptives
B. As long as patients are counseled regarding the risks of thromboembolism, it is reasonable to prescribe estrogen-containing contraceptives to patients with low-risk thrombophilias
C. Due to the increased risk of venous thromboembolism in patients with low-risk inherited thrombophilias, progestin-only pills or implants should be the only prescribed hormonal contraceptives
D. A and B
E. None of the above

Q712: Which of the following are TRUE in regard to fetal heart rate accelerations?

A. Onset is gradual
B. Prior to 34 weeks gestation, an acceleration has a peak of 10 beats per minute above baseline
C. If it lasts greater than 10 min, then it represents a change in baseline
D. B and C
E. All of the above are true

Q713: Monitoring of fetal growth is recommended for which of the following disorders?

A. Sickle cell disease
B. Beta-thalassemia major
C. Alpha-thalassemia trait
D. A and B
E. All of the above

Q714: What step should be employed next following continued bleeding in the setting of uterine atony despite use of adequate uterotonics?

A. Tamponade of the uterus
B. Exploratory laparotomy
C. Uterine artery embolization by interventional radiology
D. Bilateral uterine artery ligation

Q715: Oral acyclovir has been proven effective in reducing maternal symptoms and preventing fetal effects of congenital varicella syndrome if started within 24 h of developing a varicella-zoster-associated rash.

A. True
B. False

Q716: How long should pregnancy be delayed after administration of the last varicella vaccine dose?

A. 1 month
B. 2 months
C. 3 months
D. No delay is necessary

Q717: Hypogastric artery ligation is the most effective surgical technique to control uterine bleeding.

A. True
B. False

Q718: A 20-year-old G2P0101 presents for a new obstetric visit at 13 weeks gestation and would like to discuss the risks and benefits of having a cerclage placed now versus undergoing ultrasound monitoring. How do you counsel her?

A. Ultrasound surveillance involves monitoring cervical length starting now until 30 weeks gestational age
B. It is safer to have one placed now because 90% of women with a history of preterm delivery develop cervical effacement and will need rescue cerclage placement

C. By monitoring your cervical length, there is a 50% chance we could avoid needing to place a cerclage
D. If cerclage is placed, it would need to be removed on your due date
E. A and C

Q719: Which of the following are recommended by ACOG during cerclage placement?
A. Antibiotics are shown to decrease inflammation
B. Prophylactic tocolysis improves efficacy
C. Monitoring of cervical lengths after cerclage placement to assure efficacy
D. B and C
E. None of the above

Q720: What are the two most common indications for postpartum hysterectomy?
A. Uterine atony and uterine inversion
B. Coagulation abnormalities and uterine atony
C. Placenta accreta and uterine atony
D. Coagulation abnormalities and placenta accreta

Q721: A 32-year-old G2P0101 presents for her first obstetrical visit. In reviewing her OB history, you note that her first delivery was at 31 weeks gestational age due to intrauterine growth restriction. She asks you about the risks associated with her current pregnancy. You counsel her:
A. Her risk for stillbirth is equal to the general population risk
B. Her risk for stillbirth is greater than the general population but less than a patient who has a history of prior stillbirth
C. Her risk for stillbirth is equal to a patient who has a history of a previous stillbirth
D. Her risk for stillbirth is greater than a patient who has a history of a previous stillbirth

Q722: If an abnormal karyotype is found in association with a stillbirth, the most common abnormalities include all of the following EXCEPT:

A. Monosomy X
B. Trisomy 13
C. Trisomy 18
D. Trisomy 21
E. All of the above are common abnormalities in association with stillbirth

Q723: Expectant management in late-term and postterm pregnancies is associated with a decreased risk of cesarean delivery.

A. True
B. False

Q724: A 27-year-old G2P1001 with intrauterine gestation at 37 weeks presents for OB visit. She has a past obstetrical history significant for primary cesarean delivery at term due to non-reassuring fetal heart tones. She desires trial of labor after cesarean. Her cervix is currently closed, and her pregnancy is otherwise uncomplicated. She asks you about your policy on expectant management versus induction of labor if she goes past her estimated due date. You counsel her:

A. If she does not go into labor spontaneously before her estimated due date, she should have a repeat cesarean section due to the increased risk of uterine rupture
B. Her chances of having a successful vaginal birth after cesarean delivery decrease beyond 41 weeks gestational age
C. Use of Pitocin during an induction is associated with a greater risk of uterine rupture in late-term pregnancies compared to early-term pregnancies
D. Induction of labor is contraindicated in patients who have had a prior cesarean delivery

Q725: Which of the following is FALSE in regard to placenta accreta?

A. Antepartum ultrasound can aid in diagnosis
B. Risk is related to a history of a cesarean delivery but not the number of previous cesarean sections
C. Associated with an increased risk of postpartum hemorrhage
D. Maternal age older than 35 years is a risk factor
E. None of the above

Q726: Which of the following has been shown to be associated with preterm PROM?

A. Intra-amniotic infection
B. Prior history of preterm PROM
C. Shortened cervical length
D. A and B
E. All of the above

Q727: What is the most significant maternal consequence of term PROM?

A. Intrauterine infection
B. Abruption with hemorrhage
C. Labor dystocia
D. Impaired fetal lung maturity

Q728: Under which circumstances should a uterine artery embolization be considered in a postpartum patient with hemorrhage?

A. Continued bleeding after hysterectomy
B. In a patient with a history of a tubal ligation
C. In a patient with persistent bleeding but stable vital signs
D. A and C
E. All of the above

Q729: Which of the following describes the correct administration of misoprostol?

A. One quarter of a tablet as the initial dose, placed every 6 h, starting oxytocin 4 h after the last dose
B. One quarter of a tablet as the initial dose, placed every 2–4 h, starting oxytocin 3 h after the last dose
C. One half of a tablet as the initial dose, placed every 3–6 h, starting oxytocin 4 h after the last dose
D. One half of a tablet as the initial dose, placed every 2–4 h, starting oxytocin 4 h after the last dose
E. One quarter of a tablet as the initial dose, placed every 3–6 h, starting oxytocin 4 h after the last dose

Q730: Which of the following is FALSE regarding the PGE2 vaginal insert?

A. It should be used with caution in patients with asthma and hepatic or renal dysfunction
B. Removing the insert will usually reverse tachysystole
C. It has a 1% rate of uterine tachysystole with associated fetal heart rate changes
D. Maternal side effects are uncommon

Q731: Transfusion of 50mL of platelets increases the platelet count by ________.

A. 5000–10,000/mm³ per unit
B. 10,000–15,000/mm³ per unit
C. 15,000–20,000/mm³ per unit
D. 20,000–25,000/mm³ per unit

Q732: A 35-year-old G1P0 at 22 weeks gestation with a history of a DVT with subsequent diagnosis of antiphospholipid syndrome. Which of the following is TRUE regarding your recommendation?

A. Prophylactic anticoagulation through 12 weeks postpartum is recommended
B. Aspirin is strongly recommended
C. After delivery, anticoagulation can be continued with Coumadin

D. She should use SCDs while asleep
E. All of the above are true

Q733: What do you recommend for patients with antiphospholipid syndrome in terms of antenatal testing?
A. A detailed anatomic survey at 20 weeks gestation
B. Growth ultrasounds every 4 weeks
C. Biophysical profiles every week in the third trimester
D. Data support all of the above
E. Expert opinion supports all of the above

Q734: How is "iron deficiency" defined?
A. Increases of hemoglobin concentrations of more than 2 g/dL after iron supplementation
B. Absent bone marrow iron stores on bone marrow biopsy
C. Low total iron-binding capacity
D. None of the above
E. All of the above

Q735: What measurement has the highest sensitivity and specificity for diagnosing iron deficiency anemia?
A. Serum ferritin levels
B. Plasma total iron-binding capacity
C. Plasma iron level
D. Transferrin saturation
E. None of the above

Q736: Which of the following would be classified as a Category III fetal heart tracing?
A. Baseline 100, minimal variability, recurrent late decelerations
B. Baseline 120, absent variability, intermittent variable decelerations
C. Baseline 120, absent variability, recurrent late decelerations
D. All of the above
E. None of the above

Q737: A 22-year-old G1P0 presents for a late-term induction of labor. She is initiated on oxytocin and develops a Category III fetal heart tracing. Resuscitative measures are unsuccessful, and decision is made to proceed with cesarean delivery. All of the following is true EXCEPT:

A. Historically, the time frame from decision to incision had been 30 min
B. Expedient delivery may not improve fetal outcomes if injury has already been sustained
C. Neonatal outcomes are best when delivery can be accomplished within 15 min
D. Additional surgical preparation for maternal conditions such as morbid obesity should be accomplished
E. None

Q738: Transfusion with fresh frozen plasma involves a greater replacement of volume than cryoprecipitate.

A. True
B. False

Q739: A 40-year-old G1P0 presents to triage with a term gestation. Her baby is known to have intrauterine growth restriction. The team decides to perform a contraction stress test. Which of the following describes the correct method of performing the test?

A. Contractions may be spontaneous, produced by oxytocin or by nipple stimulation
B. An adequate test must include at least two contractions for 30 sections each in a 10 min period
C. This test relies on the premise that fetal oxygenation is worsened by contractions; hence, internal monitoring should be used to measure Montevideo units
D. A and B
E. All of the above

Q740: Two units of packed red blood cells will increase hematocrit by ______ percentage points.
A. Three
B. Four
C. Five
D. Six

Q741: Which procedure performed to reverse uterine inversion involves incising the cervical ring posteriorly?
A. Friedman procedure
B. Haultain procedure
C. Huntington procedure
D. Hasselbalch procedure

Q742: What is the recurrence risk of postpartum hemorrhage in a subsequent pregnancy?
A. 1%
B. 5%
C. 10%
D. 15%
E. 20%

Q743: Which of the following agents can be used to aid in uterine relaxation when managing a uterine inversion?
A. Magnesium sulfate
B. Halogenated general anesthetics
C. Terbutaline
D. B and C
E. All of the above

Q744: You notice on the labor and delivery schedule that there is a patient for a repeat cesarean who has had six previous cesarean deliveries. What is the risk that she will need a hysterectomy?
A. 1%
B. 3%
C. 4%
D. 5%
E. 9%

Q745: To decrease the potentially dangerous side effects associated with local anesthetics, it is important to take which precaution when using them?

A. First aspirate for blood prior to injection
B. Prehydrate patient with 500–1000 mL normal saline
C. Use a small caliber needle
D. Ensure normal electrolyte balance prior to use

Q746: What proportion of pregnant women take a psychotropic medication at some point during their pregnancy?

A. 1/10
B. 1/5
C. 1/4
D. 1/3
E. None of the above

Q747: What is the ultimate goal of fetal surveillance?

A. To detect academia
B. To detect hypoxemia
C. To assess fetal well-being in pregnancies complicated by preexisting maternal conditions and conditions which have developed
D. To prevent fetal death

Q748: Tests of fetal well-being can predict which of the following?

A. Oligohydramnios caused by decreased renal perfusion
B. Umbilical cord accidents
C. Duration of the acid-base disturbance
D. Severity of the acid-base disturbance

Q749: What proportion of psychotropic medications are present in amniotic fluid?

A. 1/10
B. 1/5
C. 1/4

D. 1/3
E. None of the above

Q750: Which of the following substances are LEAST likely to cross the placenta?
A. Thyroid antibodies in Graves' disease
B. Maternal free T4
C. Thioamide medications
D. Thyroid inhibitory antibodies

Q751: A 30-year-old pregnant patient has an elevated TSH and a low free T4. Which of the following are TRUE?
A. If she does not start treatment, she will be at risk for preeclampsia, preterm birth, and abruption
B. Regardless of treatment, her fetus is at risk for low birth rate and for impaired neuropsychologic development
C. The most likely cause for her symptoms is Hashimoto's thyroiditis
D. The most likely cause for her symptoms is Graves' disease
E. A and C

Q752: Antidepressants, psychotherapy, and electroconvulsive therapy are all treatment options for pregnant women suffering from:
A. Anxiety disorders
B. Major depression
C. Bipolar disorder
D. Schizophrenia
E. All of the above

Q753: Which of the following is FALSE regarding maternal morbidity and mortality associated with anesthesia administration during labor and delivery?
A. Regional anesthesia is preferred due to increased morbidity associated with general anesthesia
B. Complications from anesthesia account for approximately 5% of maternal deaths

C. The rate of failed intubation is higher in pregnant patients than in nonpregnant patients
D. If a patient is thought to be at increased risk for urgent cesarean delivery, it is reasonable to obtain early regional anesthesia during labor
E. None of the above

Q754: Due to the association of abnormal fetal oxygenation, maternal blood transfusion is recommended in a pregnant woman with a hemoglobin below which level?
A. 8 g/dL
B. 7 g/dL
C. 6 g/dL
D. 5 g/dL

Q755: In women with multiple gestations who are in preterm labor, which of the following are indicated?
A. Tocolysis
B. Antenatal steroids
C. Magnesium sulfate
D. B and C
E. All of the above

Q756: Which of the following patients would be a candidate for rescue dose steroid administration?
A. A patient initially given a course of steroids at 23/4 weeks gestation who represents to labor and delivery with continued concern for preterm labor at 27 weeks gestational age
B. A patient initially given a course of steroids at 24/0 weeks gestation who then begins to show signs of imminent delivery at 25/0 weeks gestation
C. A patient initially given a course of steroids at 29/0 weeks gestation who represents with concerns of labor at 34/2 weeks gestation
D. A and B
E. All of the above

Q757: All of the following should be included in a preconception counseling visit for a woman with diabetes EXCEPT:

A. Impact of euglycemia in decreasing risk for congenital anomalies to baseline population risk
B. 24 h urine protein collection
C. TSH if type II diabetic as 40% will have hypothyroidism
D. Counseling to take a multivitamin with folate due to increased risk for neural tube defects
E. All of the above are true

Q758: Following a stillbirth in one of your patients, you offer her a fetal autopsy explaining it is the most important test in evaluation of the cause of stillbirth. She declines and wants to know what other alternatives can be offered. You counsel her:

A. A head-sparing autopsy has the same benefits of a full autopsy
B. An MRI of the fetus following delivery will aid in identification of CNS, cardiac, and infectious pathology
C. Gross and microscopic placenta examination and external examination with selected biopsies will be helpful in identifying fetal infections
D. The best alternative is a fetal ultrasound performed after birth in conjunction with an external exanimation by a perinatal pathologist

Q759: Karyotype analysis is an adequate method to detect:

A. Genetic abnormalities obtained from stillbirth specimens
B. Small gene rearrangements
C. Mosaicism
D. Aneuploidies
E. All of the above

Q760: Which of the following should be considered a screening test?
A. FISH analysis
B. Microarray analysis
C. Karyotype analysis
D. None of the above

Q761: Routine maternal evaluation at the time of demise may include the following labs EXCEPT:
A. Antithrombin III deficiency
B. Anticardiolipin antibodies
C. Syphilis testing
D. Human parvovirus B19 immunoglobulin G and M antibody
E. Fetal-maternal hemorrhage screen

Q762: A type II diabetic patient presents for a new obstetric visit. She is currently taking glyburide and metformin and asks about the safety of those medications during pregnancy. You tell her:
A. Glyburide crosses the placenta but appears to be safe in retrospective studies
B. Glyburide has an onset of action of 3 h with a duration of 12 h
C. Metformin is a category A drug
D. The long-term effect of metformin on pregnancy is unknown
E. All of the above are true

Q763: A 30-year-old G1P0 presents to your office for a new obstetric visit. She reports a history of a DVT when she was 17 and was on oral contraceptives. She asks what you recommend for her in terms of anticoagulation. You recommend:
A. Prophylactic anticoagulation to continue postpartum
B. Therapeutic anticoagulation to continue postpartum
C. Prophylactic anticoagulation to stop postpartum

D. Therapeutic anticoagulation to stop postpartum
E. No anticoagulation indicated

Q764: While working in triage on labor and delivery, a patient at 20 weeks gestation presents and lists warfarin as one of her medications. Which of the following is TRUE of warfarin?

A. It is associated with embryopathy if used in the second trimester
B. All patients on warfarin should be transitioned to heparin compounds if pregnant
C. Most patients on warfarin should be transitioned to heparin compounds if pregnant
D. A and B
E. A and C

Q765: A preterm type II diabetic patient is admitted to the hospital for elevated blood pressures, and a steroid course is initiated for fetal lung maturity. She asks how long she should expect to have an increased need in her insulin dosing. You tell her:

A. 48 h
B. 72 h
C. 5 days
D. 7 days
E. 10 days

Q766: Which of the following is TRUE regarding thyroid changes in pregnancy?

A. Maternal thyroid size increases 30% by the third trimester
B. TSH increases in early pregnancy because of stimulation by b-hCG
C. Thyroid-binding globulin decreases throughout pregnancy
D. All of the above are false
E. All of the above are true

Q767: A 26-year-old presents to your office at 14 weeks gestation. Her lab values reveal an increased TSH and a decreased free T4. Which of the following is the correct diagnosis?

A. Overt hyperthyroidism
B. Subclinical hyperthyroidism
C. Overt hypothyroidism
D. Subclinical hypothyroidism
E. Additional antibody testing is required for a diagnosis

Q768: What is the preferred inhaled corticosteroid for use during pregnancy?

A. Budesonide
B. Salmeterol
C. Fluticasone
D. Theophylline

Q769: A 22-year-old G1P0 presents for her first obstetrical visit. In review of her history, she has a diagnosis of moderate asthma with a history of intubation secondary to acute asthma attack about 3 years ago. When discussing the necessary fetal surveillance for this patient, you counsel her:

A. She will need a first-trimester scan for dating and Level II ultrasound to assess for any structural abnormalities
B. She will need a first-trimester scan for dating and serial growth ultrasounds with antenatal testing to start at approximately 32 weeks
C. She will need a first-trimester scan for dating and only serial growth ultrasounds if an abnormality is found on her Level II scan
D. She will need a first-trimester scan for dating and only serial growth ultrasounds if her symptoms worsen during the course of her pregnancy

Q770: Rh positive refers to:
A. Presence of D antibody
B. Presence of D antigen
C. Neither
D. Both

Q771: Shoulder dystocia increases maternal risk for which of the following?
A. Postpartum hemorrhage
B. Fourth-degree laceration
C. Postpartum endometritis
D. A and B
E. B and C

Q772: A 34-year-old G3P2002 with intrauterine pregnancy at 32 week gestational age presents to labor and delivery in preterm labor with a cervical dilation of 3 cm. No vaginal bleeding is noted. She is Rh negative and received anti-D immune globulin prophylaxis at 28 weeks. Upon admission, she should receive:
A. Betamethasone
B. Betamethasone and 300 μg anti-D immune globulin
C. Betamethasone and 50 μg anti-D immune globulin
D. Betamethasone and 300 μg anti-D immune globulin 12 h later

Q773: With vacuum extractor use, cephalohematomas are more likely to occur as the duration of vacuum application increases. Given this finding, you:
A. Release vacuum pressure between contractions to improve outcomes
B. Alert pediatricians of vacuum application as soon as decision is made to perform an operative delivery
C. Apply rocking motion and torque with each pull to decrease time to delivery
D. A and B
E. All of the above

Q774: Potential indications for operative vaginal delivery include all of the following EXCEPT:
A. Multigravida who has been pushing for greater than 2 h without delivery of fetus
B. Fetal monitoring reveals repetitive early decelerations with each contraction
C. Primigravida with cardiac condition which prevents her from being able to Valsalva safely
D. All of the above are appropriate indications for operative vaginal delivery

Q775: Which of the following is KNOWN in regard to the effect of epidural analgesia on labor?
A. May prolong labor up to 90 min
B. It doubles the need for oxytocin administration
C. Increases the rate of cesarean section
D. A and B
E. All of the above

Q776: Which of the following is FALSE regarding asthma?
A. Airway obstruction is at least partially reversible
B. Characterized by decreased responsiveness to stimuli
C. Characterized by chronic airway inflammation
D. None of the above

Q777: What are the two most common symptoms of a DVT?
A. Pain and swelling at the extremity
B Shortness of breath and pain at the extremity
C. Shortness of breath and swelling at the extremity
D. Tachycardia and swelling at the extremity
E. Tachycardia and pain at the extremity

Q778: A 38-year-old patient presents at 38 weeks gestation with complaints concerning for a DVT. What diagnostic testing do you order?
A. Ultrasound. If negative and suspect iliac vein thrombosis, proceed with CT angiogram to evaluate for pulmonary embolism

B. D-dimer and then ultrasound if elevated
C. Ultrasound. If negative and suspect iliac vein thrombosis, proceed with anticoagulation
D. Ultrasound. If negative and suspect iliac vein thrombosis, proceed with MRI
E. C and D

Q779: A 33-year-old G1P0 presents for her new obstetrical visit at 6 weeks gestation. She has a history of moderate persistent asthma and is currently on two different medications to control her symptoms. She is concerned about how the medications will interfere with the development of her fetus. You counsel her:

A. She should stop taking all medications due to known fetal risks and that her symptoms will be treated as they arise
B. She should continue to take her current medications because there is no known fetal risk associated with them
C. She should discontinue her medications because the teratogenic risks far outweigh the risks of an asthma exacerbation
D. She should continue her current medication regimen as the benefits of well-controlled asthma symptoms clearly outweigh the potential teratogenic risks to her fetus

Q780: A 30-year-old G2P1001 at 13 weeks gestation who had a previous term delivery after cerclage placement presents for a routine obstetric visit. What type of cerclage would you offer her?

A. History indicated
B. Physical exam indicated
C. Ultrasound indicated
D. Do not offer cerclage
E. Do not offer cerclage but would offer her vaginal progesterone therapy

Q781: An 18-year-old G2P1001 at 23 weeks gestation is found to have a cervical length of 15 mm. Her cervix is found to be closed on vaginal exam. What type of cerclage would you offer her?

A. Rescue cerclage
B. Physical exam indicated
C. Ultrasound indicated
D. Do not offer cerclage
E. Do not offer cerclage but would offer her vaginal progesterone therapy

Q782: A 36-year-old G1P0 presents to her routine prenatal visit at 36 weeks gestation with questions regarding the optimal time to obtain epidural anesthesia during labor. You counsel her:

A. Due to the increased risk of cesarean section associated with early epidural, the patient should not expect to get an epidural until at least 4–5 cm dilation
B. There is no increased risk of cesarean section associated with early epidural so the patient may have the epidural placed upon her request regardless of her cervical dilation
C. Due to evidence of early epidural increasing the risk of cesarean section, it is reasonable to try and delay epidural administration until 4–5 cm dilation if possible
D. Due to the risks of prolonging labor associated with early epidural, the patient should be encouraged to delay placement until at least 6 cm dilation
E. None of the above

Q783: A 20-year-old known cocaine user presents to triage complaining of loss of fluid without vaginal bleeding at 30 weeks gestation and is found to have ruptured membranes. Documents show that she is Rh negative and received anti-D immune globulin at a previous triage visit at 26 weeks. Despite extensive counseling, she opts to leave the hospital AMA. Given her high risk of abruption, prior to leaving, she should receive:

A. No prophylaxis
B. 300 μg anti-D immune globulin
C. 50 μg anti-D immune globulin

Q784: Which of the following is FALSE regarding folic acid supplementation?

A. It is recommended that all patients of reproductive age take 400 mg of folic acid daily
B. There is limited risk to taking higher levels of folic acid
C. It may interfere with some seizure medications
D. If additional folic acid supplementation is needed, it is recommended that a patient increase the dosing of their daily prenatal vitamin
E. None of the above

Q785: Which of the following is TRUE regarding transmission of parvovirus B19?

A. Transmitted through respiratory secretions and hand-to-mouth contact
B. Risk of exposure and subsequent transmission is higher in a child care setting than in household setting
C. Prevalence of seropositivity increases with age
D. A and C
E. All of the above

Q786: Parvovirus B19 is cytotoxic to:

A. Immunoglobulin precursors
B. Neuronal precursors
C. Erythroid precursors
D. Hepatocyte precursors
E. All of the above

Q787: Your G1P0 patient has a Bishop score of 4 and requests induction. You counsel her that her risk for a cesarean section if induced as opposed to waiting for spontaneous labor is threefold. Is this:

A. True
B. False

Q788: Your patient presents for a medically indicated induction and is found to have an unfavorable cervix. Which of the following is true regarding methods of cervical ripening?

A. Foley catheter placement would significantly reduce the duration of labor
B. PGE2 gel is significantly more effective at decreasing the cesarean rate than Foley catheter placement
C. When oxytocin is added to the use of the Foley catheter, time to delivery is decreased
D. Dinoprostone is associated with more tachysystole than vaginal misoprostol
E. All of the above are false

Q789: Which patient is at an increased risk of having a child with a neural tube defect?

A. A patient taking 400 mg of folic acid supplementation prior to conception and who has a fasting blood glucose of 230 mg/dL at her first-trimester obstetrical visit
B. A patient not taking a folic acid supplementation prior to conception and who has a fasting blood glucose of 230 mg/dL at her first obstetrical visit
C. A new obstetrical patient who reports daily adherence to recommended folic acid supplementation and recent hot tub exposure while on vacation at her first obstetrical visit

D. A patient who upon review of her medications takes valproic acid and a daily prenatal vitamin
E. All of the above

Q790: All of the following are known risk factors for stillbirth EXCEPT:
A. Hispanic race
B. Advanced maternal age
C. Multiple gestation
D. Nulliparity
E. All of the above are known risk factors

Q791: In which of the following situations would cerclage removal be recommended?
A. A 32-year-old at 37 weeks gestation with no complaints at her routine office visit
B. A 25-year-old G2P0101 at 34 weeks gestation who complains of cramping
C. A 37-year-old G5P0400 at 25 weeks gestation with vaginal bleeding and painful contractions
D. A and C
E. All of the above

Q792: Cerclage should always be removed at the time of preterm premature rupture of membranes.
A. True
B. False

Q793: Which of the following is FALSE regarding obesity and the associated risk of stillbirth?
A. The risk of obesity-related stillbirth may increase with gestational age
B. Is often related to placental dysfunction
C. Is not related to early fetal loss
D. Risk may be greater with BMI greater than 30

Q794: Which of the following is NOT a medical indication for epidural analgesia during labor and delivery?
A. History of deep vein thrombosis
B. History of malignant hyperthermia
C. Concern that the patient will be a difficult intubation
D. Prevention of autonomic hyperreflexia in patients with high spinal cord lesions

Q795: A 30-year-old G2P0101 with intrauterine gestation at 31 weeks presents to your office with concerns that she has been exposed to a child at work who has parvovirus. You immediately obtain serologic screening. A few days later, the lab results return, and your patient is IgM negative but IgG positive. You call her and inform her:
A. She should be closely monitored for potential fetal infection
B. She should undergo repeat serologic testing in 4 weeks
C. She is not at risk of transplacental transmission
D. A and B

Q796: How is parvovirus fetal infection diagnosed?
A. PCR analysis of fractionated fetal blood obtained from maternal blood samples
B. PCR analysis of amniotic fluid
C. Culture of amniotic fluid
D. By ultrasonography revealing hydrops fetalis

Q797: What is the typical duration of anesthesia provided with a spinal?
A. 30–60 min
B. 60–120 min
C. 30–180 min
D. 30–250 min

Q798: Which of the following increase the risk for shoulder dystocia?
A. Epidural
B. Labor induction

C. Operative vaginal delivery
D. Obesity
E. All of the above

Q799: Which of the following is FALSE regarding methylene tetrahydrofolate reductase (MTHFR) mutations?
A. Pregnant patients should not be screened for MTHFR mutations
B. Homozygosity for MTHFR mutations is the most common cause of hyperhomocysteinemia
C. MTHFR mutations do not increase the risk for thromboembolism in nonpregnant women
D. MTHFR mutations increase the risk for thromboembolism in pregnant women
E. A and C

Q800: Which thrombophilia infers the greatest risk for thromboembolism in pregnancy regardless of history?
A. Antithrombin deficiency
B. Protein C deficiency
C. Protein S deficiency
D. Factor V Leiden homozygote
E. None of the above

Q801: Most cases of shoulder dystocia can be predicted.
A. True
B. False

Q802: A type II diabetic patient brings her glucose log for review at her prenatal visit. It is noted that her premeal glucose values are consistently elevated. Her current insulin dosing is intermediate-acting insulin 20 units BID and lispro 10 units with meals. How should her dosing be adjusted?
A. Increase nighttime intermediate-acting insulin to 25 units
B. Increase lispro to 12 units with meals
C. Increase morning intermediate-acting insulin to 22 units
D. Increase morning intermediate-acting insulin 24 units

Q803: About 75% of obstetric patients admitted to the ICU are postpartum.

A. True
B. False

Q804: Delivery in the ICU is associated with:

A. Increased likelihood of operative vaginal delivery
B. Lack of space to accommodate key pediatric equipment and providers
C. Decreased risk of nosocomial infection with drug-resistant organisms
D. A and B
E. All of the above

Q805: A 28-year-old G1P0 with pregnancy at 32 weeks gestation is admitted to the ICU for airway management due to acute sepsis related to suspected pneumonia. The ICU critical care physician is concerned about how the medications and additional workup needed for this patient will affect the fetus. You advise:

A. Necessary medications should not be withheld
B. Only non-contrast imaging studies should be ordered
C. Corticosteroids for fetal lung maturity are contraindicated in the setting of sepsis
D. A and C
E. All of the above

Q806: When increasing a patent's insulin, it is important to warn them about the risks of hypoglycemia. How do you counsel her?

A. She should have a glass of milk if she becomes hypoglycemic
B. She should have a glass of orange juice if she becomes hypoglycemic
C. Hypoglycemia is defined as a blood sugar of less than 60 mg/dL

D. A and C
E. All of the above are reasonable

Q807: A medical student expresses concern that a fetal heart tracing shows recurrent late decelerations. Which of the following is TRUE regarding recurrent late decelerations?
A. Maneuvers to promote uteroplacental perfusion should be initiated
B. Late decelerations are highly predictive of academia
C. If variability becomes absent, the tracing is Category III
D. A and B
E. A and C
F. All of the above are true

Q808: Which of the following is FALSE regarding fetal tachycardia?
A. In isolation, it is poorly predictive of fetal academia
B. Treatment should be directed at the underlying cause
C. Infection is a common cause
D. It is defined as a rate greater than 160 for 5 min or more
E. None of the above

Q809: A Rh-negative patient should be considered a candidate for anti-D immune globulin prophylaxis after all of the following events EXCEPT:
A. External cephalic version
B. Evacuation of molar pregnancy
C. Threatened abortion
D. All of the above should be considered for prophylaxis

Q810: The risk of recurrent stillbirth is greatest after 37 weeks gestational age.
A. True
B. False

Q811: All of the following criteria are most commonly cited in the diagnosis of hyperemesis gravidarum EXCEPT?
A. Other possible causes have been ruled out
B. Documented weight loss
C. Volume of emesis
D. Ketonuria
E. Electrolyte abnormalities

Q812: Which of the following would suggest a diagnosis other than nausea/vomiting of pregnancy?
A. Symptoms starting before 9 weeks gestation
B. Headache
C. Mild epigastric pain
D. A and B
E. B and C

Q813: Fetal kick counting can decrease the incidence of stillbirth.
A. True
B. False

Q814: Which of the following statements is FALSE about preimplantation genetic diagnosis?
A. Refers to the testing of an embryo for a specific genetic disorder prior to implantation
B. Can be performed on polar bodies from the oocyte and zygote
C. Can be performed using molecular or cytogenetic techniques
D. It is not recommended that results be confirmed with CVS or amniocentesis

Q815: Which of the following is NOT an absolute indication for anti-D immune globulin in a Rh-negative woman?
A. First-trimester pregnancy loss
B. Second- or third-trimester vaginal bleeding
C. Amniocentesis
D. Fetal blood sampling

Q816: Successfully performing an operative vaginal delivery has many potential benefits in comparison to performing a cesarean section such as:
A. Preventing the increased morbidity associated with repeat cesarean sections
B. Decreased cost
C. Reducing or preventing the potential exposure of intrapartum insults to the fetus
D. All of the above

Q817: Which of the following is NOT a necessary component of the clinicians' assessment prior to performing an operative vaginal delivery?
A. Estimation of fetal weight
B. Adequacy of maternal effort with pushing
C. Clinical adequacy of maternal pelvis
D. Identification of fetal station and position

Q818: Shoulder dystocia is defined as:
A. Requiring use of additional maneuvers other than downward traction on the fetal head to deliver the shoulders
B. A period or 30 s or more between delivery of the head and the shoulders
C. Use of two or more maneuvers to deliver the fetal shoulders
D. All of the above are acceptable definitions

Q819: A 19-year-old has just learned she is pregnant. At her NOB visit, you counsel her on the increased risk for complications based on her BMI of 37. She asks if she should lose weight. How do you counsel her?

A. Yes, but no more than 5 pounds a trimester
B. No, because it can lead to vitamin deficiencies
C. Yes, but only during the first trimester
D. No, because it increases the risk of a small-for-gestational-age infant

Q820: Detection of fetal anomalies by standard ultrasonography is ___ for women with a normal BMI and ____ for women with class III obesity.

A. 49%; 22%
B. 76%; 45%
C. 76%; 22%
D. 66%; 22%

Q821: Maternal fever can be a side effect of epidural analgesia, especially in nulliparous women.

A. True
B. False

Q822: Which of the following places the screening tests in correct order from lowest rate of detection for Down syndrome to highest rate of detection?

A. Ultrasound, cell-free fetal DNA, serum screening
B. Cell-free fetal DNA, ultrasound, serum screening
C. Serum screening, cell-free fetal DNA, ultrasound
D. Ultrasound, serum screening, cell-free fetal DNA

Q823: A 28-year-old G3P2002 presents for her first obstetrical visit. Her hemoglobin is 12.2 g/dL. You counsel her that the recommended daily dietary allowance of ferrous iron during pregnancy is:

A. 20 mg
B. 24 mg

C. 27 mg
D. 30 mg

Q824: Supplemental sustained-release iron preparations may be less effective because they dissolve poorly.
A. True
B. False

Q825: A nurse calls because she is concerned that a patient's contractions are too frequent. The patient is in spontaneous labor at term with five contractions in 10 min for the past 30 min. The fetus is currently Category I. How would you classify her pattern of uterine contractions?
A. Normal uterine activity
B. Tachysystole
C. Uterine hyperstimulation
D. Uterine hypercontractility
E. B and C

Q826: How often should a fetal heart rate tracing be reviewed during labor?
A. Every 30 min during the first phase and every 15 min during the second phase by a nurse or physician
B. Every 30 min during the first phase and every 15 min during the second phase by a physician
C. Every 60 min during the first phase and every 30 min during the second phase by a nurse or physician
D. Every 60 min during the first phase and every 30 min during the second phase by a physician

Q827: Which of the following is TRUE regarding inhaled anesthetic agents used during general anesthesia?
A. Some have been shown to have minimal passage across the placenta
B. They have not been associated with neonatal depression

C. They can be used as uterine relaxants in certain situations if given in high concentrations
D. Their use increases blood loss during cesarean section
E. None of the above

Q828: A woman presents to your office with quadruplets and requests information about multifetal reduction. How would you counsel her?
A. She would have a decreased risk of IUGR and decreased risk of cesarean section but an increased risk of preterm delivery
B. She would have an increased risk of IUGR, decreased risk of cesarean section, and no change in her risk of preterm delivery
C. She would have a decreased risk of IUGR, decreased risk of cesarean section, and a decreased risk of preterm delivery
D. She would have an increased risk of IUGR, decreased risk of cesarean section, and an increased risk of preeclampsia

Q829: A woman presents to your office with quadruplets. Records reveal that she has one monochorionic pair. What would you recommend in terms of reduction?
A. Reduction of one of the non-monochorionic fetuses
B. Reduction of one of the monochorionic fetuses
C. Reduction of both monochorionic fetuses
D. Recommend against reduction given the increased risks associated with it

Q830: Which selective serotonin reuptake inhibitor (SSRI) has a pregnancy risk category of D?
A. Paroxetine
B. Escitalopram
C. Citalopram
D. A and B
E. B and C

Q831: A Rh-negative woman is postpartum day #1 after a vaginal delivery and is ready for discharge. Her baby is found to be Rh negative as well. She should receive anti-D immune globulin prior to discharge.

A. True
B. False

Q832: Some of the potential benefits of using parental fentanyl for pain control during labor and delivery include:

A. Not associated with neonatal neurobehavioral depression
B. Has a short half-life
C. Associated with less nausea and vomiting
D. B and C
E. All of the above

Q833: What percentage of Rh alloimmunization occurs due to antepartum fetomaternal hemorrhage?

A. 1%
B. 5%
C. 10%
D. 15%

Q834: Following a vaginal delivery, a hemostatic first-degree laceration is noted. Which of the following are reasonable options?

A. Adhesive glue
B. Standard suture
C. No repair
D. A and B
E. All of the above

Q835: Which of the following are important considerations in choosing a suture to repair a second degree?

A. Absorbable synthetic suture may require a postpartum visit for suture removal
B. Closure of the perineal skin with adhesive glue results in decreased repair time but increased pain
C. Interrupted sutures are recommended as they achieve improved hemostasis

D. Choice of suture can impact dyspareunia at 3 months to a year
E. None of the above

Q836: Which of the following patients are candidates for anti-D immune globulin?
A. A 28-year-old at 28 weeks gestation who is Rh negative, antibody negative
B. A 28-year-old at 28 weeks gestation who is Rh negative, antibody positive
C. A 28-year-old at 28 weeks gestation who is Rh negative, sensitized, with Kell alloimmunization
D. A and C
E. All of the above

Q837: Which of the following are included in fetal valproate syndrome?
A. Asperger's syndrome
B. Developmental delay
C. Facial dysmorphology
D. B and C
E. All of the above

Q838: Which of the following is TRUE regarding antibiotic prophylaxis?
A. May need to administered for an extended period of time
B. Ideal to achieve therapeutic tissue levels prior to the end of the procedure
C. Agent chosen should be short acting and broadly focused on multiple different types of bacteria
D. Use may increase the risk of resistant flora seen postoperatively

Q839: Increases in *E. coli* sepsis and resistance are mainly seen in the preterm and low birth weight infant population.
A. True
B. False

Q840: Carbamazepine has been shown to be associated with which of the following fetal anomalies?
A. Growth restriction
B. Neural tube defects
C. Developmental delay
D. Fingernail hypoplasia
E. All of the above

Q841: Which of the following is TRUE in regard to neural tube defects?
A. Can be isolated or occur as part of a genetic syndrome
B. Affect the vertebral column and urogenital diaphragm
C. Most common congenital anomaly worldwide
D. Neural tube closure is normally complete by the end of the second week after conception (4 weeks after the last period)
E. All of the above

Q842: When counseling a patient, it is important to stress which of the following in regard to maternal morbidity and mode of delivery?
A. A VBAC carries the greatest risk to maternal morbidity
B. A scheduled repeat cesarean section carries the greatest risk to maternal morbidity
C. A scheduled repeat cesarean section has a greater risk to maternal morbidity than a failed TOLAC
D. A failed TOLAC carries the greatest risk to maternal morbidity

Q843: The outcome associated with TOLAC that most greatly increases the risk of neonatal and maternal morbidity is:
A. Endometritis
B. Arrest of descent
C. Uterine rupture
D. Cord prolapse
E. None of the above

Q844: Most cranial neural tube defects are lethal.
- A. True
- B. False

Q845: Which of the following is TRUE?
- A. Pregestational diabetes complicates 10% of all pregnancies
- B. 90% of all diabetes cases during pregnancy are pregestational
- C. Pathogenesis of type 1 diabetes includes destruction of pancreatic beta cells
- D. A and C
- E. All of the above

Q846: The primary function of mitochondria is in anaerobic metabolism.
- A. True
- B. False

Q847: During which phase of mitosis is karyotype analysis performed?
- A. Interphase
- B. Metaphase
- C. Anaphase
- D. Telophase

Q848: Late in the first trimester:
- A. Estrogen increases insulin sensitivity
- B. Estrogen decreases insulin sensitivity
- C. Progesterone decreases insulin sensitivity
- D. Progesterone increases insulin sensitivity

Q849: What percent of daily caloric intake should come from protein during pregnancy?
- A. 20%
- B. 30%
- C. 40%
- D. 50%

Q850: What is the best way to administer naloxone to a neonate?

A. Intramuscularly
B. Intravenously
C. Subcutaneously
D. Orally
E. A or B

Q851: Given the risk for shoulder dystocia and brachial plexus injury, early induction should be considered if macrosomia is discovered at 37 weeks gestation.

A. Sometimes
B. Always
C. Never

Q852: The risk of shoulder dystocia is unaffected by assisted vaginal delivery.

A. True
B. False

Q853: There is an increased relative risk of poor pregnancy outcomes associated with elevated MSAFP.

A. True
B. False

Q854: After how long should a cesarean section be considered for maternal and fetal benefit when a pregnant woman has cardiopulmonary arrest in the third trimester?

A. 2 min
B. 3 min
C. 4 min
D. 5 min

Q855: Which of the following is TRUE regarding management of sepsis in an OB patient?

A. It is critical for blood cultures to be drawn prior to the administration of antibiotics
B. It is reasonable to wait to start antibiotics until transfer to ICU has been completed

C. Broad-spectrum antibiotics should be started within 1 h of diagnosis of severe sepsis or septic shock
D. Fetal resuscitation in utero is difficult; thus, cesarean section should strongly be considered with fetal heart tone abnormalities

Q856: Which of the following are interventions that can be accomplished when a pregnant patient is being transported and fetal heart tones become non-reassuring?
A. Alert the receiving institution of possible need for delivery
B. Return to transferring facility for delivery planning if it is closer
C. Emergency cesarean delivery for Category 3 fetal heart rate tracings
D. All of the above

Q857: A 19-year-old G0 at 30 weeks gestational age is admitted to the ICU after a car accident. Her fetus is intermittently Category 2, however, predominantly Category 1. Which of the following need to be determined as soon as possible?
A. Where delivery will occur
B. Preferred mode of delivery
C. Which family members will be present
D. A and B
E. All of the above

Q858: Decreased levels of MSAFP are independently associated with an increased risk of fetal aneuploidy.
A. True
B. False

Q859: Cervical remodeling includes which of the following changes?
A. Collagen breakdown and rearrangement
B. Decreased production of cytokines

C. Red blood cell infiltration
D. All of the above

Q860: What is the average cost per premature infant in the Unites States according to the Institute of Medicine?
A. $20,000
B. $26,000
C. $40,000
D. $51,000

Q861: Preterm birth is defined as delivery between what gestational ages?
A. 20/0 and 38/6 weeks gestational age
B. 20/0 and 36/6 weeks gestational age
C. 24/0 and 38/6 weeks gestational age
D. 24/0 and 36/6 weeks gestational age

Q862: At which Bishop score is the probability of a vaginal delivery similar to that of spontaneous labor?
A. 4
B. 6
C. 8
D. Induction never obtains the same probability as spontaneous labor

Q863: Preterm premature rupture of membranes (preterm PROM) complicates ____% of pregnancies.
A. 1%
B. 3%
C. 9%
D. 12%

Q864: Preterm PROM is defined as the rupture of membranes before the onset of labor prior to:
A. 40 weeks gestational age
B. 39 weeks gestational age
C. 37 weeks gestational age
D. 34 weeks gestational age

Q865: Alloimmunization occurs when a fetal blood group factor from the ____ is not possessed by the ____.

A. Mother, father
B. Father, mother

Q866: Most shoulder dystocias occur with delivery of a:

A. Normal weight fetus
B. Macrosomic fetus with a diabetic mother
C. Macrosomic fetus with an untreated diabetic mother
D. Macrosomic fetus with a nondiabetic mother
E. B and C

Q867: Which of the following is NOT a risk factor for fetal macrosomia?

A. Positive 50 g glucose screen with normal 3 h glucose tolerance test
B. Advanced maternal age
C. Excessive gestational weight gain
D. Postterm pregnancy
E. Nulliparity

Q868: Which of the following is TRUE regarding the Fisher-Race nomenclature?

A. Includes five genetic loci each with two major alleles
B. No antiserum specific for "e" antigen has been found; thus, testing indicates absence of allelic product
C. Each Rh gene complex is described by three letters
D. Rh positive refers to the absence of "D" antigen on erythrocytes
E. None of the above

Q869: Anaphylaxis to penicillin is rare. The risk of a less severe reaction to penicillin is more common, estimated to be about _____%.

A. 5%
B. 10%
C. 20%
D. 30%

Q870: Lower serum levels of antibiotics may be seen in the pregnant patient due to all of the following physiologic changes associated with pregnancy EXCEPT:

A. Increases in glomerular filtration rate
B. Increases in plasma volume
C. Decreases in binding proteins
D. Decreases in gastric emptying time

Q871: Kell alloimmunization is diagnosed in a new obstetrical patient. How should she be counseled?

A. Kell alloimmunization is often caused by prior transfusions
B. Amniotic fluid analysis correlates with the severity of fetal anemia
C. Aggressive fetal assessment is unwarranted
D. A and B
E. All of the above

Q872: Which of the following supports the theory that hCG and estrogen can cause nausea and vomiting?

A. Lower levels of hormones caused by multiple gestations and molar pregnancies generally cause less nausea and vomiting
B. Smokers have increased levels of these hormones and are more likely to have nausea and vomiting

C. Women who experienced nausea and vomiting with combined oral contraceptive pills are more likely to have nausea and vomiting during pregnancy
D. A and C
E. All of the above

Q873: Which of the following does NOT increase the risk for nausea and vomiting of pregnancy?
A. Increased placental mass
B. Motion sickness
C. Family history of nausea and vomiting of pregnancy
D. Obesity
E. All of the above increase the risk of nausea and vomiting of pregnancy

Q874: Which of the following statements is FALSE regarding cell-free fetal DNA?
A. Cells are derived from fetal skin
B. It can be tested from 10 weeks gestation to term
C. It can identify Rh-negative babies in Rh-positive moms
D. It has the highest detection rate for Down syndrome

Answers

Q1: B, Q2: C, Q3: A, Q4: D, Q5: C, Q6: D, Q7: D, Q8: E, Q9: C, Q10: B, Q11: C, Q12: A, Q13: D, Q14: B, Q15: B, Q16: B, Q17: C, Q18: B, Q19: A, Q20: D, Q21: C, Q22: D, Q23: B, Q24: C, Q25: B, Q26: C, Q27: D, Q28: C, Q29: B, Q30: A, Q31: D, Q32: D, Q33: A, Q34: C, Q35: D, Q36: E, Q37: B, Q38: E, Q39: B, Q40: D, Q41: D, Q42: A, Q43: B,44: D, Q45: D, Q46: D, Q47: E, Q48: D, Q49: C, Q50: D, Q51: A, Q52: B, Q53: E, Q54: B, Q55: A, Q56: B, Q57: A, Q58: D, Q59: A, Q60: B, Q61: E, Q62: B, Q63: D, Q64: E, Q65: A, Q66: A, Q67: B, Q68: A, Q69: B, Q70: A, Q71: B, Q72: A, Q73: D, Q74: C, Q75: D, Q76: B, Q77: E,

Q78: C, Q79: D, Q80: D, Q81: D, Q82: E, Q83: B, Q84: C, Q85: D, Q86: A, Q87: D, Q88: D, Q89: C, Q90: E, Q91: D, Q92: B, Q93: A, Q94: C, Q95: C, Q96: E, Q97: D, Q98: B, Q99: D, Q100: B, Q101: E, Q102: C, Q103: C, Q104: D, Q105: E, Q106: A, Q107: C, Q108: A, Q109: D, Q110: B, Q111: A, Q112: A, Q113: A, Q114: D, Q115: D, Q116: E, Q117: B, Q118: D, Q119: D, Q120: B, Q121: C, Q122: B, Q123: C, Q124: C, Q125: A, Q126: C, Q127: E, Q128: D, Q129: B, Q130: B, Q131: B, Q132: A, Q133: B, Q134: A, Q135: B, Q136: B, Q137: A, Q138: D, Q139: D, Q140: B, Q141: D, Q142: C, Q143: A, Q144: E, Q145: E, Q146: D, Q147: B, Q148: B, Q149: D, Q150: A, Q151: D, Q152: E, Q153: A, Q154: D, Q155: B, Q156: B, Q157: E, Q158: B, Q159: C, Q160: A, Q161: B, Q162: A, Q163: D, Q164: C, Q165: B, Q166: B, Q167: B, Q168: B, Q169: B, Q170: C, Q171: C, Q172: E, Q173: E, Q174: A, Q175: E, Q176: B, Q177: D, Q178: D, Q179: A, Q180: D, Q181: C, Q182: D, Q183: B, Q184: B, Q185: A, Q186: C, Q187: B, Q188: A, Q189: B, Q190: B, Q191: A, Q192: A, Q193: E, Q194: E, Q195: B, Q196: A, Q197: A, Q198: C, Q199: E, Q200: A, Q201: D, Q202: B, Q203: A, Q204: B, Q205: C, Q206: B, Q207: B, Q208: A, Q209: C, Q210: B, Q211: B, Q212: C, Q213: E, Q214: E, Q215: A, Q216: E, Q217: C, Q218: D, Q219: A, Q220: A, Q221: A, Q222: D, Q223: B, Q224: D, Q225: E, Q226: E, Q227: D, Q228: A, Q229: D, Q230: E, Q231: D, Q232: B, Q233: B, Q234: D, Q235: E, Q236: C, Q237: C, Q238: C, Q239: B, Q240: B, Q241: A, Q242: E, Q243: D, Q244: A, Q245: C, Q246: B, Q247: D, Q248: B, Q249: E, Q250: A, Q251: A, Q252: B, Q253: D, Q254: D, Q255: C, Q256: B, Q257: D, Q258: C, Q259: D, Q260: D, Q261: C, Q262: E, Q263: B, Q264: D, Q265: C, Q266: B, Q267: D, Q268: D, Q269: D, Q270: B, Q271: C, Q272: C, Q273: A, Q274: E, Q275: B, Q276: D, Q277: E, Q278: C, Q279: A, Q280: A, Q281: B, Q282: B, Q283: D, Q284: B, Q285: E, Q286: B, Q287: C, Q288: B, Q289: A, Q290: B, Q291: C, Q292: A, Q293: C, Q294: D, Q295: D, Q296: B, Q297: D, Q298: B, Q299: E, Q300: B, Q301: C, Q302: B, Q303: E, Q304: B, Q305: D 306: B, Q307: B, Q308: A, Q309: E, Q310: D, Q311: E, Q312: E, Q313: E, Q314: B, Q315: D, Q316: B, Q317: F, Q318: F, Q319: A, Q320: B, Q321: C, Q322: B, Q323: D, Q324: A, Q325: A, Q326: C, Q327: C, Q328: A,

Q329: B, Q330: B, Q331: B, Q332: B, Q333: D, Q334: A, Q335: D, Q336: A, Q337: A, Q338: D, Q339: E, Q340: B, Q341: B, Q342: E, Q343: B, Q344: E, Q345: C, Q346: B, Q347: C, Q348: A, Q349: D, Q350: B, Q351: E, Q352: B, Q353: A, Q354: A, Q355: A, Q356: B, Q357: B, Q358: C, Q359: C, Q360: C, Q361: E, Q362: C, Q363: A, Q364: B, Q365: B, Q366: A, Q367: B, Q368: D, Q369: E, Q370: C, Q371: D, Q372: D, Q373: E, Q374: D, Q375: D, Q376: E, Q377: D, Q378: A, Q379: A, Q380: A, Q381: E, Q382: C, Q383: A, Q384: D, Q385: D, Q386: D, Q387: B, Q388: E, Q389: B, Q390: E, Q391: B, Q392: D, Q393: C, Q394: D, Q395: A, Q396: B, Q397: B, Q398: E, Q399: C, Q400: A, Q401: A, Q402: E, Q403: B, Q404: D, Q405: C, Q406: D, Q407: D, Q408: D, Q409: B, Q410: E, Q411: C, Q412: A, Q413: A, Q414: E, Q415: A, Q416: D, Q417: A, Q418: B, Q419: B, Q420: C, Q421: B, Q422: C, Q423: B, Q424: D, Q425: D, Q426: D, Q427: A, Q428: B, Q429: E, Q430: A, Q431: D, Q432: C, Q433: D, Q434: A, Q435: B, Q436: A, Q437: E, Q438: C, Q439: A, Q440: D, Q441: A, Q442: A, Q443: D, Q444: D, Q445: A, Q446: B, Q447: B, Q448: D, Q449: B, Q450: D, Q451: A Q452: A, Q453: B, Q454: A, Q455: B, Q456: D, Q457: B, Q458: A, Q459: C, Q460: C, Q461: C, Q462: B, Q463: B, Q464: B, Q465: B, Q466: A, Q467: E, Q468: A, Q469: D, Q470: B, Q471: D, Q472: B, Q473: B, Q474: A, Q475: B, Q476: A, Q477: A, Q478: D, Q479: D, Q480: E, Q481: E, Q482: E, Q483: A, Q484: B, Q485: A, Q486: B, Q487: A, Q488: B, Q489: E, Q490: C, Q491: C, Q492: A, Q493: E, Q494: A, Q495: E, Q496: A, Q497: E, Q498: A, Q499: D, Q500: D, Q501: D, Q502: D, Q503: B, Q504: C, Q505: D, Q506: C, Q507: D, Q508: D, Q509: E, Q510: E, Q511: A, Q512: B, Q513: A, Q514: A, Q515: B, Q516: B, Q517: A, Q518: B, Q519: D, Q520: D, Q521: A, Q522: B, Q523: E, Q524: D, Q525: A, Q526: B, Q527: B, Q528: B, Q529: D, Q530: C, Q531: E, Q532: A, Q533: A, Q534: C, Q535: D, Q536: D, Q537: B, Q538: B, Q539: B, Q540: C, Q541: A, Q542: D, Q543: D, Q544: B, Q545: A, Q546: D, Q547: C, Q548: E, Q549: B, Q550: B, Q551: D, Q552: B, Q553: E, Q554: C, Q555: A, Q556: C, Q557: D, Q558: A, Q559: C, Q560: D, Q561: B, Q562: D, Q563: B, Q564: B, Q565: D, Q566: C, Q567: E, Q568: C, Q569: D, Q570: A, Q571: B, Q572: B, Q573: C, Q574. D, 575: B, Q576:

B, Q577: A, Q578: E, Q579: A, Q580: B, Q581: A, Q582: B, Q583: A, Q584: A, Q585: D, Q586: B, Q587: C, Q588: D, Q589: B, Q590: B, Q591: D, Q592: D, Q593: B, Q594: A, Q595: D, Q596: B, Q597: B, Q598: D, Q599: E, Q600: C, Q601: B, Q602: B, Q603: B, Q604: C, Q605: B, Q606: E, Q607: B, Q608: C, Q609: B, Q610: D, Q611: E, Q612: B, Q613: B, Q614: D, Q615: C, Q616: E, Q617: B, Q618: C, Q619: B, Q620: D, Q621: A, Q622: B, Q623: C, Q624: C, Q625: B, Q626: D, Q627: E, Q628: A, Q629: C, Q630: B, Q631: B, Q632: C, Q633: A, Q634: E, Q635: E, Q636: D, Q637: E, Q638: A, Q639: C, Q640: E, Q641: A, Q642: E, Q643: F, Q644: C, Q645: B, Q646: D, Q647: A, Q648: D, Q649: B, Q650: A, Q651: A, Q652: D, Q653: B, Q654: A, Q655: E, Q656: C, Q657: C, Q658: A, Q659: B, Q660: C, Q661: B, Q662: A, Q663: A, Q664: E, Q665: B, Q666: E, Q667: D, Q668: B, Q669: A, Q670: D, Q671: A, Q672: D, Q673: D, Q674: C, Q675: D, Q676: A, Q677: A, Q678: D, Q679: B, Q680: C, Q681: D, Q682: D, Q683: D, Q684: E, Q685: C, Q686: D, Q687: E, Q688: E, Q689: A, Q690: B, Q691: D, Q692: C, Q693: B, Q694: B, Q695: C, Q696: B, Q697: A, Q698: D, Q699: B, Q700: B, Q701: A, Q702: B, Q703: D, Q704: A, Q705: D, Q706: E, Q707: B, Q708: C, Q709: C, Q710: E, Q711: C, Q712: C, Q713: D, Q714: A, Q715: B, Q716: A, Q717: B, Q718: C, Q719: E, Q720: C, Q721: D, Q722: E, Q723: B, Q724: B, Q725: B, Q726: E, Q727: A, Q728: D, Q729: E, Q730: C, Q731: A, Q732: C, Q733: E, Q734: B, Q735: A, Q736: C, Q737: C, Q738: A, Q739: A, Q740: D, Q741: B, Q742: C, Q743: E, Q744: E, Q745: A, Q746: D, Q747: D, Q748: A, Q749: E, Q750: D, Q751: E, Q752: B, Q753: E, Q754: C, Q755: D, Q756: D, Q757: C, Q758: C, Q759: D, Q760: A, Q761: A, Q762: D, Q763: A, Q764: C, Q765: C, Q766: A, Q767: C, Q768: A, Q769: B, Q770: B, Q771: D, Q772: A, Q773: B, Q774: B, Q775: D, Q776: B, Q777: A, Q778: E, Q779: D, Q780: A, Q781: E, Q782: C, Q783: A, Q784: D, Q785: D, Q786: C, Q787: B, Q788: A, Q789: E, Q790: A, Q791: D, Q792: B, Q793: C, Q794: A, Q795: C, Q796: B, Q797: D, Q798: E, Q799: D, Q800: A, Q801: B, Q802: D, Q803: A, Q804: D, Q805: A, Q806: D, Q807: E, Q808: D, Q809: D, Q810: B, Q811: C, Q812: B, Q813: B, Q814: D, Q815: B, Q816: D, Q817: B, Q818: A, Q819: D, Q820: D, Q821: A, Q822: D, Q823:

C, Q824: A, Q825: A, Q826: A, Q827: C, Q828: C, Q829: C, Q830: A, Q831: B, Q832: E, Q833: A, Q834: E, Q835: A, Q836: D, Q837: E, Q838: D, Q839: A, Q840: D, Q841: A, Q842: D, Q843: C, Q844: A, Q845: C, Q846: B, Q847: B, Q848: A, Q849: A, Q850: B, Q851: C, Q852: B, Q853: A, Q854: C, Q855: C, Q856: A, Q857: D, Q858: B, Q859: A, Q860: D, Q861: B, Q862: C, Q863: B, Q864: C, Q865: B, Q866: A, Q867: E, Q868: C, Q869: B, Q870: C, Q871: A, Q872: C, Q873: D, Q874: A.

Index

K.C. Arnold, C.J. Flint, *Obstetrics Essentials*,
DOI 10.1007/978-3-319-57675-6

P

R

S